Sexually Transmitted Diseases in Women

Sexually Transmitted Diseases in Women

Sebastian Faro, M.D., Ph.D.

Clinical Professor
Department of Obstetrics, Gynecology, and
Reproductive Sciences
Houston Health Sciences Center
University of Texas
Attending Physician
The Woman's Hospital of Texas
Houston, Texas

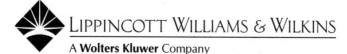

LIPPINCOTT WILLIAMS & WILKINS
A **Wolters Kluwer** Company
Philadelphia · Baltimore · New York · London
Buenos Aires · Hong Kong · Sydney · Tokyo

Acquisitions Editor: Lisa McAllister
Developmental Editor: Joanne Bersin
Production Editor: Karina Mikhli
Manufacturing Manager: Colin Warnock
Cover Designer: Christine Jenny
Compositor: Lippincott Williams & Wilkins Desktop Division
Printer: Maple-Vail

Library of Congress Cataloging-in-Publication Data

Sexually transmitted diseases in women / editor, Sebastian Faro.—1st ed.
    p. ; cm.
    Includes bibliographical references and index.
    ISBN 0-397-51303-8
    1. Sexually transmitted diseases. 2. Women—Diseases. I. Faro, Sebastian.
    [DNLM: 1. Sexually Transmitted Diseases. 2. Women's Health. WC 140 S51785 2003]
    RA644.V4S3779 2003
    616.95′1′0082—dc21

                                                                                2003044602

Care has been taken to confirm the accuracy of the information presented and to describe generally accepted practices. However, the author and publisher are not responsible for errors or omissions or for any consequences from application of the information in this book and make no warranty, expressed or implied, with respect to the currency, completeness, or accuracy of the contents of the publication. Application of this information in a particular situation remains the professional responsibility of the practitioner.

The author and publisher have exerted every effort to ensure that drug selection and dosage set forth in this text are in accordance with current recommendations and practice at the time of publication. However, in view of ongoing research, changes in government regulations, and the constant flow of information relating to drug therapy and drug reactions, the reader is urged to check the package insert for each drug for any change in indications and dosage and for added warnings and precautions. This is particularly important when the recommended agent is a new or infrequently employed drug.

Some drugs and medical devices presented in this publication have Food and Drug Administration (FDA) clearance for limited use in restricted research settings. It is the responsibility of the health care provider to ascertain the FDA status of each drug or device planned for use in their clinical practice.

10 9 8 7 6 5 4 3 2 1

To Abe Mikal, M.D., 1912–2001, who will always be remembered by the numerous medical students and residents whose education and personal lives he has influenced over the years. Dr. Mikal will especially be remembered and missed by those who had the good fortune to work with him. He was not only a teacher and mentor, but also an inspiration—constantly encouraging one to uncover the simplest of facts to better understand the disease process. Dr. Mikal was instrumental in the development of the subspecialty of infectious diseases in obstetrics and gynecology by demonstrating his own interest in the field and by encouraging and physically supporting obstetricians and gynecologists. Additionally, he furthered the subspecialty by assisting in the development of the medical infectious disease program and laboratory at Louisiana State University Medical Center. I am personally grateful to Dr. Mikal for his patience, guidance, and for taking an interest in me.

Contents

Preface

Sexually transmitted diseases are still associated with significant morbidity and cost. These infections are prevalent among young women, especially those between 15 and 25 years of age. However, all sexually active women are at risk to contract a sexually transmitted infection. Both bacterial and viral infections continue to be prevalent. Trichomoniasis does appear to be on the decline, but this may be because of the heavy use of metronidazole to treat conditions such as bacterial vaginosis. Agents of sexually transmitted disease may exist as co-infections within the same host, thus increasing the morbidity, and tend to be and to remain asymptomatic while progressing to cause significant morbidity.

This book was written for physicians, residents in training, nurse practitioners, and nurse midwives responsible for providing medical care to women. Each chapter conveys the essential information (e.g., epidemiology, microbiology, diagnosis, and management) for the common sexually transmitted diseases and vulvovaginal conditions that may co-exist with these infections. The reader will not only obtain the necessary background information to help the patient understand the means of transmission and acquisition, but will also acquire assistance to prevent reinfection. The reader will also be able to quickly retrieve information regarding methods to establish a diagnosis and to provide a sound management program that includes appropriate treatment options.

An infection that begins in the cervix can result in devastating consequences even though it remains asymptomatic until the patient attempts to achieve pregnancy. The infertile patient is often faced with the information that an infection in her past has resulted in her being infertile. Another common occurrence is that a Pap smear result informs the patient that she has dysplasia and human papillomavirus. This is a double shock, especially if she repeatedly had normal Pap smears and now, at age 36 and after 10 or more years of marriage, she learns that she has a sexually transmitted disease.

This book should enable the physician or nurse practitioner to understand the epidemiology and microbiology of these diseases, which will allow them to assist the patient in understanding when and how she may have acquired the infection. This information will also facilitate the patient's understanding of the types of treatments available and what to expect from such treatment.

Each physician can make a significant contribution in reducing the prevalence of sexually transmitted diseases by simply understanding that all sexually active women and men are at risk for acquiring and transmitting these infections.

Sexually Transmitted Diseases in Women

1

Neisseria Gonorrhoeae

"And it was so, that after they had carried it about, the hand of the Lord was against the city with a very great destruction: and he smote the men of the city, both small and great, and they had emerods in their secret parts." I Samuel 6:19

INTRODUCTION

Gonorrhea is an ancient disease whose clinical manifestations have been described in the ancient writings of the Chinese, Japanese, Egyptians, Romans, and Greeks (1,2). The disease has also been referred to in the Old Testament and the Talmud as exudates from the genital tract (3). Galen (130 to 200 A.D.) described a purulent urethral discharge that was probably due to gonococcal infection but mistakenly thought to be a seminal discharge and termed this "gonorrhea" from the Greek *rheowhich* meaning discharge and *gnos* meaning semen. Taken together they mean "flow of seed" (1).

In 1879, Neisser identified the bacterium for the first time in stained smears from urethral discharge and specimens from patients with ophthalmia neonatorium (4). The bacterium was first successfully cultured in 1882 and treated for the first time in the 1930s. However, since its first description and successful treatment, gonorrhea continues to be a major public health problem because of its ability to evolve strains resistant to a variety of antibiotics. *Neisseria gonorrhoeae* knows no racial, socioeconomic, or geographic boundaries. Men, women, and children are all susceptible to this organism and its sequelae. The ease with which people can travel across great distances has enabled the gonococcus to be distributed across the globe and mobilize resistance factors with ease.

EPIDEMIOLOGY

For the past 30 years, gonococcal infection has been a reportable disease in the United States. Sexually transmitted diseases (STDs) have also been reported to central health agencies in Sweden and the United Kingdom. The Centers for

Disease Control and Prevention (CDC) in Atlanta, Georgia, reported that cases of gonococcal infection rose steadily until 1975, then they plateaued in 1982. After this time, the incidence of the disease decreased (Fig. 1-1) (5). Currently, it appears that the prevalence of gonorrhea has stabilized at 300 cases per 100,000 people (6). This bacterium has been identified in every state, with those east of the Mississippi River reporting the highest rates of infection (Fig. 1-2). It should be pointed out, however, that this data is likely to be inaccurate because retrieval of this information is dependent on physicians reporting the cases to their local public health department. Because of the characteristic profiles of patients seen in a private practice setting, it is unlikely that the physician, who is likely to make judgments based on the dress and socioeconomic status of the patient, will screen the patient appropriately unless given cause by the patient. However, the physician should be taking a detailed history to determine the sexual behavioral pattern of the patient. This should lead to appropriate screening of the more common STDs. Therefore, it has always been assumed that the number of cases reported most likely represents approximately ⅓ of the actual number of cases. The underreporting of cases does not, and should not, detract from the significance of this easily acquired STD. The physician should always be alert to the possibility of the presence of this organism in the community, because of the significant sequelae associated with unrecognized gonococcal disease or inappropriate treatment of this infection. Knowing the epidemiologic characteristics of the disease within a given community is extremely important

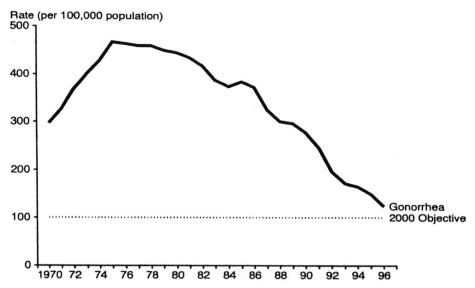

FIG. 1-1. Gonorrhea—reported rates in the Unites States from 1970 to 1996 and the Healthy People year 2000 objective. Georgia did not report gonorrhea statistics in 1994. (From *Sexually Transmitted Disease Surveillance, 1996*, U.S. Department of Health and Human Services, Centers for Disease Control, Atlanta, GA, with permission.)

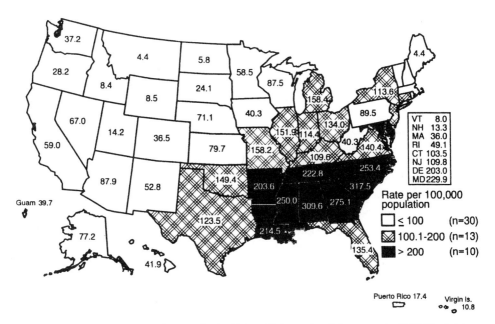

FIG. 1-2. Gonorrhea—rates by state in the Unites States and outlying areas in 1996. The total rate of gonorrhea for the United States and outlying areas (including Guam, Puerto Rico, and Virgin Islands) was 122.4 per 100,000 population. The Healthy People year 2000 objective is 100 per 100,000 population. (From *Sexually Transmitted Disease Surveillance, 1996*, U.S. Department of Health and Human Services, Centers for Disease Control, Atlanta, GA, with permission.)

to determine and administer appropriate treatment, as well as to contain the spread of the disease.

N. gonorrhoeae occurs primarily in individuals between the ages of 15 and 29 years (Fig. 1-3). However, the physician should remember that the infection can occur in any female who is sexually active. The fact that the patient may have had a hysterectomy does not give her immunity to infection. In the female population, the disease is most prevalent among the 15 to 19 year olds. In a study of unmarried 15- to 19-year-old women conducted in 1979, approximately 50% had experienced coitus (7). The incidence of gonorrhea among this group of individuals was 2,938 per 100,000 or approximately 3%; whereas in the 20- to 24-year-old population with 95% of the group reporting sexual activity, the incidence was 1,612 cases per 100,000 or 1.6%. Thus, although the older individuals tend to be more sexually active, they tend to limit the number of partners and are less sexually promiscuous. Therefore, when young women, especially those who are 19 years of age or younger, are seen in the office, health clinics, or emergency rooms for complaints relating to the pelvic organs, they should be asked questions regarding their sexual practices and screened appropriately.

Acquisition of gonorrhea appears to be seasonally dependent, with the highest incidence occurring in late summer and the lowest rates in winter and spring

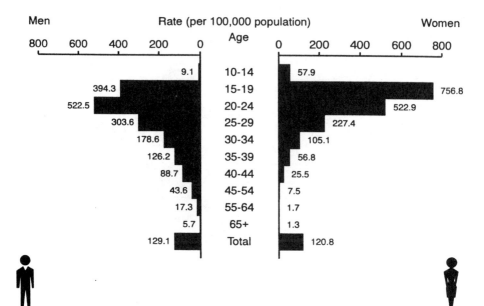

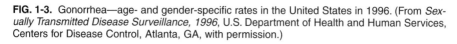

FIG. 1-3. Gonorrhea—age- and gender-specific rates in the United States in 1996. (From *Sexually Transmitted Disease Surveillance, 1996*, U.S. Department of Health and Human Services, Centers for Disease Control, Atlanta, GA, with permission.)

(8). However, this data may be inaccurate because it will be dependent on geographical location, the ease with which the individual can access the medical system, and the affordability of medical care. The warmer weather may allow the individual more mobilization creating a greater opportunity for sexual encounters, therefore increasing her exposure to the pool of infected individuals.

Risk factors for the acquisition of gonorrhea are listed in Table 1-1 (9). Examination of these risk factors reveals that women who are younger than 25 years are more likely to have several of these risk factors; however, these factors are not confined to this age group. Therefore, any individual who fits the profile, regardless of age, should be considered at risk. Black Americans appear to be at greater risk for acquiring gonorrhea than Caucasian Americans (Fig. 1-4). This

TABLE 1-1. *Risk factors for acquiring gonorrhea*

Socioeconomic level
City dwelling
Early age of first sexual intercourse
Unmarried and sexually active
Multiple sexual partners
Failure to use barrier contraception
Sexual partner known to have an STD
History of having had an STD
History of being treated for *Neisseria gonorrhoeae*

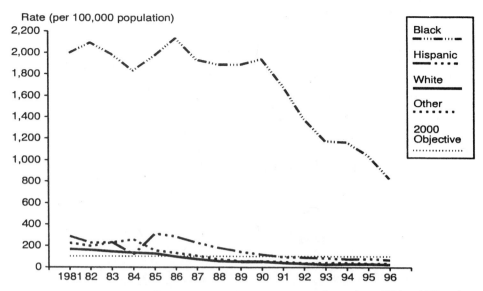

FIG. 1-4. Gonorrhea—rates by race and ethnicity in the United States from 1981 to 1996 and the Healthy People year 2000 objective. "Other" includes Asia/Pacific Islander and American Indian/Alaska Native populations. Georgia did not report gonorrhea statistics in 1994. (From *Sexually Transmitted Disease Surveillance, 1996*, U.S. Department of Health and Human Services, Centers for Disease Control, Atlanta, GA, with permission.)

may be an artifact of reporting because black Americans are more likely to attend public health clinics, public hospitals, and emergency rooms to obtain treatment. In a study conducted in Nashville, Tennessee, 34.1% of 1,549 women attending a venereal disease clinic were infected with *N. gonorrhoeae*. Black Americans were 27.1% to 36.7% more likely to be infected than Caucasian Americans. These investigators attributed this to the fact that black women were more likely to be exposed to infected black men than white women were to be exposed to infected white men and not to any differences in any other factors (10).

Therefore, the need for screening and monitoring the prevalence of infection is important not only to obtain precise information concerning the frequency of infection but also to determine adequate treatment guidelines. When providing wellness care for the patient, it is important that the physician begin a prevention and screening program as early as possible. A thorough history should be obtained at each visit, especially if the patient is presenting with complaints of vaginitis. Programs should be ongoing in each community, and a central laboratory should monitor the antibiotic sensitivity pattern of all isolates. The incidence of antibiotic resistant strains has been steadily increasing. The second increase in overall isolation rates began in 1985 and decreased in 1987 (Figs. 1-5 and 1-6). In 1985, approximately 1% of the isolates were resistant to the com-

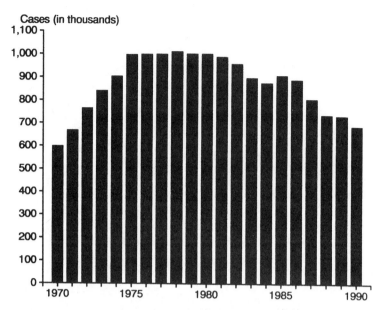

FIG. 1-5. Gonorrhea—reported cases in the United States from 1970 to 1990. (From *Sexually Transmitted Disease Surveillance, 1996*, U.S. Department of Health and Human Services, Centers for Disease Control, Atlanta, GA, with permission.)

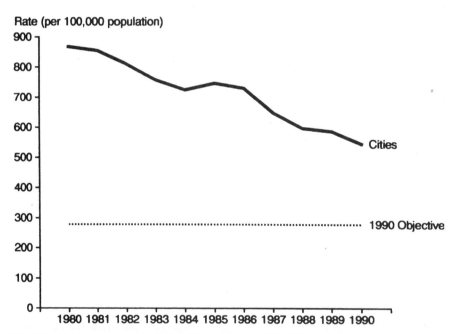

FIG. 1-6. Gonorrhea—rates in United States cities of >200,000 population from 1980 to 1990 and the 1990 objective. (From *Sexually Transmitted Disease Surveillance, 1996*, U.S. Department of Health and Human Services, Centers for Disease Control, Atlanta, GA, with permission.)

monly used antibiotics, and in 1989, the rate rose to 8.5% (Figs. 1-7 and 1-8). The isolation of *N. gonorrhoeae,* resistant to penicillins and tetracycline, continued to rise until 1993 (Figs. 1-7 and 1-8). The rate of isolation of *N. gonorrhoeae* resistant to penicillin and tetracycline, plasma-mediated, plateaued in 1994 (Fig. 1-7). Penicillinase-producing strains of *N. gonorrhoeae* (PPNG) were first isolated in the United States in 1976 (11). Most cases were identified among military personnel and overseas travelers. The increase in PPNG cases in the 1980s was derived mainly from endemic areas (e.g., Korea, Vietnam, the Philippines, and Africa) (12). In 1982 and 1983, spectinomycin-resistant gonococcal strains were isolated from American servicemen stationed in Korea (13). Earlier studies have shown that individuals who began having sex at an early age were more likely to have multiple partners (14). This would increase their risk for exposure to the pool of individuals infected with the gonococcus and, thereby, increase the possibility for acquiring a resistant strain.

In the United States, the Gonococcal Isolate Surveillance Project reported that the incidence of isolates of PPNG rose from 3.2% in 1988 to 7.4% in 1989 (Fig. 1-8) (15). Significant increases occurred in Atlanta, Georgia; Birmingham, Alabama; San Antonio, Texas; and New Orleans, Louisiana. There also appeared to be an increase in the incidence of plasmid-mediated tetracycline resistance as well as high-level chromosomally mediated resistance (16). During the years 1976 through 1989, there were 105 cases of PPNG infections, representing 0.5%

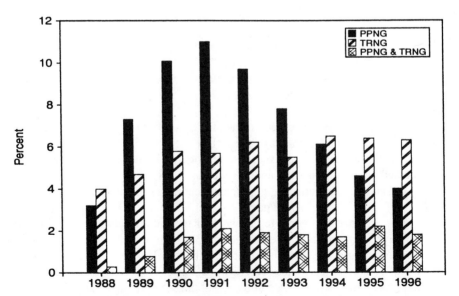

FIG. 1-7. Gonococcal Isolate Surveillance Project (GISP)—trends in plasmid-mediated resistance to penicillin and tetracycline from 1988 to 1996. PPNG, penicillinase-producing *Neisseria gonorrhoeae*; TRNG, tetracycline-resistant *N. gonorrhoeae;* refer to plasmid-mediated resistance to penicillin and tetracycline, respectively. (From *Sexually Transmitted Disease Surveillance, 1996,* U.S. Department of Health and Human Services, Centers for Disease Control, Atlanta, GA, with permission.)

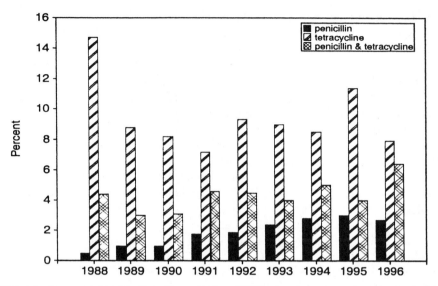

FIG. 1-8. Gonococcal Isolate Surveillance Project (GISP)—trends in chromosomally mediated resistance to penicillin and tetracycline from 1988 to 1996. Chromosomally mediated resistance to penicillin denotes a minimum inhibitory concentration (MIC) of greater than or equal to 2 μg penicillin/mL and beta-lactamase negative; chromosomally mediated resistance to tetracycline corresponds to a MIC of greater than or equal to 2 μg tetracycline/mL without plasmid-mediated tetracycline resistance. (From *Sexually Transmitted Disease Surveillance, 1996*, U.S. Department of Health and Human Services, Centers for Disease Control, Atlanta, GA, with permission.)

of all gonococcal cases in Colorado Springs, Colorado. In 1990, 56 cases of PPNG were reported in Colorado Springs. This study revealed the presence of a core group or pool that accounted for 70% of the 56 cases. Overall, the pool and their sexual partners accounted for 261 (22%) of the 1,170 cases of gonococcal infections (17).

Although quinolones have been in use for a number of years, they were not used frequently in the treatment of gonorrhea until ciprofloxacin became available. In 1990, there was no resistance to ciprofloxacin; however, resistance was documented beginning in 1971 and has increased (Fig. 1-9).

N. gonorrhoeae resistance to quinolones occurs via mutation of the A and B subunits of DNA gyrase or the par C subunit structure of topoisomerase (18). The degree of resistance is related to whether the mutation has occurred in the GyrA or GyrB subunits and whether the par C subunit is involved. For example, mutations involving the GyrB subunit only have a low level of resistance; if GyrA is affected, the resistance levels can be higher (19). Resistance may be of a higher level when both GyrA and par C subunits are mutated (20).

The use of quinolones for the treatment of gonorrhea has increased significantly since the mid-1980s. This use has resulted in increased resistance to the quinolones and has been reported from various countries around the world

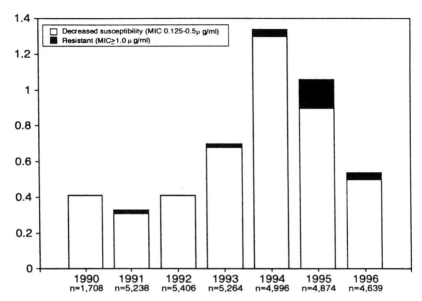

FIG. 1-9. Gonococcal Isolate Surveillance Project (GISP)—prevalence of *Neisseria gonorrhoeae* with decreased susceptibility of resistance to ciprofloxacin from 1990 to 1996. Numbers of isolates with decreased susceptibility are given in the bars. There were fourteen resistant isolates: one in 1991, one in 1993, two in 1994, eight in 1995, and two in 1996. (From *Sexually Transmitted Disease Surveillance, 1996*, U.S. Department of Health and Human Services, Centers for Disease Control, Atlanta, GA, with permission.)

including the United States. Treatment failures have been reported with use of ciprofloxacin (500 mg), ofloxacin (400 mg), and norfloxacin (600 mg) (21–25). Although resistance is uncommon in the United States, the incidence of isolates with decreased susceptibility to ciprofloxacin rose from 0.4% in 1990 to 1.3% in 1994 (26). The fact that resistant strains, as well as strains with decreased susceptibility to quinolones, have been isolated necessitates that the empiric use of quinolones should be avoided in areas where these strains have been isolated. In addition, when quinolones are used, they should be administered in high doses as a single dose. Although the fluoroquinolones have good activity against *Chlamydia trachomatis,* multidosing regimens are required (e.g., treatment for 7 days). Long-term use favors induction of resistance.

In a study of gonococcal isolates from Nicaragua, 89% (16/18) were found to be resistant to penicillin and ampicillin and 78% were penicillinase-producing strains. Eight (44%) isolates were resistant to tetracycline, 4 (22%) were resistant to chloramphenicol, 2 (11%) were resistant to erythromycin, and 5 (28%) were resistant to cefamandole. All isolates were sensitive to ceftriaxone, spectinomycin, cefazolin, cefoxitin, and rifampin. However, the cephalosporins, spectinomycin, and rifampin are not available in Nicaragua. Penicillin, chloramphenicol, erythromycin, and cefamandole have been used in abundance and likely account for the selection of resistant strains among the population (27).

MICROBIOLOGY

N. gonorrhoeae is a gram-negative bacterium, which belongs to the family Neisseriaceae. *N. gonorrhoeae* typically exists as diplococci resembling two kidney-shaped beans with their indented surfaces opposed. In clinical specimens, the bacteria appear as two organisms adjacent to each other within vacuoles in white blood cells (WBCs), typically polymorphonuclear leukocytes (Fig. 1-10). There are four genera within the family Neisseriaceae: *Neisseria, Branhamella, Moraxella,* and *Acinetobacter.* All but *Acinetobacter* are oxidase positive. The species of *Neisseria* are *N. gonorrhoeae, Neisseria meningitidis, Neisseria sicca, Neisseria subflava, Neisseria flavescens,* and *Neisseria mucosa.* Only *N. gonorrhoeae* and *N. meningitidis* are pathogenic in humans.

Kellog et al. (28,29) demonstrated in the 1960s that variation in colony morphology could be correlated with pathogenesis. Four colony types were described: T1, T2, T3, and T4. Colony types 1 and 2 were small in diameter, possessed pili, and tended to be opaque. Types 3 and 4 did not possess pili but were opaque. Kellog et al. (28,29) also demonstrated stability in colony morphology in isolates obtained from the cervix and rectum and showed that the organisms maintained their virulence. They found that after subculturing the specific types 440 times, types 1 and 2 retained their virulence and were able to infect volunteers (28,29). However, when types 1 and 2 were transferred and subcultured

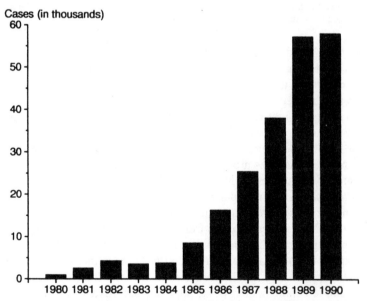

FIG. 1-10. Antibiotic-resistant gonorrhea—reported cases in the United States from 1980 to 1990. More than 95% of reported antibiotic-resistant cases are due to penicillinase-producing strains of *Neisseria gonorrhoeae* (PPNG). (From *Sexually Transmitted Disease Surveillance, 1996,* U.S. Department of Health and Human Services, Centers for Disease Control, Atlanta, GA, with permission.)

nonselectively, there was a transformation from T1 and T2 to T3 and T4 colony morphotypes. In the transformation process, the transformed strains lost their pili (30–33). The cell surface of the gonococcus is complex, consisting of a membrane and a rigid peptidoglycan layer. The existence of a capsule has been strongly suspected and evidence suggests that a capsule is present. Staining the organism with India ink and the Quellung reaction supports the existence of a capsule (34–36). The presence of a capsule was also suggested by the uptake of Alcian blue stain, indicating that the capsule is made of an acidic polysaccharide (35). The capsule does not appear to be stable but is transient. It is only demonstrated on a freshly isolated specimen but cannot be detected on specimens that have been subcultured. The capsule may play a significant role in preventing phagocytosis by polymorphonuclear leukocytes (37). However, confirmation of the existence of a capsule has not been established because the chemical structure of this material is unknown.

The outer membrane of the gonococcus is actually a complex structure, referred to as OMC, and is composed of protein, lipid, and lipopolysaccharide (LPS) (38,39). The outer protein maintains the integrity of the cell and plays a role in the pathogenicity of the bacterium. The major protein, Protein I, accounts for approximately 60% of the total weight of the outer protein and has been termed the principal outer membrane protein. There appears to be variation of the structure of Protein I, based on molecular weight. These variants of Protein I have been designated as low, intermediate, and high molecular weight protein strains. Low molecular weight strains appear to be associated with disseminated gonococcal infection and are usually resistant to killing by the patient's serum (40–42). High molecular weight Protein I is usually found in complex with Protein III. Together these proteins form pores in the outer membrane complex referred to as porins (43).

Protein II is a series of proteins termed minor proteins, referred to as protein 2, protein 2+, protein II, protein II+, opacity-associated protein, leukocyte-associated protein 60, and heat modified protein (42,43). The major function of Protein II is to serve as the site of attachment of bacteria to each other and receptors on the host cell.

Protein III has a lower molecular weight than Protein I and has the same molecular weight for all colony types of a given strain of *N. gonorrhoeae*. The main function of Protein III is its association with Protein I in the function of porins. There are other proteins found in the outer membranes that have not been fully characterized.

The LPS, also known as endotoxin, is clinically one of the most important surface structures of *N. gonorrhoeae* and other gram-negative bacteria. LPS plays an important role in the pathogenesis of this bacterium because it imparts virulence to *N. gonorrhoeae*. The LPS of *N. gonorrhoeae* is similar to the endotoxin of *Escherichia coli* and *Salmonella* species (44). The LPS is anchored to the outer membrane via a hydrophilic fraction, termed lipid A, which, in turn, is linked to a core oligosaccharide. The main component of the core oligosaccharide is sugar known as 3-deoxy-octulosonic acid, commonly referred to as KDO-containing core is bound to an "O" antigenic polysaccharide. Six antigenically distinct gonococcal LPSs have been identified (45,46). The carbohydrate side chains are responsible for the difference in antigenicity. The toxicity of LPS is most likely because of the lipid A moiety, causing fever, alterations in WBC count, and overall toxicity.

The gonococcus also produces IgA protease that is excreted and can be detected in the growth medium (46,47). This enzyme is important clinically because it is capable of splitting IgA1 at the union of its two arms, directly in the middle of the molecule. This renders the patient's IgA inactive, thus facilitating the bacterium's ability to establish an infection (48).

The remaining components of the cell envelop hairlike projections, termed pili, and are composed of repeating identical subunits (pilins). These structures are found on the surface of pathogenic strains and not on saprophytic species. Pilins of *N. gonorrhoeae* are similar to those found in *Moraxella nonliquefaciens, Moraxella bovis, Pseudomonas aeruginosa, Pseudomonas putida, Bacteroides nodosa, Dichelobacter nodosus,* and *Vibro cholerae* (49–51). Pili consist of repeating protein subunits and small amounts of carbohydrates and phosphates (52,53). The pili molecule consists of three segments, designated as CB-1, CB-2, and CB-3. CB-1 represents the *N*-terminal portion that contains seven amino acids that do not appear to differ between strains. CB-2 is the central portion, contains amino acids 8 to 96, and is similar in all strains. The central portion, CB-2, binds to red blood cells and is believed to be the mechanism that enables the gonococcus to adhere to host epithelial cells. CB-3 provides heterogeneity that is found in the gonococcal pili. It is this segment that stimulates the host immune system and, therefore, is responsible for the differences in the host immune response (53,54).

The piliated strains are able to undergo transformation, the process by which one bacterium is able to receive DNA from another bacterium. Once the DNA is taken into the cell, the new DNA is integrated into the recipient genome and expression of the new genes is possible. The gonococcus also contains extra-chromosomal DNA termed plasmids. A plasmid consists of double-stranded DNA, circular in configuration, separate from the main DNA chromosome, and capable of autonomous replication. The gonococcus contains three types of plasmids: R plasmids responsible for the production of beta-lactamases, conjugative plasmids that are self-transmissible from one cell to another receptive cell, and a third whose function is unknown (55). Bacterial cells that are able to possess ananea on the cell surface while under conjugation can synthesize a sex pilus. A unique characteristic of R plasmids is their ability to be transported between different genera of bacteria. This may be the mechanism by which the gonococcus acquired the gene for the production of penicillinase, which is identical to the gene found in *Haemophilus parainfluenzae* (56).

There are several species of the genus that all grow optimally in an atmosphere of 5% to 10% CO_2. Therefore, if the specimen is not placed in an appropriate transport system, retrieval of the gonococcus will be unlikely. *N. gonorrhoeae* is distinguished from other species by its ability to not only metabolize glucose but also to metabolize maltose, sucrose, or lactose as well. Gonococcal strains are differentiated by their nutritional requirements and have been termed auxotypes. The gonococci have been typed according to their amino acid requirements (auxotypes) (57,58). Auxotyping has been useful in epidemiologic studies tracking particular strains to determine if a predominance of one or several strains exists in a geographical area.

PATHOGENESIS

In order for bacterial infection to exist several events must occur. There must be an appropriate inoculum size; that is, the numbers of bacteria present must be sufficient to overcome the host's defensive mechanisms. The bacteria must have the ability to adhere to the host's epithelial cells, which allows the bacteria to invade the host's tissue. Once inside the host, the bacteria must be able to reproduce while overcoming the host defenses that will attempt to eradicate the bacteria. The primary site of gonococcal infection in the female patient is the endocervix, although any surface lined by columnar epithelial cells may be infected. The endocervix is a prime target because it is readily accessible, presents a large surface area, and comes into direct contact with an opposing infected site during sexual intercourse. Because the male penis constantly strikes the cervix during intercourse, it is likely to traumatize the columnar epithelium of the cervix, thus increasing the likelihood of establishing an infection.

The columnar epithelium of the cervix is often present on the exocervix [e.g., in women taking oral contraceptive pills, in those who are pregnant, in those who have cervical inflammation, and in those who were exposed to diethylstilbestrol (DES) in utero]. These conditions all favor the acquisition and establishment of a gonococcal infection when exposed to this bacterium. The gonococcus has the ability to adhere to the columnar epithelium and ascend along this tissue that lines the endocervix, the uterus, and the fallopian tubes. Another factor that may impede the infectious process is the state of the vaginal ecosystem with its own endogenous microflora. Growth of *N. gonorrhoeae* is inhibited by *Lactobacillus* as well as other gram-positive and gram-negative bacteria (59,60). The endocervix also contains mucus-secreting cells that provide a physical and chemical barrier inhibiting microorganisms from gaining entrance to the upper genital tract. The endocervical mucus is rich in carbohydrates, and the sugar moieties can, and in some instances do, bind to the bacteria. These sugars occupy receptor sites on the bacterial surface that prevents their adherence to the host epithelial cells. The mucus also contains substances, such as lactoferrin that inhibits the growth of bacteria. Other antibacterial substances are also present in the endocervical mucus, such as lysozyme and antibodies (e.g., IgA), that all potentially interfere with the growth of bacteria and their ability to cause infection.

The mucus also provides opsonins (compounds that are necessary to facilitate phagocytosis).

Lysozyme is an enzyme found in the endocervical mucus and in vacuoles contained within the cytoplasm of polymorphonuclear leukocytes. Lysozyme hydrolyzes beta-1-4-linkages in the cell walls of bacteria. This action weakens the bacterial cell wall, thus causing the bacterium to loose its characteristic shape and develop into a spheroplast, that is, a cell whose outermost structure is a membrane. The bacterial cell looses its ability to maintain fluid balance and undergoes osmotic lysis (61). Lactoferrin, an iron-binding protein, competes with bacteria for iron and thereby slows or inhibits bacterial growth. Investigators have postulated that those organisms that are poor competitors for iron are less likely to produce disseminated infection (e.g., *N. gonorrhoeae*) (62). Specifically, the Arg⁻Hyx⁻Ura⁻ strain of the gonococcus usually produces asymptomatic infection and does not have good capability of retrieving iron from lactoferrin (63). It has also been postulated that these strains are more likely to inflict disease at the time of menses because iron becomes more readily available from hemin and transferrin. Therefore, the bacteria do not have to compete with lactoferrin.

Antibodies are also found in the mucus secreted by the columnar epithelium lining the endocervix. Antibodies function in several ways: they can interfere with bacterial adhesion, act with compliment to effect bactericidal activity, and opsonize bacteria facilitating phagocytosis. The following antibodies can be found in the endocervical mucus: IgA, IgG, and IgM. Both IgA and IgG interfere with gonococcal adhesion to the endocervical epithelial cells.

Although the endocervix has a number of specific defensive mechanisms to abate infection, the large surface of endocervical columnar epithelium provides an ideal site for inoculation. The risk of a woman acquiring a gonococcal infection after a single exposure to an infected male is approximately 90%, whereas a male exposed to an infected female has approximately a 20% chance of developing an infection. After an uninfected male has had four repeated exposures, the risk of acquiring an infection is approximately between 60% and 80% (64). The use of hormonal contraception may or may not increase the risk of acquiring a gonococcal infection.

CLINICAL PRESENTATION AND DIAGNOSIS

Female infection by *N. gonorrhoeae* can be asymptomatic or symptomatic, may be limited to one site or involve several sites, or may be disseminated (Table 1-2). Asymptomatic infection tends to occur when the site is the urethra, endocervix, rectum, or pharynx. Although symptomatic infection may also occur when any combination of these sites is infected, it is important that the physician ask the patient about her sexual practices. This is necessary to determine the appropriate sites for culture. The incubation period in the female patient is not known but is thought to be approximately 10 days (65). It is common to find

TABLE 1-2. *Clinical spectrum of gonococcal infection*

Urethritis	Skene's gland infection
Cervicitis	Bartholin's gland infection
Proctitis	Endosalpingitis
Pharyngitis	Salpingitis
Lymphangitis	Septic abortion
Chorioamnionitis	Bacteremia
Arthritis	Endocarditis
	Skin infection

both periurethral and urethral infection in women with gonococcal endocervicitis. In women who have had a hysterectomy, the urethra is the most common site of infection (66).

It is important that the physician be alert in suspecting either a gonococcal or other bacterial infection in patients presenting with vague symptomology (Table 1-2). The index of suspicion should be increased when the patient presents with any of the conditions listed in Table 1-2 or states that she has recently developed a foul-smelling vaginal discharge. The patient may either present with one or more symptoms or not have any symptoms, but the cervix may appear hypertrophic and erythematous during the pelvic examination. On gently palpating the cervix with a cotton-tipped applicator, it begins to bleed briskly (67).

Symptoms may be present but are unknown to the patient or are so vague that the patient does not relate them to the possible presence of an STD. However, recent onset of vaginitis associated with a foul odor may be an indication that an STD is present (Fig. 1-11). An example of this would be the STD trichomoniasis. Patients presenting with *Trichomonas vaginalis,* especially if sexually active, should be evaluated for the presence of a second STD. *T. vaginalis* can be found in 62% of women with gonorrhea (68). Studies have shown that the prevalence of gonorrhea is almost two times higher in women with trichomoniasis than without this infection. Thus, it is important that patients who present with vaginitis be counseled about the possibility and significance of other STDs. The patient who complains of burning, vulvovaginal itching, or dyspareunia at the introitus should be examined for the presence of human papillomavirus (HPV) infection. The presence of HPV, either in its subtle form or frank *condyloma acuminata,* should alert the physician to the possible presence of other STDs. Table 1-3 lists the characteristics of vaginal discharge that may indicate the presence of a STD. The physician should recognize that an abnormal vaginal discharge may be an indication of the presence of a significant infection. The presence of a foul-smelling discharge in a patient who is sexually active, although the patient may believe she is in a monogamous relationship, may indicate a STD. However, this does not imply that all individuals who are in a monogamous relationship should be screened for a STD. If the history suggests that the patient or the patient's partner may have behavioral practices that place them at risk, strong consideration for evaluation of the existence of a STD must be made.

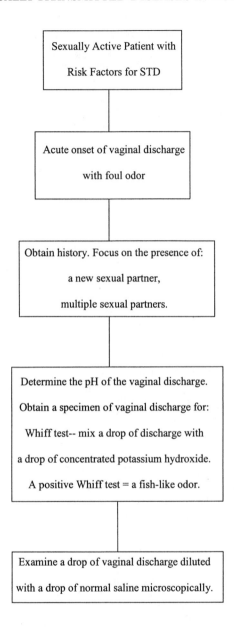

FIG. 1-11. Algorithm for evaluating vaginal discharge.

TABLE 1-3. *Evaluation of vaginal discharge*

Color of the vaginal discharge	pH	Whiff test	Clue cells	WBC	Dominant bacterial morphotype
Healthy vaginal ecosystem					
Slate-gray to white	3.8 to 4.2	Negative	Absent	Rare	Uniform bacilli
Bacterial vaginosis					
Dirty-gray	≥4.5	Positive	Present	Rare	None
Trichomoniasis					
Dirty-gray to green	≥4.5	Positive	Present	Positive	None
Candidiasis					
White	<4.5	Negative	Absent	May be present	Uniform bacilli
Nonspecific					
White to green	≥4.5	Negative	Absent	Present	None

The cervix should be closely examined for the presence of mucopus that may be grossly apparent or detected by sampling the endocervical canal with a Dacron or cotton-tipped applicator. Patients suspected of having cervicitis should be evaluated as described in Fig. 1-12. The specimen should be examined microscopically by diluting it with 1 to 2 mL of normal saline and placing a drop on a glass slide, overlaid with a glass cover slip. The specimen should be examined microscopically under 40× magnification. If the specimen contains fewer than 10 squamous epithelial cells per microscopic field, it can be considered as representative of endocervical discharge and not contaminated by vaginal fluid. The presence of 10 or more WBCs and the absence of any microbe may be interpreted as a possible chlamydial or gonococcal infection. If the specimen is gram stained and no microbes are seen but more than 10 WBCs are present, then a chlamydial infection should be suspected. The presence of intracellular gram-negative diplococci should be taken as indicative of gonococcal infection. A specimen should be obtained for culture, or another specific test (e.g., Gyn-Probe, etc.) for the detection of *C. trachomatis* or *N. gonorrhoeae* should be performed. Other characteristics that may suggest the presence of these two STDs are hypertrophy of the endocervical columnar epithelium, brisk bleeding when the cervix is gently touched with a cotton-tipped applicator, and the presence of inflammation on the Papanicolaou smear.

The patient should be treated with one of the following:

1. Ceftriaxone 125 mg IM once + doxycycline 100 mg orally BID × 7 days
2. Ceftriaxone 125 mg IM once + azithromycin 1 g orally in a single dose
3. Ofloxacin 300 mg orally BID × 7 days
4. Trovafloxacin 200 mg orally × 7 days
5. Cefixime 400 mg orally one time + doxycycline 100 mg BID × 7 days
6. Cefixime 400 mg orally one time + azithromycin 1 g orally in a single dose
7. Spectinomycin 2 g IM in a single dose + doxycycline 100 mg BID × 7 days

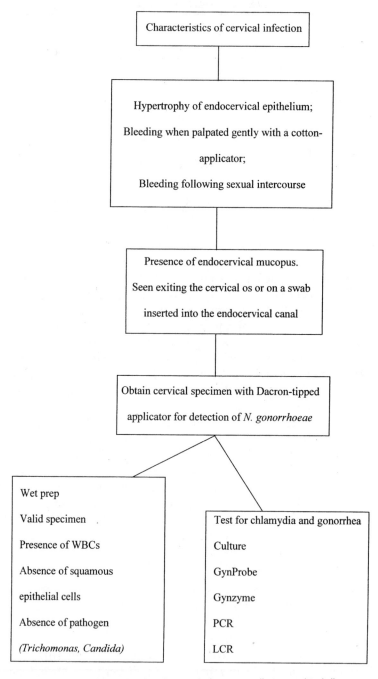

FIG. 1-12. Algorithm for evaluating the cervix for a sexually transmitted disease.

TABLE 1-4. *Clinical clues to possible gonococcal infection*

Vague lower abdominal pain
Intramenstrual spotting
Breakthrough bleeding on OCPs
Recent onset of postcoital bleeding
Bacterial vaginitis
Trichomoniasis
Recent development of dyspareunia
Recent development of dysmenorrhea

OCPs, oral contraceptive pills.

8. Spectinomycin 2 g IM in a single dose + azithromycin 1 g orally in a single dose

No patient should be told that she has a STD unless it has been confirmed by a specific test. However, treatment should not be withheld if there is strong clinical evidence suggesting infection. This should be clearly discussed with the patient because the objectives are (a) eradication of the offending organism(s) and (b) prevention of upper genital tract infection. The latter is of particular concern because most women patients, when infected with either gonococcus and/or chlamydia, do not have symptoms. If confirmation is indeed obtained, which can be accomplished within 24 hours, the patient should be brought back to the office and a discussion held concerning the rationale for testing for syphilis, hepatitis B, and human immunodeficiency virus (HIV).

Upper genital tract infection may be, and usually is, subtle in its presentation, thus often unnoticed by the patient. Symptoms are often confused with normal variances experienced by the patient, which are not severe enough to cause her to seek medical attention. There may be a variety of vague symptoms that occur in the pelvis that can be overlooked (Table 1-4).

TREATMENT

Treatment of gonococcal disease should always include treatment for chlamydial infection. The CDC recommends using two antibiotics for the treatment of these two STDs, namely ceftriaxone and doxycycline (Table 1-5). However, there are alternatives that are just as efficacious and may result in better compliance by the patient. Many treatment regimens are based on short-term administration of antibiotics. The assumption is that when treating cervicitis, the infection has not advanced to the genital tract. (The CDC uses this assumption in their recommendations, extrapolating their treatment recommendations instead of basing them on proven data.) Urethral infection in the male is not similar to cervical infection in the female. In addition, because pelvic infection in women tends to be asymptomatic, there is likely to be a significant delay in establishing that a pelvic infection exists. Therefore, not knowing how long the infection has

TABLE 1-5. *Treatment regimens for gonococcal and chlamydial cervicitis[a]*

Ceftriaxone 125 mg IM in a single dose + doxycycline 100 mg orally BID × 7 days
Cefixime 400 mg orally in a single dose + doxycycline 100 mg orally BID × 7 days
Ofloxacin 300 mg orally BID × 7 days (effective against both *N. gonorrhoeae* and *C. trachomatis)*
Trovafloxacin 200 mg orally QD × 7 days (effective against both *N. gonorrhoeae* and *C. trachomatis)*
Ceftizoxime 500 mg IM in a single dose + doxycycline 100 mg orally BID × 7 days
Cefotaxime 500 mg IM in a single dose + doxycycline 100 mg orally BID × 7 days
Cefotetan 1 g IM in a single dose + doxycycline 100 mg orally BID × 7 days
Cefoxitin 2 g IM in a single dose + doxycycline 100 mg orally BID × 7 days
Cefuroxime axetil 1 g orally in a single dose + doxycycline 100 mg BID × 7 days
Cefpodoxime 200 mg orally in a single dose + doxycycline 100 mg BID × 7 days
Amoxicillin/clavulanic acid 500 mg orally TID × 7 days
Spectinomycin 2 g IM in a single dose + doxycycline 100 mg BID × 7 days

[a]Adapted from Centers for Disease Control. Sexually transmitted diseases treatment guidelines, 1993. *MMWR* 1993;42:56–60, with permission.

existed raises significant concerns for those physicians delivering medical care to women.

The first concern is whether the organism has had an opportunity to migrate to the upper genital tract to involve the fallopian tubes. A second concern is if the infection has progressed to a point at which the endogenous pathogenic bacteria of the vaginal microflora have become involved in the infectious process. The combination of the gonococcus, chlamydia, and facultative and obligate anaerobic bacteria can be very destructive to tissue. Therefore, choosing an antibiotic combination such as ceftriaxone and doxycycline may not be in the best interest of the patient in an attempt to protect her fertility. Ceftriaxone does not have a good spectrum of activity against anaerobic bacteria, especially *Bacteroides,* and would not offer the patient any protection against ascending infection if it should be polymicrobial. There is no doubt about the efficacy of ceftriaxone in treating gonococcal infection, including PPNG strains. However, no existing data indicates that a single dose of ceftriaxone prevents upper genital tract infection or potential damage to the fallopian tubes; neither does any existing data address the efficacy of ceftriaxone plus doxycycline in the prevention or subsequent development of pelvic inflammatory disease. This concern is supported by the fact that the number of cases of ectopic pregnancy and infertility are rising. The rise in the number of ectopic pregnancies is likely due to the use of broad-spectrum antibiotics, which has reduced the mortality rate. However, the problem may rest in one or more areas: (a) most cases resulting in ectopic pregnancy or infertility may be secondary to asymptomatic infection; (b) when the patient presents for treatment, tubal damage has already begun or occurred; (c) the choice of antibiotic and duration of treatment is inappropriate; and (d) a large number of patients have asymptomatic infection.

Both pregnant and nonpregnant patients allergic to penicillin can be treated with spectinomycin (Table 1-5). Second- and third-generation cephalosporins should not be substituted for ceftriaxone. The former agents do have activity against the gonococcus but do not have a long enough serum half-life and are more rapidly excreted in the urine. Ceftriaxone has a half-life of 7 to 8 hours and, therefore, is not rapidly excreted in the urine. In addition, the second- and third-generation cephalosporins have not been extensively tested when administered in a single dose for the treatment of gonococcal cervicitis. However, some of these agents [e.g., cefotetan, cefoxitin, ceftizoxime, and cefotaxime (Claforan)] have been shown to be effective in the treatment of pelvic inflammatory disease when used in conjunction with an agent that has activity against *C. trachomatis*.

Two areas are of great concern when considering treatment of gonococcal cervicitis. The first is the nonpregnant patient: treatment should not be solely based on the eradication of localized infection but on treating the potential ascending component of the disease. As pointed out earlier, the patient found to have cervical infection is not likely to present with symptoms and, therefore, discovery of the infection is likely to be based on history, related to the patient's contact with an individual known to or suspected of having an STD, physical findings uncovered during a routine examination, or pure serendipity. Therefore, the goals of therapy are (a) eradication of the organism from all infected sites and (b) prevention of tubal damage. The physician must assume that the patient found to have cervicitis is likely to have some degree of upper genital tract infection. There are no significant studies that have addressed the possibility that patients with cervicitis may have upper genital tract infection nor have there been any follow-up studies to determine the status of the fallopian tubes. Furthermore, existing studies do not determine the incidence of ectopic pregnancy or infertility in a group of patients previously treated for gonococcal or chlamydial cervicitis.

The second concern is the pregnant patient with gonococcal cervicitis. This patient is most likely to have symptomatic infection that is detected, again, by serendipity. It must be considered that this patient may well have already developed ascending infection involving the decidua and/or chorionic membranes. Existing data does not explain the relationship between treatment of gonococcal cervicitis, eradication of the gonococcus from the endocervix, and ultimate short-term outcome of the pregnancy. Because of the potential for significant posttreatment morbidity, perhaps single-dose therapy should not be relied on in women patients with gonococcal or chlamydial cervicitis.

When considering alternative treatment regimens, the physician should remember that although several antibiotics have been shown to be effective not all regimens are equal. Overall, chromosomally mediated resistance to penicillin and tetracycline is 2.6%, tetracycline resistance alone is 8.5%, and penicillin alone is 1%. Plasmid-mediated resistance to penicillin and tetracycline is 0.9%, tetracycline alone is 4.9%, and penicillin alone is 7.4% (69,70). It is important for the physician to keep abreast of the available information concerning antibiotic resistance patterns in *N. gonorrhoeae* in the community. This will prevent the use of antibiotics that are ineffective in the treatment of gonococcal infection.

TABLE 1-6. *Quinolones: Treatment of gonococcal and chlamydial cervicitis[a]*

Agent	Effective against N. gonorrhoeae	Effective against C. trachomatis
Ofloxacin	Yes	Yes
Trovafloxacin	Yes	Yes
Ciprofloxacin	Yes	Yes (relapse rate high)
Norfloxacin	Yes	No
Lomefloxacin	Yes	No
Enoxacin	Yes	No

[a]Quinolones are not effective in treating *Treponema pallidum.*

New agents such as the fluorinated quinolones have been shown to have good activity *in vitro* against the gonococcus. However, not all quinolones are equal in their activity or suitability for treatment (Table 1-6). Ciprofloxacin is known to have activity against both the gonococcus and chlamydia, as well as other gram-positive and gram-negative bacteria. Resistance in the gonococcus has been increasing and relapse in treatment of chlamydial infection is not uncommon (71,72). Although when initially available the quinolones were thought to become the agents of choice in treating gonococcal infection, especially the PPNG-producing strains, this has not been the case. Treatment failures have been reported to single-dose treatment with ciprofloxacin in the United Kingdom since 1990 (73–76). Failures have also been reported with administration of ofloxacin in the United Kingdom, Australia, Canada, Hong Kong, and the United States (77). Interestingly, resistance has been demonstrated in gonococcal strains producing beta-lactamase as well as strains with chromosomally mediated resistance to penicillin and tetracycline. Resistance to quinolones is infrequently found in strains that are not resistant to penicillin and tetracycline (78,79). Quinolones should not be administered to treat pregnant and breast-feeding women.

Because the primary treatment regimen recommended by the CDC (Table 1-5), ceftriaxone and doxycycline, does not provide adequate coverage against anaerobic bacteria, there is concern that this regimen may not be appropriate for the female patient. In addition, tetracyclines, including doxycycline and minocycline, should not be administered to the pregnant patient. There is no doubt that this treatment regimen can eradicate both the gonococcus and chlamydia from the endocervix. However, the concerns expressed earlier over the existing infection, and the progressive nature of this disease make these recommendations suspect. It may be appropriate to administer an antibiotic regimen that will maintain a greater period of adequate serum levels and have a broader spectrum of activity. This can be accomplished in the nonpregnant patient by administering any of the agents listed in Table 1-5.

Augmentin (amoxicillin/clavulanic acid) and amoxicillin have been shown to be effective in the treatment of *C. trachomatis* (80,81). However, the use of amoxicillin without the beta-lactamase inhibitor would raise concern over its efficacy against *N. gonorrhoeae,* if a PPNG should be present. Therefore, the use of Augmentin provides activity against *C. trachomatis* and *N. gonorrhoeae* and against PPNG strains. Another advantage of Augmentin is its activity against gram-negative and gram-positive facultative, as well as obligate anaerobes. Thus, Augmentin has the potential of providing the broad spectrum of activity to prevent or treat upper genital tract infection. In addition, it can be used to treat the pregnant patient. The combinations of antibiotics listed in Table 1-5 not only provide the spectrum of activity required to prevent tubal damage but also the necessary activity against both the gonococcus and chlamydia. Clindamycin would appear preferable to metronidazole because it has activity against *Chlamydia.* The fact that clindamycin and ofloxacin exert their antibacterial activity differently, this may result in a synergistic effect. It is important to emphasize that all studies evaluating the effectiveness of an antibiotic with regard to *N. gonorrhoeae* and *C. trachomatis* have not considered any long-term sequelae. Therefore, obstetricians/gynecologists or any physicians who assume the primary care of women and who are concerned about their overall wellness should consider potential long-term sequelae when treating these STDs.

Whichever treatment regimen is selected, it is important that the patient be reevaluated within 48 to 72 hours of initiating treatment. The patient should be advised that sexual activity should be withheld until the entire treatment course and follow-up has been completed. If this is not possible, then the patient should be educated as to the transmissibility of these bacteria and the consequences of inappropriate management and noncompliance. On the initial examination, the physician should conduct a thorough pelvic examination, meticulously noting both visual and palpation findings. This is important because the follow-up examinations, at 48 to 72 hours and 14 and 21 days following the termination of therapy, will be compared to the initial examination. These return visits are important because they provide the physician with the opportunity to determine if the educational process and therapy are having a positive effect. At the tenth and fourteenth day visits, the patient should be recultured or tested to determine if there has been eradication of the organisms or if there has been a failure of therapy. At the twenty-first to twenty-fifth day visit, the patient should be recultured or tested to determine if the educational process has been effective or not and if reinfection has occurred.

At the initiation of therapy, if the patient is not already taking oral contraceptive pills, the patient should begin taking them. This is recommended to prevent infection of the ovaries if the infection has already migrated to the upper genital tract. Infection of the ovaries can be prevented by suppressing ovulation, thereby preventing rupture of an ovarian follicle. Preventing a break in the ovarian cortex will prevent bacteria from entering the ovary proper. The mucus produced by patients taking oral contraceptive pills tends to be thick and tenacious, which is unfavorable to the ascent of bacteria along the endocervical canal. It is important that this aspect of management be considered even if the patient is planning pregnancy in the very near future. It would seem prudent to recommend a course of oral contraceptive therapy for 1 to 3 months to allow sufficient time for complete therapy, determine the likelihood of reinfection or relapse, and allow for an educational process to take place in preventing the patient from exposing herself to serious infection.

During the course of the return visits, the physician has the opportunity to reevaluate the patient's history and to determine if the patient is at risk for tubal damage. It also allows for the development of rapport between the patient and the physician, thus providing an opportunity to learn more about the behavioral pattern of the patient. In order for the patient to understand the significance of being infected with regard to transmitting the diseases to her sex partner and the possible adverse effect of the infection on her reproductive capability, it is important that the patient realize both how the infection is transmitted and the sequelae associated with an STD. This latter concept is extremely important because every physician should be concerned about the cause of STDs. It is important to note that the educational process should include the patient's sexual partner. Patients whose behavior exposes them to an STD should also be evaluated for syphilis, hepatitis B, and HIV. Another significant STD that the patient should be evaluated for is HPV and, perhaps, hepatitis C.

SUMMARY

Treatment of *N. gonorrhoeae* infection of the cervix should always include *C. trachomatis*. Although this appears to be a simple or uncomplicated infection, it should be approached as one that is complex and not equated with urethritis in the male. Infection of the cervix is likely to be associated with coinfection of the urethra, Skene's glands, Bartholin's glands, and/or the endometrium. Progression of infection may well have advanced to the fallopian tubes even though the patient is asymptomatic. Exposure of an uninfected woman to an infected man is more likely to result in infection than when an uninfected man is exposed to an infected woman. Sequelae are more likely to occur in the female because of the lymphatic and vascular nature of the female reproductive tract. Infection in women tends to be asymptomatic; therefore, they are less likely to seek treatment.

Follow-up examinations are an important constituent of the treatment of STDs, which must include an educational program for the patient and partner. STDs are nondiscriminatory and, therefore, individuals from the middle and upper socioeconomic classes are at risk for contracting an infection if their behavior places them at risk. Contraction of one STD, regardless of which one it is, places the patient at risk for acquiring gonorrhea and/or chlamydia. This, in turn, contributes to the pool of STDs in the community.

REFERENCES

1. Rosebury T. *Microbes and morals.* New York: Viking Press, 1971:10.
2. Kamal HA. *Dictionary of pharaonic medicine,* Cairo, Egypt: National Publication House, 1967.
3. Preuss J. *Biblical and Talmudic Medicine* (originally published in 1911). New York: Sanhedrin Press, 1978. Rossener F, translator.

4. Kampeier RH. Identification of the gonococcus by Albert Neisser. *Sex Transm Dis* 1978;5:71.
5. *Sexually Transmitted Disease Surveillance*, 1991. U.S. Department of Health and Human Services, Centers for Disease Control, Atlanta, GA.
6. Magabab WI, Lutz FB. Randomized study of cefotaxime versus ceftriaxone for uncomplicated gonorrhoeae. *South Med J* 1984;87:461.
7. Zelnik M, Kanter JF. Sexual activity, contraception and pregnancy among metropolitan area teenagers: 1971–1979. *Fam Plann Perspect* 1980;12:230.
8. Wright RA, Judson FN. Relative and seasonal incidence of sexually transmitted diseases: a two year statistical review. *Br J Vener Dis* 1978;53:443.
9. Pedersen AHB, Bonin P. Screening females for asymptomatic gonorrhea infection. *North Med* 1971;70:255.
10. Quinn RW, O'Reilly KR, Khaw M. Gonococcal infection in women attending the venereal disease clinic in Nashville Davidson County Metropolitan Health Department 1984. *South Med J* 1988;81:851.
11. Jaffe HJ, Biddle JW, Johnson SP et al. Infection due to penicillinase-producing *Neisseria gonorrhoeae* in the United States, 1976–1980. *J Infect Dis* 1980;144:191.
12. Brown S, Warnnissor T, Biddle J. Antimicrobial resistance of *Neisseria gonorrhoeae* in Bangkok. Is single-drug resistance passe? *Lancet* 1982;2:1366–1368.
13. Jones O, Strohmeyer G, Brockett J. Spectinomycin-resistant penicillinase producing *Neisseria gonorrhoeae*. *MMWR* 1983;35:51.
14. Zelink M, Kanter JF. Sexual and contraceptive experience of young unmarried women in the United States 1971 and 1976. *Fam Plann Perspect* 1976;9:55.
15. Centers for Disease Control. Plasma mediated antimicrobial resistance in *Neisseria gonorrhoeae*—United States, 1988 and 1989. *MMWR* 1990;39:284.
16. Schwarcz SK, Zenilman JM, Schell D, et al. National surveillance of antimicrobial resistance in *Neisseria gonorrhoeae*. *JAMA* 1990;264:1413.
17. Centers for Disease Control. Gang related outbreak of penicillinase-producing *Neisseria gonorrhoeae* and other sexually transmitted diseases—Colorado Springs, Colorado. *MMWR* 1993;42:25.
18. DiCarlo RP, Martin DH. Use of the quinolones in sexually transmitted diseases. In: Andriole VT, ed. *The quinolones*. New York: Academic Press, 1998;203–213.
19. Deguchi T, Yasuda M, Makano M, et al. Uncommon occurrence of mutations in the gyrB gene associated with quinolone resistance in clinical isolated *Neisseria gonorrhoeae*. *Antimicrob Agents Chemother* 1996;40:2437–2438.
20. Deguchi T, Yasuda M, Nakano M, et al. Quinolone-resistance to *Neisseria gonorrhoeae*. Correlation of alterations in the GyrA subunit of DNA gyrase and the Par C subunit of topoisomerase IV with antimicrobial susceptibility profiles. *Antimicrob Agents Chemother* 1996;40:1020–1023.
21. Tapsall SW, Shultz TR, Lovett R, et al. Failure of 500 mg ciprofloxacin therapy in male urethral gonorrhea. *Med J Aust* 1992;156:143.
22. Jephcott AE, Turner A. Ciprofloxacin resistance in gonococci. *Lancet* 1990;335:164.
23. Anonymous. Fluoroquinolone resistant *Neisseria gonorrhoeae*—Colorado and Washington. *MMWR* 1995;20:761-64.
24. Kam KM, Wong PW, Cheung MM, et al. Quinolone-resistant *Neisseria gonorrhoeae* in Hong Kong. *Sex Transm Dis* 1996;23:103–108.
25. Kam KM, Lo KK, Lai CF, et al. Ofloxacin susceptibilities of 5,667 *Neisseria gonorrhoeae* strains isolated in Hong Kong. *Antimicrob Agents Chemother* 1993;37:2007–2008.
26. Fox KK, Knapp JS, Holmes KK, et al. Antimicrobial resistance in *Neisseria gonorrhoeae* in the United States, 1988–94: the emergence of decreased susceptibility to the fluoroquinolones. *J Infect Dis* 1997;175:1396–1403.
27. Castro I, Bergeron G, Chamberland S. Characterization of multiresistant strains of *Neisseria gonorrhoeae* isolated in Nicaragua. *Sex Transm Dis* 1993;20:314.
28. Kellog DS, Peacock WL, Deacon WE, et al. *Neisseria gonorrhoeae*. I. Virulence genetically linked to colonial variation. *J Bacteriol* 1963;85:1274.
29. Kellog DS, Cohen IR, Norins LC, et al. *Neisseria gonorrhoeae*. II. Colonial variation and pathogenicity during 35 months in vitro. *J Bacteriol* 1968;96:596.
30. Sparling PF, Yobs AR. Colonial morphology of *Neisseria gonorrhoeae* isolated from males and females. *J Bacteriol* 1967;93:513.
31. Kovalchik MT, Kraus SJ. *Neisseria gonorrhoeae*. Colonial morphology of the isolates. *Appl Microbiol* 1972;23:986.
32. Swanson J, Kraus SJ, Gotschlich EC. Studies on infection. I. Pili and zones of adhesion: their relation to gonococcal growth patterns. *Exp Med* 1971;34:886.

33. Jephcott AE, Reyan A, Birch-Andersen A. *Neisseria gonorrhoeae*. II. Demonstration of presumed appendages to cells from different colony types. *Acta Path Microbiol Scand* (Section B) 1971;79:437.
34. Hendly JO, Powell KR, Jordan JR, et al. Capsule of *Neissria gonorrhoeae*. In: Brooks GF, Gotschlich EC, Holmes KK, et al., eds. *Immunology of Neisseria gonorrhoeae*. Washington DC: American Society of Microbiology, 1978:116.
35. Hendley JO, Powell KR, Rodewald R, et al. Demonstration of a capsule on *Neisseria gonorrhoeae*. *New Engl J Med* 1977;296:608.
36. James JF, Swanson J. The capsule of the gonococcus. *J Exp Med* 1978;145:1082.
37. Richardson WP, Sadoff JC. Production of a capsule by *Neisseria gonorrhoeae*. *Infect Immun* 1977;15:663.
38. Johnson KH, Gotshlich EC. Isolation and characterization of the outer membrane of *Neisseria gonorrhoeae*. *J Bacteriol* 1974;119:250.
39. Swanson J. Cell wall outer membrane variants of *Neisseria gonorrhoeae*. In: Brooks GF, Gotschlich EC, Holmes KK, et al., eds. *Immunobiology of Neisseria gonorrhoeae*. Washington DC: American Society of Microbiology, 1978:130.
40. Heckals JE. The outer membrane of *Neisseria gonorrhoeae*: evidence that protein I is a transmembrane protein. *FEMS Microbiol Lett* 1979;6:325.
41. Douglas JT, Lee MD, Nikado H. Protein I of *Neisseria gonorrhoeae* outer membrane is porin. *FMS Microbiol Lett* 1981;12:305.
42. Walstad DL, Guymon LF, Sparling PF. Altered outer membrane protein in different colonial types of *Neisseria gonorrhoeae*. *J Bacteriol* 1977;129:1623.
43. Swanson J. Studies on gonococcus infection. XIV. Cell wall protein differences among color/opacity colony variants of *Neisseria gonorrhoeae*. *Infect Immun* 1978;21:292.
44. Brooks GF. Structure and characteristics of the gonococcal cell wall. In: Broeeks GF, Donegan EA, eds. *Gonococcal infection*. London, UK: Edward Arnold, 1985:9.
45. Apicella MA, Bennett KM, Hermath CA, et al. Monoclonal antibody analysis of lipopolysaccharide from *Neisseria gonorrhoeae* and *Neisseria meningitidis*. *Infect Immun* 1981;34:75.
46. Kornfeld SJ, Plaut AG. Secretory immunity and bacterial IgA. *Rev Infect Dis* 1981;3:521.
47. Swanson J. Studies on gonococcus infection. XVI. Purification of *Neisseria gonorrhoeae* immunoglobulin A1 protease. *Infect Immun* 1981;22:350.
48. Plaut AG, Gilbert JV, Wistar R. Loss of antibody activity in human immunoglobulin A exposed to extracellular immunoglobulin A proteases of *Neisseria gonorrhoeae* and *Streptococcus sanguis*. *Infect Immun* 1977;17:130.
49. Nassif X, So M. Interaction of pathogenic Neisseriae with nonpathogenic cells. *Clin Microbiol* 1995;8:376.
50. Darlrymple BP, Mattick JS. An analysis of the organization and evolution of type 4 (MePhe) fimbrial subunit proteins. *J Mol Evol* 1987;25:261.
51. Mattick JS, Anderson J, Cox PT, et al. Gene sequences and comparison of the fimbrial subunits representative of *Bacteroides nodosus* serotypes A to I: class I and class II strains. *Mol Microbiol* 1991;5:561.
52. Swansin J, Kraus SJ, Gotschlich EC. Studies on gonococcus infection. I. Pili and zones of adhesion; their relation to gonococcal growth patterns. *J Exp Med* 1975;141:1470.
53. Buchanan TM. Antigenic heterogeneity of gonococci pili. *J Exp Med* 1975;11:1450.
54. Schoolink GK, Tai JY, Gotschlich EC. The human erythrocyte binding domain of gonococcal pili. In Weinstein L, Fields BN, eds. *Seminars in infectious diseases. IV. Bacterial vaccines*. New York: Thieme-Stratton, 1982:172.
55. Pearce WA, Buchanan TM. Attachment role of gonococcal pili. Optimum conditions and quantitation of adherence of isolated pili to human cells *in vitro. J Clin Invest* 1978;68:931.
56. Roberts M, Elwell L, Falkow D. Introduction to the mechanisms of genetic exchange in the gonococcus: plasmids and conjugation in *Neisseria gonorrhoeae*. In: Brooks GF, Gotschlich EC, Holmes KK, et al., eds. *Immunobiology of Neisseria gonorrhoeae*. Washington DC: American Society of Microbiology, 1978:44.
57. Sparling PF, Sox TE, Mohammed W, et al. Antibiotic resistance in the gonococcus: diverse mechanisms of coping with a hostile environment, In: Brooks GF, Gotschlich EC, Holmes KK, et al., eds. *Immunobiology of Neisseria gonorrhoeae*. Washington DC: American Society of Microbiology, 1978:44.
58. Carifo K, Caatlin BW. *Neisseria gonorrhoeae* auxotyping: differentiation of clinical isolates based on growth responses on chemically defined media. *Applied Microbiol* 1973;26:223.
59. Caatlin BW. Nutritional profiles of *Neisseria gonorrhoeae, Neisseria meningitidis* and *Neisseria lac-*

tamica in chemically defined media and the use of growth requirements for gonococcal typing. *J Infect Dis* 1973;128:178.

60. Kaye D, Levinson ME. In-vitro growth inhibition of *Neisseria gonorrhoeae* by genital micro-organisms. *Sex Transm Dis* 1977;4:1.

61. Saigh JH. Inhibition of *Neisseria gonorrhoeae* by aerobic and facultatively anaerobic components of the endocervical flora: evidence for a protective effect against infection. *Infect Immun* 1978;19:704.

62. Strominger JL, Ghuysen JM. Mechanism of enzymatic bacteriolysis. *Science* 1967;156:213.

63. Payne SM, Finkelstein RA. The critical role of iron in host bacterial interactions. *J Clin Invest* 1978;61:1428.

64. Misckelsen PA. Ability of *Neisseria gonorrhoeae, Neisseria meningitidis* and commensal *Neisseria* species to obtain iron from lactoferrin. *Infect Immun* 1982;35:915.

65. Hooper RR. Cohort study of venereal disease: I. The risk of gonorrhea transmission from infected women to men. *Am J Epidemiol* 1978;108:136.

66. Wallin J. Gonorrhea in 1972: a 1 year study of patients attending the VD unit in Uppsala. *Br J Vener Dis* 1974;31:41.

67. Judson FN, Ruder MA. Effect of hysterectomy on genital infections. *Br J Vener Dis* 1979;55:434.

68. Curran JW. Female gonorrhea: its relationship to abnormal uterine bleeding, urinary tract symptoms and cervicitis. *Obstet Gynecol* 1975;454:195.

69. Judson FN. The importance of coexisting syphilitic, chlamydial, mycoplasmal and trichomonal infections in the treatment of gonorrhoeae. *Sex Transm Dis* 1979;6:112.

70. Faruki H, Kohmescher RN, McKinney WP. A community based outbreak of infection with penicillin resistant *Neisseria gonorrhoeae* not producing penicillinase (chromosomal mediated resistance). *N Engl J Med* 1985;313:607.

71. Morse SA, Johnson SR, Biddles JW, et al. High level tetracycline resistance in *Neisseria gonorrhoeae* is a result of acquisition of streptococcal the M determinant. *Antimicrob Agents Chemother* 1986; 30:664.

72. Grandsden WR, Warren CA, Phillips I. Decreased susceptibility of *N. gonorrhoeae* to ciprofloxacin. *Lancet* 1990;335:51.

73. Knapp JS, Fox KK, Trees DL, et al. Fluoroquinolone resistance in *Neisseria gonorrhoeae. Emerging Infect Dis* 1997;3:33.

74. Gransden WR, Warren CA, Phillips I, et al. Decreased susceptibility of *Neisseria gonorrhoeae* to ciprofloxacin. *Lancet* 1990;335:51.

75. Jephcott AE, Turner A. Ciprofloxacin resistance in gonococci. *Lancet* 1990;335:165.

76. Nirley H, McDonald P, Carvey P, et al. High level ciprofloxacin resistance in *Neisseria gonorrhoeae. Genitourin Med* 1994;70:292.

77. Gransden WR, Warren C, Phillips I. 4-Fluoroquinolone resistant *Neisseria gonorrhoeae* in the United Kingdom. *J Med Microbiol* 1991;34:23.

78. Anonymous. Fluoroquinolone resistance in *Neisseria gonorrhoeae*—Colorado and Washington, 1995. *MMWR* 1995;20:761.

79. Knapp JS, Mesola V, Neal SW, et al. Molecular epidemiology in 1994 of *Neisseria gonorrhoeae* in Manila and Cebu City, Republic of Philippines. *Sex Transm Dis* 1997;24:1.

80. Cromblehome WR, Schachter J, Grossman M, et al. Amoxicillin therapy for *Chlamydia trachomatis* in pregnancy. *Obstet Gynecol* 1990;75:752.

81. Mann MS, Faro S, Maccato M, et al. Treatment of cervical Chlamydial infection with amoxicillin/clavulanate potassium. *Inf Dis Obstet Gynecol* 1993;1:104–107.

2

Chlamydia

INTRODUCTION

Chlamydia trachomatis is the most common sexually transmitted bacteria infecting men and women. *C. trachomatis* and *Neisseria gonorrhoeae* are the most common causes of pelvic inflammatory disease (PID), and it is estimated that 10% to 15% of reproductive age women have had at least one episode of PID (1). *C. trachomatis* accounts for approximately 4 million cases of genital infection each year (2,3). Although *C. trachomatis* occurs predominantly among individuals 15 to 25 years of age, all women who are sexually active are at risk for infection (4,5). The prevalence among sexually active women ranges from 5% to 20%, and approximately 80% are asymptomatic (6,7). Once the organism has invaded the cervical columnar epithelium, it can evade the host immune system and remain in a state of latency. It can also ascend to the upper genital tract without causing symptoms (8). Infection of the fallopian tubes can result in infertility and ectopic pregnancy (9).

MICROBIOLOGY

Chlamydia is a member of the order Chlamydiales and the family Chlamydiaceae, which contain a single genus, *Chlamydia*. There are three species: *Chlamydia pneumoniae, Chlamydia psittaci,* and *C. trachomatis. C. trachomatis* is a gram-negative bacterium that is a true parasite. It requires an exogenous source of adenosine triphosphate (ATP). There are three stages in the life cycle of *Chlamydia*: the elementary body (EB), the intermediate body, and the reticulate body (RB).

The elementary and reticulate bodies of *C. trachomatis* resemble gram-negative bacteria because they contain both an inner cytoplasmic membrane and an outer membrane (10–13). However, the chlamydial envelope differs from the outer cell wall of typical gram-negative bacteria in that the former lacks a peptidoglycan layer between the outer and inner membranes (13). Chemical analysis demonstrates that there is no muramic acid or any other amino sugars present (14,15). *C. trachomatis* has retained vestiges of peptidoglycan as demonstrated by the presence of penicillin-binding proteins that are similar in location, size, and affinity for penicillins to those found in gram-negative bacteria (14). The affinity for penicillins is demonstrated by the inhibition by penicillin of the growth and division of RBs, as well as their reorganization into EBs (16). Further evidence of the relationship to gram-negative bacteria is founded in the fact that D-cycloserine blocks the growth and multiplication of *C. trachomatis* and *C. psittaci* (16,17). D-Cycloserine, like penicillin, blocks peptidoglycan synthesis. D-Cycloserine blocks the formation of D-alanine from L-alanine and the synthesis of D-alanine-D-alanine cross linkages (18). Penicillin blocks transpeptidation, thus preventing the development of cross-links in peptidoglycan (18,19).

All isolates of *C. psittaci* and *C. trachomatis* possess a group-specific antigen similar to the lipopolysaccharide (LPS) found in the outer membrane in typical gram-negative bacteria. The LPS of *Chlamydia* strongly resembles the LPS of true gram-negative bacteria in location, chemical structure, and activity (20–24).

LIFE CYCLE

The infectious particle, EB, attaches to the host cell via two mechanisms that have not been completely elucidated. Attachment of *Chlamydia* is believed to occur through a nonspecific physical attraction. This action is thought to occur through contact between *Chlamydia* and filopodia or microvilli on the surface of the host cell (25) (Fig. 2-1). The organism can also gain entrance into the host cell via receptors on the host cell. Two proteins have been identified on the surface of *C. trachomatis* EBs (infectious bodies) but not on RBs. It is hypothesized that once the chlamydial cell binds to the host cell via the receptor, there is continuity established between the membrane of the parasite and the host (26).

Once the bacterium has established contact with the host cell, it gains entrance into the cell either by phagocytosis, which is an energy-dependent process, or a microfilament-independent process by which chlamydiae are converted into clathrin-coated vesicles via receptor-mediated endocytosis (27–31). This mechanism allows the host cell to capture the organism by permitting the host membrane to coat the bacterium. Clathrin-dependent mechanisms are the processes by which the host cell, via micropinocytotic uptake, takes in receptor-bound hormones and interferon (Fig. 2-2).

Once in the host cell, foreign bodies are at risk for dissolution by lysosomal enzymes; however, *Chlamydia* remains safely within the endosomal vacuole. It has been demonstrated that *C. psittaci* can block the fusion of the lysosome with the endosome containing *Chlamydia* (32–35). Whether or not the same mechanism holds for *C. trachomatis* is not known. There is evidence to suggest that some strains of *C. trachomatis,* as well as *C. psittaci,* fail to grow in certain host cells; that is, infection is unsuccessful because the bacteria do not have the ability to block the fusion of the chlamydial-containing vacuole and the lysosome (36).

A few hours after the EB has entered the host cell, it begins the first of two morphogeneses of its life cycle and differentiates into an RB. The deoxyribonu-

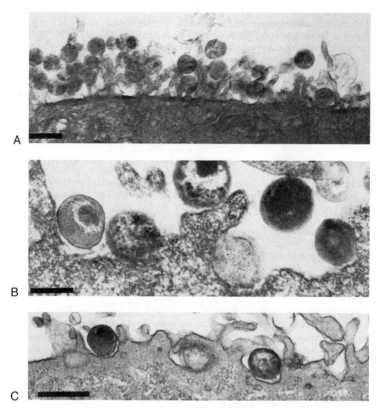

FIG. 2-1. Attachment and uptake of *Chlamydia trachomatis* L2. **A:** Initial chlamydial attachment is with microvilli projecting from host cell surface. In this thick (approximately 1.0 μm) section for transmission electron microscopy at 125 kV, microvilli enfold both sides of the adherent chlamydiae. **B:** *Chlamydia* make contact with the cell surface at the base of the microvilli. **C:** Internalization 5 minutes after inducing uptake of attached chlamydiae by warming to 36°C. Organisms are deeply enfolded by the host cell surface or within endosomes. In these electron micrographs, the bars represent 1 and 0.25 μm, respectively. (From Barron AL, ed. *Microbiology of chlamydia.* Boca Raton, FL: CRC, 1988, with permission.)

FIG. 2-2. Uptake of *Chlamydia trachomatis* L2 initiated as described in Fig. 2-1. **A:** An internalized *Chlamydia* in an endosome. Note the relative size of the clathrin-coated vesicle (*arrow*) that still retains its connection with the cell surface. **B:** When many organisms are internalized, endosomes containing multiple chlamydiae are observed, presumably derived from fusion of individual endosomes. Staining of the host cell glycocalyx with colloidal thorium demonstrated that these chlamydiae were not lying in an invagination of the host cell surface. **C:** The host cell was challenged at a ratio of 2,000 elementary bodies per cell; 30 minutes after stimulating uptake, numerous chlamydiae can be seen in tight-fitting endosomes. The bars represent 0.25 μm, respectively. (From Barron AL, ed. *Microbiology of chlamydia.* Boca Raton, FL: CRC, 1988, with permission.)

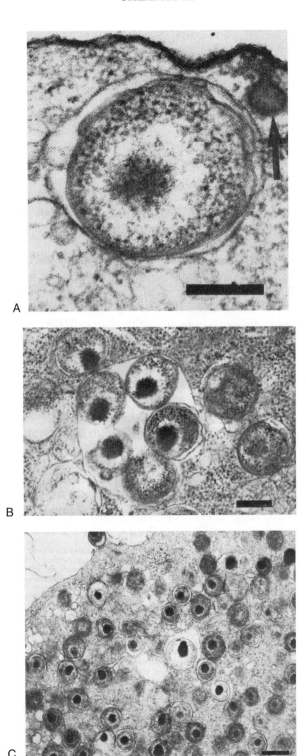

A

B

C

cleic acid (DNA) becomes less dense, the rigidity of the cell envelope is relaxed, the cytoplasm is much more granular because of the production of ribosomes, and the bacterium enlarges. This transformation takes approximately 9 hours. The RB divide by binary fission but lack cytochromes and other key elements of cellular respiration. Therefore, they cannot synthesize ATP but must derive this from the host cell (37,38). Penicillin inhibits the growth of the RB and reproduction, as well as its morphogenesis back to an EB (39). Delays in the development of *Chlamydia* can arise from exposure to antibiotics, the unavailability of essential nutrients, or interferon (40,41).

In the absence of treatment, genital tract infection caused by *C. trachomatis* may persist for months (42,43). Detection of *C. trachomatis* from the cervix of women who had sexual contact with men known to have gonococcal urethritis was dependent on two factors: (a) chlamydial infection or colonization in the male and (b) acute gonococcal infection in the female (43).

Approximately 18 to 20 hours following initial infection, the RBs begin morphogenesis to form EBs. The initial step is the formation of a central core of DNA. A single RB may contain multiple sites of DNA condensation, enabling a single RB to give rise to multiple EBs.

Twenty to 30 hours following infection of the host cell, the cellular organelles develop progressive degeneration and necrosis. The host cell exhibits a loss of ribosomes, vesiculation of the endoplasmic reticulum, and loss of microvilli (44). Once the nutrients of the host have been expended, the cytoplasmic membrane lysis releases EB.

Chlamydia may cause an asymptomatic, latent infection that can persist for months (43,45). Detection of *C. trachomatis* from the cervix of female contacts of males with gonococcal urethritis was dependent on the presence of chlamydiae in the male and acute gonococcal infection in the female (43). The hypothesis is that acute gonococcal infection that activates the latent chlamydiae to produce acute chlamydial infection.

The greatest activity with regard to active chlamydia infection occurs in host cells that are metabolically active and dividing (46). The most active cells are those responding to trauma or infection. In cells that are not growing and dividing there is the possibility that *Chlamydia* will not be detected because only the superficial host cells become infected. Those are sloughed off as part of the normal cycle of host epithelium. However, if *Chlamydia* can gain access to the deeper tissue, then the infection may become either asymptomatic or acute. The potential for asymptomatic infection is probably the one most important aspect of infection caused by *C. trachomatis*. Approximately 80% of infections in women are asymptomatic; therefore, these women will not seek medical assistance, and the disease process is likely to continue (47,48).

CLINICAL MANIFESTATIONS

The propensity to cause asymptomatic infection led to the recommendation for universal screening of all sexually active women, especially between the ages

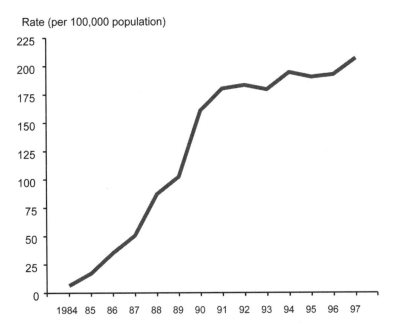

FIG. 2-3. Chlamydia—reported rates in the Unites States from 1984 to 1997. (From *Sexually Transmitted Disease Surveillance, 1997*, Centers for Disease Control, Atlanta, GA, with permission.)

of 15 to 25. This recommendation is reinforced by the fact that approximately 4 million urogenital infections caused by *Chlamydia* occur annually in the United States (Fig. 2-3) (47,49). The prevalence nationwide has been reported to be between 5% and 20% (50). This recommendation, however, will result in screening many more women than necessary and raise the cost significantly. Perhaps a more logical approach is to obtain an in-depth history to determine a risk profile for each patient and screen those who fulfill the risk criteria. A study was conducted in the U.S. military to determine the prevalence of *C. trachomatis*. A total of 13,204 new female recruits were screened using ligase chain reaction and risk factor data assessment (51). The investigators found that the prevalence was 9.2% among all recruits and 12.2% among 17 year olds. A list of risk factors obtained from this study is located in Table 2-1. These authors concluded that a

TABLE 2-1. *Risk factors for acquisition of genital chlamydial infection*

Risk factor	Odds ratio
Having ever had vaginal intercourse	5.9
≤25 years of age	3.0
African American	3.4
≥1 sex partner in the previous 90 days	1.4
A new partner within 90 days	1.3
Partner not using a condom	1.4
Ever having had an STD	1.2

screening program for subjects ≤ 25 years of age (which made up 88% of the sample) would have identified 95.3 % of the infected women (51).

The need to screen sexually active women for chlamydial infection is based on two facts: (a) infection tends to be asymptomatic and (b) the progressive nature of this infection results in cervicitis, endometritis, and salpingitis, which can result in infertility, ectopic pregnancy, and tubo-ovarian abscess. Ectopic pregnancy continues to be a major cause of morbidity and mortality among women. It accounts for 9% of all pregnancy-related deaths and is the major cause of those that occur in the first trimester (52,53). The ectopic pregnancy rate increased from 1980 until 1989 then steadily decreased, with approximately 38,000 cases reported in 1996 (Fig. 2-4). Although the overall rate of ectopic pregnancy has decreased, the risk of having an ectopic pregnancy increases proportionally with the number of chlamydial infections. Hillis et al. (53), demonstrated that the risk of a woman having an ectopic pregnancy increases significantly when a woman has two (odds ratio 2.1, 95% confidence interval 1.3 to 3.4) and three or more chlamydial infections (odds ratio 4.5, 95% confidence interval 1.8 to 5.3).

Although usually asymptomatic, chlamydial infection of the cervix does have subtle signs and symptoms. The patient may note spotting or bleeding following

Number of Ectopic Pregnancies

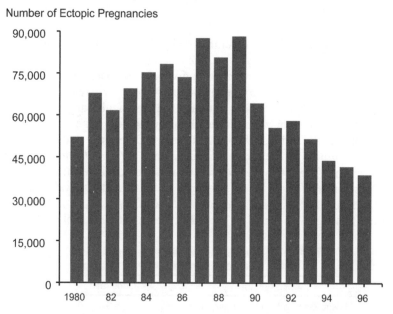

FIG. 2-4. Ectopic pregnancy—hospitalization of women 15 to 44 years of age in the United States from 1980 to 1996. Some variations in 1981 and 1988 numbers may be due to changes in sampling procedures. The relative standard error for these estimates ranges from 8% to 12%. (From *National Hospital Discharge Survey*, National Center for Health Statistics, Centers for Disease Control, Atlanta, GA, with permission.)

vaginal intercourse or the recent onset of dyspareunia. On speculum examination, the physician may note that the cervix appears erythematous (may even appear dark red and have a velvet-like appearance), which is caused by hypertrophy of the endocervical columnar epithelium. When obtaining a Papanicolaou (Pap) smear the cervix also bleeds briskly. Another sign of a possible chlamydial infection is the presence of endocervical mucopus. This is usually not noted to be free-flowing endocervical discharge but is thick mucus detected by placing a Dacron or cotton swab in the endocervical canal. If present, the purulent mucus will adhere to the swab when it is withdrawn. If any of these signs are present a specimen should be obtained for the detection of *C. trachomatis* and *N. gonorrhoeae.* It is extremely important that these clues to chlamydial infection not be overlooked or be interpreted as minor or insignificant because chlamydial infection, although "asymptomatic," will progress to cause upper genital disease.

There are 15 serovars of *C. trachomatis,* A, B, and C, are usually associated with trachoma, and D through K are frequently found to cause genital and neonatal infection (54). It appears that the serovar causing infection may have variable expressions of virulence. Workowski et al. (55) found that women infected with serovar F tended to be asymptomatic but were associated with easily induced cervical bleeding, hypertrophy of the endocervical columnar epithelium, and the presence of endocervical mucopus. In addition, they did not find any association between a specific serovar and PID. This data implies that there may be other serovars that appear less virulent, thereby causing asymptomatic infection, but all appear capable of causing salpingitis. The distribution of serovars found among women with PID were: serovar E 14%, D 11%, B 1%, F 11%, G 2%, J 10%, K 1%, Ia 5%, and H 1% (57).

A variety of tests are available for the detection of *Chlamydia* (Table 2-2). The particular test employed is dependent on the objective and the cost. If large populations are to be screened, an economical test with a low false-negative rate is necessary. Using an expensive, relatively complicated test would not yield the turn-around time to effectively render treatment.

The problem facing medical providers is not taking the time to determine who should be screened and who does not need to be screened. Another problem is that many insurance carriers, especially health maintenance organizations

TABLE 2-2. *Diagnostic tests for detecting chlamydia trachomatis*

Culture
Antigen detection based on fluorescein-conjugated
    monoclonal antibodies
Enzyme immunoassay tests
DNA probes
PCR
LCR

LCR, ligase chain reaction; PCR, polymerase chain reaction.

(HMOs), will not reimburse physicians for screening patients for sexually transmitted diseases (STDs). This is a tragic commentary on health care in the United States with more than 300 cases/100,000 population or greater than 4 million diagnosed cases a year (56,57). Washington et al. (58) estimates that chlamydial infections in women cost Americans approximately $1.106 million of the $1.4 million spent annually on chlamydial infections in the general population (58). These investigators estimated that if the rate of infection projected in 1987 (~75 cases/100,000 population) persisted (1996 ~340 cases/100,000 population) the cost for chlamydial disease, including its sequelae, will exceed $2.18 billion (58).

Chlamydial infection is unique in that the sequelae leading to salpingitis render the patient infertile or at risk for ectopic pregnancy. The prevalence of chlamydial disease among young women has lead to the development of various recommended strategies for screening and treating patients at risk. However, these strategies are either not cost effective or subject the patients to the unnecessary exposure of antibiotic treatment. One strategy that has been proposed is to screen individuals using a direct antigen test, either an immunofluorescence or enzyme-linked immunosorbent assay (ELISA) (59–61). In this study, Nettleman and Jones (62) proposed comparing microimmunofluorescence to detect antibody to *C. trachomatis* that had a sensitivity of 97% and a specificity of 64% with an indirect fluorescent antibody assay that had a sensitivity of 87% and a specificity of 64%. Microimmunofluorescence was also compared with an enzyme-linked immunoassay with a sensitivity of 84% and a specificity of 51%. Nettleman and Jones concluded that screening with a serologic test was not highly predictive of active infection. Screening with a direct antigen test would be cost effective; however, only 54% of patients with positive test results would actually be infected. They concluded that direct antigen testing would be an acceptable approach and a cost-effective alternative to either testing or treating (62). This does not seem to be an acceptable alternative to physicians not screening their patients because it will encourage the misuse of antibiotics. The physician must accept the responsibility of screening patients at risk for STD.

The insidious nature of chlamydial infection and its low prevalence in non-high-risk groups lulls physicians into downplaying the significance of this STD. Phillips et al. (63) reported the prevalence of cervical *C. trachomatis* infection, in a study of 1,141 women, divided between a hospital based practice (530) and a private practice setting (611). They found 24 of the 503 women (4.5%) and 17 of the 611 women (2.8%) to be infected. Among the infected individuals, 61% (25) were symptomatic. Analysis of the women revealed the group most likely to be infected had the following characteristics: were sexually active and 18 to 35 years of age, had a high school education or less, had a sex partner who had other sexual partners during the prior 3 months, and experienced endocervical bleeding when the cervix was palpated with an endocervical swab (63). This model was tested and found valid in 611 patients via a questionnaire, examination, and culture. The mean age was 30.6 ±6.6, 71% completed college, 86% were Caucasian, 2.2% had a positive culture, and 70% of the infected patients were asymptomatic (63). These investigators found that in women with one or more risk factors the prevalence of infection was 5.8% (95% confidence interval, 4.0 to 8.6) compared with 0.9% of patients without these risk factors ($p = 0.005$) (63).

In a high-risk population, the risk factors associated with infection are age 24 or younger, vaginal sex with a new partner within the preceding 2 months, mucopurulent endocervical pus, bleeding of the endocervix when gently touched with a swab, and failure to use barrier contraception (64). The presence of endocervical mucopus appears to be highly associated with endocervicitis caused by *C. trachomatis.* Katz et al. (65) investigated the use of Gram stain and culture in 214 women. Approximately 24% of the Gram stains were not suitable. Isolation of *C. trachomatis* was statistically significant from women with valid smears and 10 or more polymorphonuclear leukocytes per smear (44% vs. 19%, $p = 0.0008$). This finding was independent of the presence of gonococcal infection (65).

Although chlamydial infection has been detected on cytologic specimens, that is, Pap smear and Giemsa stain, the sensitivity and specificity has not been high and, therefore, is not reliable. Purola and Paavonen (66) reported that the changes seen, cytologically, in cells retrieved from the cervix were not specific for chlamydia infected cells but could also be seen in association with inflammatory conditions not solely restricted to chlamydial infection. However, 38% of women infected with *C. trachomatis* (93/240) had atypia compared with 18% of women not infected with *C. trachomatis* (147/240) (66). Carr et al., (67) using an immunofluorescent stain to determine the presence of anti-chlamydial antibodies in cervical secretions, found 15 of 33 patients (45%) to be positive. Eleven of the 15 patients (73%) had abnormal Pap smears [Class II or Class III probably equivalent to high-grade squamous intraepithelial lesion (HSIL)] and had anti-chlamydial antibodies. Only 3 of 18 patients without anti-chlamydial antibodies had similar Pap smears. Although there appears to be an implication between chlamydial infection and cervical cell abnormalities, this relationship has not been validated. However, when a patient's Pap smear reveals acute or chronic inflammation, atypia, or perhaps low-grade squamous intraepithelial lesion (LSIL), *Chlamydia* should be suspected and appropriate tests performed. If *C. trachomatis* is found, appropriate treatment should be instituted.

Traditionally, chlamydial detection depended on culturing the organism in tissue culture. This is a costly and laborious task and is often logistically difficult to carry out. Several different tests have been developed relying on antigen detection, nucleic acid detection, and DNA amplification, which has increased the sensitivity and specificity of chlamydial detection. The first important step in determining if *C. trachomatis* is present in clinical specimens is obtaining the specimen. The cytobrush was compared with a Calgiswab and Dacron-tipped applicator. The cytobrush was found to be superior for collecting cervical specimens for the purpose of isolating *C. trachomatis* (68). The cytobrush improved the culture results. Detection with Calgiswab was 69% versus 100% with cytobrush; when using the direct fluorescent antibody test, Calgiswab detected 68%

versus 85% detected with cytobrush (68). These investigators also compared these two collecting systems in antigen detection employing an ELISA with comparable results (68). Thus, the cytobrush appears to be a better tool for the collection of endocervical cells.

Using culture to detect chlamydial infection is laborious, requires less than 72 hours to obtain results, and, therefore, is not practical. Cytology is unreliable because of its lack of specificity. Other modalities have been developed to decrease the time required from obtaining the specimen to obtaining the results, as well as decreasing the cost.

One such test is based on antigen detection. There are two approaches to detecting the presence of chlamydial antigen; one is to use the direct monoclonal fluorescent antibody test (MicroTrak, Syva Co, Palo Alto, CA), and the other is an enzyme immunoassay or ELISA (Chlamydiazyme, Abbott Laboratories, North Chicago, IL). The direct fluorescent antibody test has a sensitivity of 55.9% to 100% when cervical specimens are tested, and the enzyme immunoassay system has a sensitivity of 44.4% to 100% (69). The physician can increase the accuracy of the test by removing cervical mucus and secretion from the cervix before obtaining the specimen. The specimen must contain columnar epithelial cells from the endocervix because the organism does not infect squamous epithelial cells. The specimen should not be collected following the use contraceptive foams, creams, suppositories, or unprotected vaginal intercourse. Both seminal fluid and the contraceptive agents are toxic to chlamydial cells (70). When collecting a cervical specimen, cotton or calcium alginate swabs should not be used because they have been found to be toxic to *Chlamydia*. Because a wooden shaft is also toxic, a Dacron or rayon fabric on a plastic or aluminum shaft should be used (71–74).

Other factors that influence the sensitivity and specificity of the tests used (e.g., culture, direct fluorescence antigen detection, or enzyme immunoassay) are the number of columnar epithelial cells sampled, and the number of chlamydial inclusions present. In comparing the nonculture assays with culture, many of the false-positive antigen results were actually true positives that were associated with false-negative culture results (75, 76). The gold standard, before the use of polymerase chain reaction (PCR), has been culture; however, because culture has a sensitivity of less than 100%, the antigen detection systems are actually similar or identical to culture methods (77–79).

Another factor to consider when evaluating data to determine which test to use for the detection of *C. trachomatis* is the threshold for detecting the organism: the lower the threshold, that is, the number of inclusions, the higher the sensitivity of the test. In addition, the threshold will have a significant bearing on the outcome depending on whether the population is at a high or low risk for contracting a STD. The test would have a high positive predictive value if the prevalence of *Chlamydia* was high and a low positive predictive value if the prevalence was low. The direct fluorescent antigen and enzyme immunoassay tests are highly sensitive and specific. The direct fluorescent antigen test reacts with the outer membrane of the EB, so the test can be positive even if the chlamydial cells are dead. The enzyme immunoassay test reacts with chlamydial LPS (80–82). These two methods have been reported to yield false-positive results when gram-positive (e.g., *Staphylococcus aureus, Streptococcus agalactiae, Peptostreptococcus* species) and gram-negative (e.g., *N. gonorrhoeae, Acinetobacter* species, *Salmonella* species, *Escherichia coli,* and *Gardnerella vaginalis*) bacteria are present (83–86).

DNA probes have also been used to detect *C. trachomatis* and *N. gonorrhoeae.* DNA probes appear to have no increased sensitivity over that of cell culture. DNA amplification or PCR appears to be the most sensitive and specific in detecting *C. trachomatis.* Use of PCR has enabled investigators to detect *C. trachomatis* in specimens that were negative by culture (87–89). Witkin (90) found that PCR was more sensitive than culture in detecting *C. trachomatis* from the cervices of women with salpingitis.

SEQUELAE OF CHLAMYDIA INFECTION

The asymptomatic nature of chlamydial infection makes this one of the most significant infections of the reproductive tract. It has the ability to cause a spectrum of disease in nonpregnant and pregnant patients (Table 2-3). Asymptomatic colonization can lead to progressive upper genital infection and go unnoticed by the patient. Unfortunately, unless a detailed history is obtained the physician is not likely to suspect that the patient is infected.

CHLAMYDIAL INFECTION AND PREGNANCY

Women found to have a chlamydial cervical infection at the time of delivery were more likely to experience postpartum febrile morbidity following tubal ligation than women not infected (91). The prevalence of chlamydial cervicitis has been reported to be between 8% and 21% (92). Todd et al. (91) screened 1,447 women for cervical chlamydial infection, before delivery, who then underwent a postpartum tubal ligation. They found 1,411 women to be negative (97.5%) and 36 positive (2.5%) for *C. trachomatis* by DNA probe (Pace 2, GenProbe, San

TABLE 2-3. *Sequelae of chlamydial infection*

Nonpregnant	Pregnant
Cervicitis	Cervicitis
Endometritis	Septic abortion
Salpingitis	Salpingitis
Pyosalpinx	Chorioamnionitis
Ovarian abscess	Premature rupture of amniotic membranes
	Premature labor
	Postpartum endometritis
	Postpartum salpingitis

Diego, CA). 41 women experienced febrile morbidity exclusive of pneumonia, urinary tract infection, mastitis, or cellulitis. Fever was defined as 38°C or higher for more than 24 hours. 8/36 or 22% of the chlamydial-positive women had febrile morbidity and 33/1411 or 2% of the chlamydial-negative group also experienced febrile morbidity. The association of febrile morbidity and chlamydial cervicitis was significant ($p > 0.0001$, relative risk 9.5, 95% confidence interval 4.5 to 20.1) (91).

Chlamydial infection of the cervix in women undergoing delivery, especially those delivered vaginally, is also associated with postpartum endometritis and febrile morbidity (92–94). *C. trachomatis* appears to be an infrequent cause of postpartum endometritis, and this is related to the low prevalence of this bacterium in pregnant women. Postpartum endometritis occurs in 20% to 55% of women delivered by cesarean section and in 2% to 5% of those delivered vaginally (94). Greater than 95% of the cases of postpartum endometritis are caused by gram-negative and gram-positive bacteria that make up the endogenous microflora of the lower genital tract (95, 96). The polymicrobial nature of postpartum endometritis raises the question of the role of *C. trachomatis* in this infection. However, it may appear that *C. trachomatis* plays a role in late, up to 6 weeks, endometritis (97).

Rosene et al. (98) recovered *C. trachomatis* alone from 4% (2/51) of patients. Although *C. trachomatis* does not appear to be associated with early postpartum endometritis, it would appear to be in the patients' best interest to screen for this bacterium in those developing postpartum febrile morbidity. Because of the low prevalence of *C. trachomatis* in the general population, a practical and cost effective approach would be to screen only those patients with a risk profile for contracting a STD.

C. trachomatis has been linked to other complications of pregnancy (e.g., abortion, prematurity, and premature rupture of amniotic membranes). *C. trachomatis* can lead to asymptomatic infection resulting in significant damage to the fallopian tubes with an increased incidence in tubal infertility and ectopic pregnancy (99–101). Witkin and Ledger (99) found a relationship between high-titer immunoglobulin G antibodies to *C. trachomatis* and recurrent spontaneous abortion. These investigators also examined the possible role of other antibodies (e.g., cytomegalovirus, cardiolipin, nuclear antigens, lactoferrin, and spermatozoa) but could not find any relationship to spontaneous abortion. They found that 7/17 (41%) women with three abortions and 6/10 (60%) women with four abortions had chlamydial antibodies compared with 20/148 (13.5%) with no abortions, 6/47 (12.8%) with one abortion, and 4/33 (12.1%) with two abortions ($p > 0.01$) (99). The incidence of three or more spontaneous abortions among women with high-titer ($\geq$1:128) chlamydial antibodies was 31.8%, and among seronegative women, the incidence was 7.5% (99).

The role of chlamydial infection in pregnancy remains somewhat of a controversy; however, the data strongly supports the findings that infection during pregnancy places the mother in jeopardy of compromising her pregnancy. Chlamydial infection of the cervix during pregnancy can result in the organism infecting the amniotic fluid and/or decidua. This, in turn, can lead to premature labor, premature rupture of membranes, premature delivery, stillbirth, and death. Sweet et al. (100) reported that among 270 pregnant women with documented endocervical chlamydial infection and match controls of 270 pregnant women, no differences were found in premature rupture of membranes, preterm delivery, amnionitis, intrapartum fever, infants found to be small for gestational age, postpartum endometritis, and neonatal sepsis. A subset of pregnant women positive for endocervical chlamydial infection was found to have significant IgM antibody levels. There were 166/270 (61%) women with positive IgM antibodies to *C. trachomatis,* of which 67/166 (40%) women had significant levels of IgM antibodies (100). Comparing two groups of chlamydial positive women, those with IgM antibodies to *C. trachomatis* were significantly more prone to have premature rupture of amniotic membranes 13/67 versus 8/99 ($p = 0.03$) and preterm delivery 13/67 versus 8/99 ($p = 0.03$) (100). Although there was no direct evidence that the patients with elevated levels of IgM antibodies had any more significant disease, these investigators hypothesized that these patients may have had upper genital tract infection compared with those individuals with only endocervical infection. Martin et al. (101) found that chlamydial endocervical infection during pregnancy was correlated with a significant increase in perinatal mortality, preterm delivery, and lower mean birth weights. There is general agreement that chlamydial infection occurring during pregnancy can have a significantly negative impact on the pregnancy. Therefore, there is also general agreement among obstetricians/gynecologists specializing in infectious diseases that all pregnant women should be evaluated for the presence of *C. trachomatis* in the endocervix. Currently, the Centers for Disease Control and Prevention (CDC) recommends universal screening for all pregnant women. Perhaps the obstetrician, family practitioner, or other medical care providers rendering obstetrical services should assess the patient's degree of risk to determine whether or not screening is indicated. If the risk cannot be assessed then the patient should be screened. It is important to remember that in addition to reducing the risk of premature delivery, chlamydial infection of the cervix can result in postpartum endometritis and neonatal infection, specifically ophthalmic infection and pneumonia.

CHLAMYDIAL INFECTION AND INFERTILITY

Once again it must be emphasized that chlamydial infection is more than likely to be asymptomatic. The asymptomatic nature of this infection places the patient in harm's way because there is a significant likelihood that the infection will go unnoticed and result in significant progressive disease. The result is damage to the fallopian tubes, which prohibits normal function causing the patient, if she is able to conceive, to either develop an ectopic pregnancy or to be infertile. The patient with progressive infection to the upper genital tract can also develop a tubal abscess (pyosalpinx) or tubo-ovarian abscess.

Many patients postpone the start of their family. Marriage may also be delayed because of career development or economic reasons. During this period, and before beginning a family, sexual abstinence is not the general rule and various methods of birth control are used. Individuals who have not practiced the use of condoms (either male or female) are exposed to the risk of STDs. One of the most common forms of birth control is the oral contraceptive pill (OCP). However, the OCP does not afford the patient protection against chlamydial or gonococcal infection.

Infection of the cervix can be detected, or at least the physician's index of suspicion can be raised, by noting the presence of follicular cervicitis. Follicular cervicitis is discussed in many gynecologic textbooks but is only given superficial treatment. This may be because follicular cervicitis and its relationship to chlamydial infection has not been firmly established. Roberts and Ng (102) described the presence of lymphocytic cervicitis in 6.7% of 450 consecutive hysterectomy specimens and found that 2.4% of the specimens contained lymphoid follicles. Dunlop et al. (103) described follicular cervicitis using colposcopic examination. Dunlop et al. (104–106) reported on a significant number of women, found to have follicular cervicitis, who were diagnosed as having nongonococcal genital infections, as well as asymptomatic women known to have male sex partners with nongonococcal urethritis. Hare et al. (107) found 15 (44%) of 34 women examined colposcopically to have follicular cervicitis. These women were known to have male sex partners diagnosed with nongonococcal urethritis. Twenty-six (76.5%) were proven, by culture, to have *C. trachomatis* urethritis. Cervical cultures obtained from these women revealed that 11 (73%) were chlamydial positive and had follicular cervicitis. There was no correlation found between the presence of *Mycoplasma hominis* or *Ureaplasma urealyticum*.

Hare et al. (107) described follicular cervicitis as "creamy white, raised, rounded swellings, up to 1 mm in diameter." Typically, the follicles lie beneath ectopic columnar epithelium and immature squamous metaplasia (107). Painting the cervix with acetic acid or iodine solution does not alter the characteristics of follicular cervicitis.

In contrast to the data supporting the association between follicular cervicitis and chlamydial infection, Paavonen et al. (108) studied 144 women and isolated chlamydia in 13 or 9%. These investigators examined these women colposcopically and did not find any evidence of follicular cervicitis (108). However, the significant clinical findings suggesting chlamydial infection are as follows: hypertrophy of the endocervical epithelium, bleeding when the cervix is gently touched with a Dacron or cotton-tipped applicator, and a Pap smear revealing an inflammatory reaction. The importance of such clinical findings become significant if indeed the patient does have a chlamydial infection because the duration of infection cannot be determined. Therefore, the extent of the infection may have progressed to involve the upper genital tract and remains undetected. Improper treatment can result in the patient being infertile or at risk for ectopic pregnancy. The first opportunity to prevent the sequelae of chlamydial infection is to recognize the clinical manifestations of chlamydial cervicitis.

As mentioned, although *Chlamydia* is often referred to as causing an asymptomatic infection, it frequently causes symptoms that are often overlooked. Chlamydial endometritis is usually mistaken for irregular uterine bleeding or breakthrough bleeding occurring in patients taking OCPs. Chlamydial endometritis is also a common component of PID (109). In the absence of salpingitis, chlamydial endometritis does occur and is associated with irregular uterine bleeding, central lower abdominal pain, and an elevated body temperature. However, in cases in which the pain extends bilaterally and there is significant elevation in the patient's body temperature, it may not be possible to distinguish endometritis from endometritis-salpingitis. Chlamydial endometritis can be established by performing an endometrial biopsy and dividing the specimen into two parts. One aliquot is processed for the detection of *Chlamydia* and the other for histologic examination. Chlamydial inclusion can be detected in endometrial cells and plasma cells during the follicular or ovulatory phase of the menstrual cycle (110–113). Persistent chlamydial endometritis, even though the woman is menstruating regularly, indicates that the organism penetrates deep into the endometrium and raises concern that standard treatment regimens may not be sufficient. Patients with chronic endometritis may not experience irregular bleeding but instead report menorrhagia (114–116). Thus, patients with acute, subchronic, or chronic endometritis may have menorrhagia or irregular uterine bleeding without having evidence of salpingitis (117).

In a study of 65 women taking OCPs and reporting irregular uterine bleeding, 19 tested positive for *C. trachomatis* (116). In this study, 10.1% of patients on OCPs were found to be positive for *Chlamydia* but were not spotting or bleeding compared with 29.2% who were ($p < .01$) (116). Jones et al. (117) reported isolating *Chlamydia* from the endocervix of 26 of 60 (43%) women attending a STD clinic. They also isolated *Chlamydia* from the endometrium of 12 (20%) of the women. Chlamydial infection, because of its asymptomatic nature, may result in approximately 1/3 of the patients developing clinical salpingitis (118). Women found to have tubal infertility and serologic or cultural documentation of chlamydial infection usually have no recollection of ever having had clinical salpingitis (119–121). This data suggest and support the hypothesis that progressive infection does occur shortly after cervical infection.

Paavonen et al. (122) reported on 35 women who underwent endometrial biopsies and found 40% had plasma cell endometritis; they recovered *C. trachomatis* from 86% of these women. In contrast, 48% of the women were positive for *Chlamydia* but did not have endometritis. The data reveal that women in the reproductive age group who are sexually active and present with lower abdominal pain, with or without adnexal tenderness, with irregular uterine bleeding, and with or without endocervical mucopus should be evaluated for the presence of endometritis. These women should be considered to have upper genital tract involvement and, therefore, should not be treated with a single-dose antibiotic regimen.

INFERTILITY

Chlamydial infection has the capability of stimulating the human host to produce both humoral and cellular immunity. Infection can be limited via the production of IgM, IgG, and secretory IgA antibodies. It is hypothesized that chlamydial infection can become chronic, causing an inflammatory response via cellular immune activation resulting in the production of cytokines. Bacteria share a common antigen that belongs to the 60-kD family of heat shock proteins (hsp60). Human beings also produce hsp60 under stressful conditions such as fever and inflammation. hsp60 functions to prevent protein denaturation and inappropriate aggregation, thus allowing the cell to survive (123). Bacterial hsp60 is a significant immunogen in humans and, following an acute infection, microorganism-specific hsp60 epitopes are released (124). Upper genital tract chlamydial infection, chronic or repeated, may result in prolonged exposure to hsp60 epitopes (125–127). An autoimmune response may be facilitated in sensitized women to self-hsp60 similar to the autoimmune response seen in obese diabetic mice and adjuvant arthritis in rats (128–129). Chlamydial infection of the fallopian tubes resulting in occlusion may well be caused by an immune response to the chlamydial hsp60 (130,131). There is no doubt that chlamydial infection induces an immune response, both humoral and cell mediated. The immune response to chlamydial infection appears to be complete with the formation of antibodies, cytokines, helper T cells, and cytotoxic T cells (132–137). Chlamydial infection either progresses from acute to chronic or, more likely, begins as an asymptomatic infection that, in all likelihood, becomes chronic. Persistent infection can be induced via the effect of cytokines, such as interferon-gamma (INFγ), which causes the depletion of tryptophan and subsequently stresses the bacterium initiating the development of abnormal chlamydial forms accompanied by elevated levels of stress response proteins (138,139). Persistence of these abnormal forms has been documented in tissue, including submucosa of the fallopian tubes (140,141). Because these abnormal forms present altered antigens to the host, its immune reaction is maintained. The chlamydial stress proteins (e.g., hsp60) initiate a host-delayed hypersensitivity and result in a continued susceptibility to the inflammatory reaction (142). During this continued inflammatory reaction, fibrin is produced resulting in the formation of adhesion causing disruption of the architecture of the fallopian tubes, as well as damage to the ciliated cells lining the inner surface of the fallopian tubes. This results in agglutination of the fimbria, adhesions within the lumen of the tube, and adhesions between the fallopian tubes structure of the pelvis. These alterations within the tube can lead to the development of ectopic pregnancy or infertility.

Chlamydial infection can lead to one of two sequelae with regard to pregnancy: infertility and abortion or failure to achieve successful implantation of a fertilized ovum. Chlamydial infection may play a significant role, via the production of IgA antibodies to chlamydial hsp60, in interfering with implantation of the embryo. This phenomenon has been demonstrated in women undergoing in-vitro fertilization (IVF) (143). Because hsp50 are produced by microbes, among the first proteins produced by embryogenesis, human decidua and trophoblast exposure to *C. trachomatis,* as well as other microorganisms, induces immune sensitization in women so exposed (144–146). Witkin et al. (143) demonstrated that women undergoing IVF who were sensitized to hsp60 were more likely to experience failure of implantation than women who had not been sensitized. These investigators demonstrated that the presence of cervical IgA reactive to chlamydial hsp60 in women undergoing IVF were more likely to experience implantation failure following embryo transfer. Additional analysis of women in the reproductive age group revealed cervical IgA antibody to chlamydial hsp60 was present in 13 of 91 (14%) of individuals with primary infertility ($p = 0.003$) (143). Further study demonstrated that the presence of cervical anti-hsp60 significantly correlated with the presence of INFγ ($p = 0.001$) and tumor necrosis factor-α ($p = 0.02$) in the cervix (143). These investigators also demonstrated that in women with a history of two or more spontaneous abortions there was a higher prevalence of IgG antibodies to human hsp60 ($p = 0.01$) 36.8% compared with fertile women (matched controls) 11.8% or women with primary infertility 11.1%. Thus, these investigators conclude that immune sensitization to epitopes expressed by human hsp60 can reduce the chance of achieving a successful pregnancy. The mechanism through which this interference occurs is via activation of hsp60 previously sensitized lymphocytes, initiation of the proinflammatory response (induction and liberation of cytokines) that blocks or interferes with implantation.

SUMMARY

C. trachomatis causes, for the most part, asymptomatic infection. A significant concern is that abnormal chlamydial forms can result from improper treatment regimens that can persist in the tissue stimulating an immune response. Repeated exposure to hsp60 can initiate a proinflammatory response that can cause tissue damage and prevent or interfere with embryogenesis and/or implantation. Until further therapeutic evidence is produced, it is probably in the best interest of the patient infected with *C. trachomatis* to have the physician administer antibiotics that are not only effective but also are given for at least 7 days (Table 2-4).

TABLE 2-4. *Treatment regimens for C. trachomatis cervicitis[a]*

Preferred antibiotic regimens for uncomplicated infection
    Azithromycin 1 g orally in a single dose
    Doxycycline 100 mg twice a day for 7 days
Alternative antibiotic choices
    Erythromycin base 500 mg orally four times a day for 7 days
    Erythromycin ethylsuccinate 800 mg four times a day for 7 days
    Ofloxacin 300 mg orally twice a day for 7 days
    Levofloxacin 500 mg orally once a day for 7 days
Antibiotic regimens for the pregnant patient
    Erythromycin base 500 mg orally four times a day for 7 days
    Amoxicillin 500 mg orally three times a day for 7 days
    Erythromycin base 250 mg four times a day for 7 days
    Erythromycin ethylsuccinate 800 mg orally four times a day for 7 days
    Erythromycin ethylsuccinate 400 mg four times a day for 14 days
    Azithromycin 1 g orally in a single dose

[a]Centers for Disease Control and Prevention. Sexually transmitted diseases treatment guidelines, 2002.*MMWR* 2002;51:32-34.

REFERENCES

1. Anonymous. Pelvic inflammatory disease. Research directions in the 1990. Expert Committee on Pelvic Inflammatory Disease. *Sex Transm Dis* 1991;18(1):46–64.
2. Washington AE, Johnson RE, Sanders II Jr. Chlamydia trachomatis infections in the United States: what are they costing us? *JAMA* 1987;257:2070–2072.
3. Piot P, Anneke J, Van den Hoek R, et al. Epidemiology and control of genital chlamydial infection. Epidemiology and control of genital chlamydial infection. In: Orfila J, Byrne GI, Chernesky MA, et al., eds. *Proceedings of the eighth international symposium on human chlamydial infection.* Bologna, Italy: Societa Editrice Esculapio, 1994:7–16.
4. Stamm WE, Holmes KK. Chlamydia trachomatis infections of the adult. In: Holmes KK, Mardh PA, Sparling PF, et al., eds. *Sexually transmitted diseases,* 2nd ed. New York McGraw-Hill, 1990; 181–193.
5. Stamm WE. Diagnosis of Chlamydia trachomatis genitourinary infections. *Ann Intern Med* 1988;108:710–717.
6. Anonymous. Recommendations for the prevention and management of Chlamydia trachomatis infections, 1993. Centers for Disease Control and Prevention. *MMWR* 1993;42(RR-12):1–39.
7. Quinn TC, Gaydos C, Shepard M, et al. Epidemiologic and microbiologic correlates of Chlamydia trachomatis in sexual partnerships. *JAMA* 1996;276:1737–1742.
8. McCormack WM, Alpert S, McComb DE, et al. Fifteen month follow-up study of women infected with Chlamydia trachomatis. *N Engl J Med* 1979;300:123–125.
9. Sweet RL. Chlamydial salpingitis and infertility. *Fertil Steril* 1982;38:530–533.
10. Higashi N. Electron microscopic studies on the mode of reproduction of trachoma virus and psittacosis virus in cell cultures. *Exp Mol Pathol* 1965;4:24.
11. Friis RR. Interaction of L cells and Chlamydia psittaci: entry of the parasite and host responses to its development. *J Bacteriol* 1972;110:706–721.
12. Tamura A, Matsumoto A, Manire GP, et al. Electron microscopic observations on the structure of the envelopes of mature elementary bodies and developmental reticulate forms of Chlamydia psittaci. *J Bacteriol* 1971;105:355–360.
13. Caldwell HD, Kromhout J, Schachter J. Purification and partial characterization of the major outer membrane protein of Chlamydia trachomatis. *Infect Immun* 1981;31:1161–1176.
14. Barbour AG, Amano KI, Hackstadt T, et al. Chlamydia trachomatis has penicillin-binding proteins but not detectable muramic acid. *J Bacteriol* 1982;151:420–428.
15. Garrett AJ, Harrison MJ, Manire GP. A search for the bacterial mucopeptide component, muramic acid, in Chlamydia. *J Gen Microbiol* 1974;80:315–318.
16. Matsumoto A, Manire GP. Electron microscopic observations on the effects of penicillin on the morphology Chlamydia psittaci. *J Bacteriol* 1970;101:278–285.

17. Moulder JW, Novasel DL, Officer JE. Inhibition of the growth of agents of the psittacosis group by D-cycloserine and its specific reversal by D-alanine. *J Bacteriol* 1963;85:707.
18. Gale EF, Cundliffe E, Reynolds PE, et al. *The molecular basis of antibiotic action,* 2nd ed. New York: John Wiley & Sons, 1981.
19. Frere JM, Joris B. Penicillin-sensitive enzymes in peptidoglycan biosynthesis. *Crit Rev Microbiol* 1985;11:299–396.
20. Reeve P, Taverne J. Some properties of the complement-fixing antigens of the agents of trachoma and inclusion blennorrhea and the relation of the antigen to the developmental cycle. *J Gen Microbiol* 1962;27:501.
21. Dhir SP, Boatman ES. Location of polysaccharide on Chlamydia psittaci by silver-methenamine staining and electron microscopy. *J Bacteriol* 1972;111:267–271.
22. Dhir SP, Hakomori S, Kenny GE, et al. Immunochemical studies on chlamydial group antigen (presence of a 2-keto-3-deoxy-carbohydrate as immuno dominant group). *J Immunol* 1972;109:116–122.
23. Nurminen M., Wahlstrom E, Kleemola M, et al. Immunologically related ketodeoxyoctonate-containing structures in Chlamydia trachomatis, Re mutants of Salmonella species, and Acinetobacter calcoaceticus var. anitratus. *Infect Immun* 1984;44:609–613.
24. Nurminen M, Rietschel ET, Brade H. Chemical characterization of Chlamydia trachomatis lipopolysaccharide. *Infect Immun* 1985;48:573–575.
25. Becker Y. The chlamydia: molecular biology of procaryotic obligate parasites of eucaryocytes. *Microbiol Rev* 1978;42:274–306.
26. MacDonald AB. Antigens of Chlamydia trachomatis. *Rev Infect Dis* 1985;7:731–736.
27. Byrne GI. Requirements for ingestion of Chlamydia psittaci by mouse fibroblasts (L cells). *Infect Immun* 1976;14:645–651.
28. Byrne GI, Moulder JW. Parasite-specified phagocytosis of Chlamydia psittaci and Chlamydia trachomatis by L and HeLa cells. *Infect Immun* 1978;19:598–606.
29. Aggeler J, Werb Z. Initial events during phagocytosis by macrophages viewed from outside and inside the cell: membrane-particle interactions and clathrin. *J Cell Biol* 1982;94:613–623.
30. Goldstein JL, Anderson RG, Brown MS. Coated pits, coated vesicles, and receptor-mediated endocytosis. *Nature* 1979;279:679–685.
31. Pastan I, Willingham MC. Receptor-mediated endocytosis: coated pits, receptosomes and the Golgi. *Trends Biochem Sci* 1983;8:251.
32. Brownridge E, Wyrick PB. Interaction of Chlamydia psittaci reticulate bodies with mouse peritoneal macrophages. *Infect Immun* 1979;24:697–700.
33. Eissenberg LG, Wyrick PB. Inhibition of phagolysosome fusion is localized to Chlamydia psittaci-laden vacuoles. *Infect Immun* 1981;32:889–896.
34. Jones TC, Hirsch JG. The interaction between Toxoplasma gondii and mammalian cells. II. The absence of lysosomal fusion with phagocytic vacuoles containing living parasites. *J Exp Med* 1972;136:1173–1194.
35. Kordova N, Wilt JC, Sadiq M. Lysosomes in L cells infected with Chlamydia psittaci 6BC strain. *Can J Microbiol* 1971;17:955–959.
36. Prain CJ, Pearce JH. Endocytosis of chlamydiae by McCoy cells: measurement and effects of centrifugation. *FEMS Microbiol Lett* 1985;26:233.
37. Hatch TP, Al-Hossainy E, Silverman JA. Adenine nucleotide and lysine transport in Chlamydia psittaci. *J Bacteriol* 1982;150:662–670.
38. Moulder JW. Looking at chlamydiae without looking at their host. *ASM News* 1984;50:353.
39. Kramer MJ, Gordon FB. Ultrastructural analysis of the effects of penicillin and chlortetracycline on the development of a genital tract Chlamydia. *Infect Immun* 1971;3:333.
40. Hatch TP. Competition between Chlamydia psittaci and L cells for host isoleucine pools: a limiting factor in chlamydial multiplication. *Infect Immun* 1975;12:211–220.
41. Allan I, Pearce JH. Amino acid requirements of strains of Chlamydia trachomatis and C. psittaci growing in McCoy cells: relationship with clinical syndrome and host origin. *J Gen Microbiol* 1983;129(pt. 7):2001–2007.
42. Hanna L, Dawson CR, Briones O, et al. Latency in human infections with TRIC agents. *J Immunol* 1968;101:43–50.
43. Oriel JD, Ridgeway GL. Studies of the epidemiology of chlamydial infection of the human genital tract. In: Mardh PA, Holmes KK, Oriel JD, et al., eds. *Chlamydial infection.* Amsterdam: Elsevier, 1982:425.
44. Todd WJ, Doughri AM, Storz J. Ultrastructural changes in host cellular organelles in the course of the chlamydial developmental cycle. *Zbl Bakt Hyg I Abt Orig* 1976;236:359–373.

45. Richmond SJ. Division and transmission of inclusions of Chlamydia trachomatis in replicating McCoy cell monolayers. *FEMS Microbiol Lett* 1985;29:49.
46. Quinn TC, Cates W Jr. Epidemiology of sexually transmitted disease in the 1990a. In: Quinn TC, ed. *Sexually transmitted diseases. Advances in host defense mechanisms,* vol. 8. New York: Raven Press, 1992:1–37.
47. Quinn TC, Gaydos, C, Sheperd M, et al. Epidemiologic and microbiologic correlates of Chlamydia trachomatis infection in sexual partnerships. *JAMA* 1996;276:1737–1742.
48. Stamm WE, Holmes KK. Chlamydia trachomatis infections of the adult. In: Holmes KK, Mardh PA, Sparling PF, et al., eds. *Sexually transmitted diseases,* 2nd ed. New York: McGraw Hill, 1990: 181–193.
49. Stamm WE. Diagnosis of Chlamydia trachomatis genitourinary infections. *Ann Inter Med* 1988: 108:710–717.
50. National Center for Health Statistics. *Advanced report of final mortality statistics.* Hyattsville, MD: U.S. Department of Health and Human Services, Public Health Service, Centers for Disease Control and Prevention, *Monthly Vital Statistics Report* 1994;43(6 Suppl).
51. Gaydos CA, Howell MR, Pare B, et al. Chlamydia trachomatis infections in female military recruits. *N Engl J Med* 1998;339:739–744.
52. Goldner TE, Lawson HW, Xia Z, et al. Surveillance for ectopic pregnancy—United States, 1970–1989. *MMWR CDC Surveill Summ* 1993;42(SS-6):73–85.
53. Hillis SD, Owens LM, Marchbanks PA, et al. Recurrent chlamydial infections increase the risk of hospitalization for ectopic pregnancy and pelvic inflammatory disease. *Am J Obstet Gynecol* 1997; 176:103–107.
54. Quinn TC, Goodell SE, Mkrtichian E, et al. Chlamydia trachomatis proctitis. *N Engl J Med* 1981;305:195–200.
55. Workowski KA, Stevens CE, Suchland RJ, et al. Clinical manifestations of genital infection due to Chlamydia trachomatis in women: differences related to serovar. *Clin Inf Dis* 1994;19:756–760.
56. *Sexually Transmitted Disease Surveillance,* 1996. U.S. Department of Health and Human Services, Centers for Disease Control, Atlanta, GA; 9.
57. Washington AE, Johnson RE, Sanders LL, et al. Incidence of Chlamydia trachomatis infections in the United States: using reported Neisseria gonorrhoeae as a surrogate. In: Oriel JD, Ridgeway GL, Schather J, et al., eds. *Chlamydia trachomatis infections: proceedings of sixth international symposium on human Chlamydia trachomatis infections.* New York: Cambridge University Press, 1986:487–490.
58. Washington AE, Johnson RE, Sanders LL Jr. Chlamydia trachomatis infections in the United States. What are they costing us? *JAMA* 1987;257:2070–2072.
59. Tam MR, Stamm WE, Handsfield HH, et al. Culture-independent diagnosis of Chlamydia trachomatis using monoclonal antibodies. *N Engl J Med* 1984;310:1146–1150.
60. Lipkin ES, Moncada JV, Shafer MA, et al. Comparison of monoclonal antibody staining and culture in diagnosing cervical chlamydial infection. *J Clin Microbiol* 1986;23:114–117.
61. Stamm WE, Harrison HR, Alexander ER, et al. Diagnosis of Chlamydia trachomatis infection by direct immunofluorescence staining of genital secretions: a multicenter trial. *Ann Inter Med* 1984; 101:638–641.
62. Nettleman MD, Jones RB. Cost-effectiveness of screening women at moderate risk for genital infections caused by Chlamydia trachomatis. *JAMA* 1988;260:207–213.
63. Phillips RS, Hanff PA, Holmes MD, et al. Chlamydia trachomatis cervical infection in women seeking routine gynecologic care: criteria for selective testing. *Am J Med* 1989;86:515–520.
64. Handsfield HH, Jasman LL, Roberts PL, et al. Criteria for selective screening for Chlamydia trachomatis infection in women attending family planning clinics. *JAMA* 1986;255:1730–1734.
65. Katz BP, Caine VA, Jones RB. Diagnosis of mucopurulent cervicitis among women at risk for Chlamydia trachomatis infection. *Sex Transm Dis* 1989;16:103–136.
66. Paavonen J, Purola E. Cytologic findings in cervical chlamydial infection. *Med Biol* 1980; 58:174–178.
67. Carr MC, Hanna L, Jawetz E. Chlamydiae, cervicitis, and abnormal Papanicolaou smears. *Obstet Gynecol* 1979;53:27–30.
68. Moncada J, Schachter J, Shipp M, et al. Cytobrush in collection of cervical specimens for the detection of Chlamydia trachomatis. *J Clin Microbiol* 1989;27:1863–1866.
69. Kellogg JA. Clinical and laboratory considerations of culture vs antigen assays for detection of Chlamydia trachomatis from genital specimens. *Arch Pathol Lab Med* 1989;113:453–460.

70. Embil JA, Thiebaux HJ, Manuel FR, et al. Sequential cervical specimens and the isolation of Chlamydia trachomatis: factors affecting detection. *Sex Transm Dis* 1983;10:62–66.
71. Mardh PA, Colleen S, Sylwan J. Inhibitory effect on the formation of chlamydial inclusions in McCoy cells by seminal fluid and some of its components. *Invest Urol* 1980;17:510–513.
72. Kallings I, Mardh PA. Sampling and specimen handling in the diagnosis of genital Chlamydia trachomatis infections. *Scand J Infect Dis Suppl* 1982;32:21–24.
73. Mahony JB, Chernesky MA. Effect of swab type and storage temperature on the isolation of Chlamydia trachomatis from clinical specimens. *J Clin Microbiol* 1985;22:865–867.
74. Mardh PA, Zeeberg B. Toxic effect of sampling swabs and transportation test tubes on the formation of intracytoplasmic inclusions of Chlamydia trachomatis in McCoy cell cultures. *Br J Vener Dis* 1981;57:268–272.
75. Ryan RW, Kwasnik I, Steingrimsson O, et al. Rapid detection of Chlamydia trachomatis by an enzyme immunoassay method. *Diagn Microbial Infect Dis* 1986:5:225–234.
76. Baselski VS, McNeeley SG, Ryan G, et al. A comparison on nonculture-dependent methods for detection of Chlamydia trachomatis infections in pregnant women. *Obstet Gynecol* 1987;70:47–52.
77. Ridgway GL, Oriel JD, Mumtaz G, et al. Comparison of methods for detecting Chlamydia trachomatis. *J Clin Pathol* 1986;39:232–223.
78. Graber CD, Williamson O, Pike J, et al. Detection of Chlamydia trachomatis infection in endocervical specimens using direct immunofluorescence. *Obstet Gynecol* 1985;66:727–730.
79. Le Febvre J, La Perriere H, Rousseau H, et al. Comparison of three techniques for detection of Chlamydia trachomatis in endocervical specimens from asymptomatic women. *J Clin Microbiol* 1988;26:726–731.
80. Amortegui AJ, Meyer MP. Enzyme immunoassay for detection of Chlamydia trachomatis from the cervix. *Obstet Gynecol* 1985;65:523–526.
81. Howard LV, Coleman PF, England BJ, et al. Evaluation of Chlamydiazyme for the detection of genital infections caused by Chlamydia trachomatis. *J Clin Microbiol* 1986;23:329–332.
82. Moi H, Danielsson D. Diagnosis of genital Chlamydia trachomatis infection in males by cell culture and antigen detection test. *Eur J Clin Microbiol* 1986:5:569–572.
83. Krech T, Gerhard-Fsadni D, Hofmann N, et al. Interference of Staphylococcus aureus in the detection of Chlamydia trachomatis by monoclonal antibodies. *Lancet* 1985;1(8438):1161–1162.
84. Taylor-Robinson D, Thomas BJ, Osborn MF. Evaluation of enzyme immunoassay (Chlamydiazyme) for detecting Chlamydia trachomatis genital tract specimens. *J Clin Pathol* 1987;40:194–199.
85. Rompalo AM, Suchland RJ, Price CB, et al. Rapid diagnosis of Chlamydia trachomatis rectal infection by direct immunofluorescence staining. *J Infect Dis* 1987;155:1075–1076.
86. Saikku P, Puolakkainen M, Leinonen M, et al. Cross-reactivity between Chlamydiazyme and Acinetobacter strains. *N Engl J Med* 1986;314:922–923.
87. Bobo L, Coutlee F, Yolken RH, et al. Diagnosis of Chlamydia trachomatis cervical infection by detection of amplified DNA with an enzyme immunoassay. *J Clin Microbiol* 1990;28:1968–1973.
88. Class HC, Wagenvoort JH, Niesters HG, et al. Diagnostic value of the polymerase chain reaction for Chlamydia detection as determined in a follow-up study. *J Clin Microbiol* 1991;29:42–45.
89. Naher H, Drzonek H, Wolf J, et al. Detection of C. trachomatis in urogenital specimens by polymerase chain reaction. *Genitourin Med* 1991;67:211–214.
90. Witkin SS, Jeremias J, Toth M, et al. Detection of Chlamydia trachomatis by the polymerase chain reaction in the cervices of women with acute salpingitis. *Am J Obstet Gynecol* 1993;168:1438–1442.
91. Todd CS, Jones RB, Golichowski A, et al. Chlamydia trachomatis and febrile complications of postpartum tubal ligation. *Am J Obstet Gynecol* 1997;176:100–102.
92. Ryan GW Jr., Abdella TN, McNeeley SG, et al. Chlamydia trachomatis infection in pregnancy and the effect of treatment on outcome. *Am J Obstet Gynecol* 1990;162:34–39.
93. Black-Payne C, Ahrabi MM, Bocchini JA Jr, et al. Treatment of Chlamydia trachomatis identified with Chlamydiazyme during pregnancy: impact on perinatal complications and infants. *J Reprod Med* 1990;35:362–367.
94. Wager GP, Martin DH, Koutsky L, et al. Puerperal infectious morbidity: relationship to route of delivery and to antepartum Chlamydia trachomatis infection. *Am J Obstet Gynecol* 1980;138:1028–1033.
95. Eschenbach DA, Wager GP. Puerperal infections. *Clin Obstet Gynecol* 1980;23:1003–1037.
96. Faro S. Chlamydia trachomatis infection in women. *J Reprod Med* 1985;30(Suppl 3)273–278.
97. Watts DH, Eschenbach DA, Kenny GE. Early postpartum endometritis: the role of bacteria, genital mycoplasmas, and Chlamydia trachomatis. *Obstet Gynecol* 1989;73:52–60.

98. Rosene K, Eschenbach DA, Tompkins LS, et al. Polymicrobial early postpartum endometritis with facultative and anaerobic bacteria, genital mycoplasmas, and Chlamydia trachomatis: treatment with piperacillin or cefoxitin. *J Infect Dis* 1986;153:1028–1037.

99. Witkin SS, Ledger WJ. Antibodies to Chlamydia trachomatis in sera of women with recurrent spontaneous abortions. *Am J Obstet Gynecol* 1992;167:135–139.

100. Sweet RL, Landers DV, Walker C, et al. Chlamydial trachomatis infection and pregnancy outcome. *Am J Obstet Gynecol* 1987;156:824–833.

101. Martin DH, Koutsky L, Eschenbach DA, et al. Prematurity and perinatal mortality in pregnancies complicated by maternal Chlamydia trachomatis infections. *JAMA* 1982;247:1585–1588.

102. Roberts TH, Ng AB. Chronic lymphocytic cervicitis: cytologic and histopathologic manifestations. *Acta Cytol* 1975;19:235–243.

103. Dunlop EM, Jones BR, al-Hussaini MK. Genital infections associated with TRIC virus infection of the eye. *Br J Vener Dis* 1964;40:33–42.

104. Dunlop EM, Harper JA, al-Hussaini MK, et al. Relation of TRIC agent to "non-specific genital infection." *Br J Vener Dis* 1966;42:77–87.

105. Dunlop EM, Hare MJ, Darougar S, et al. Detection of Chlamydia (Bedsonia) in certain infections in man II. Clinical study of genital tract, eye, rectum, and other sites of recovery of Chlamydia. *J Infect Dis* 1969;120:463–470.

106. Dunlop EM, Vaughan-Jackson JD, Darougar S, et al. Chlamydial infection: incidence of "non-specific" urethritis. *Br J Vener Dis* 1972;48:425–428.

107. Hare MJ, Toone E, Taylor-Robinson D, et al. Follicular cervicitis—colposcopic appearances and association with Chlamydia trachomatis. *Br J Obstet Gynecol* 1981;88:174–180.

108. Paavonen J, Saikku P, Vesterinen E, et al. Genital chlamydial infections in patients attending a gynecological outpatient clinic. *Br J Vener Dis* 1978;54:257–261.

109. Mardh PA, Moller BR, Ingerslev HV, et al. Endometritis caused by Chlamydia trachomatis. *Br J Vener Dis* 1981;57:191–195.

110. Brudenell JM. Chronic endometritis and plasma cell infiltration of the endometrium. *J Obstet Gynecol Br Emp* 1955;62:269.

111. Moller BR, Westrom L, Ahrons S, et al. Chlamydia trachomatis infection of the fallopian tube; histologic findings in two patients. *Br J Vener Dis* 1979;55:422–428.

112. Ingerslev HJ, Moller BR, Mardh PA. Chlamydia trachomatis in acute and chronic endometritis. *Scand J Infect Dis Suppl* 1982;32:59–63.

113. Runge H. Gonorrhoe der weiblicher Geschlechtsorgane. In: Setz L, Amreich A, eds. *Biologie und Pathologie des Weibes.* Berlin: Urban & Schwarzenberg, 1953:445.

114. Buttner HH, Barter G. [Histological and diagnostic criteria and incidence of endometritis in abrasion material.] *Zentralbl att fur Gynakologic* 1976;98:1515–1517.

115. Dumoulin JG, Hughesdon PE. Chronic endometritis. *J Obstet Gynecol Br Emp* 1951;58:222.

116. Krettek JE, Arkin SI, Chaisilwattana P, et al. Chlamydia trachomatis in patients who used oral contraceptives and had intermenstrual spotting. *Obstet Gynecol* 1993;81:728–731.

117. Jones RB, Mammel JB, Shepard MK, et al. Recovery of Chlamydia trachomatis from the endometrium of women at risk for chlamydial infection. *Am J Obstet Gynecol* 1986;155:35–39.

118. Stamm WE, Guinan ME, Johnson C, et al. Effect of treatment regimens for Neisseria gonorrhoeae on simultaneous infection with Chlamydia trachomatis. *N Engl J Med* 1984;310:545–549.

119. Jones RB, Ardery BR, Hui SL, et al. Correlation between serum antichlamydial antibodies and tubal factor as a cause of infertility. *Fertil Steril* 1982;38:553–558.

120. Henry-Suchet J, Catalan F, Loffredo V, et al. Microbiology of specimens obtained by laparoscopy from controls and from patients with pelvic inflammatory disease or infertility with tubal obstruction: Chlamydia trachomatis and Ureaplasma urealyticum. *Am J Obstet Gynecol* 1980;138:1022–1025.

121. Cleary RE, Jones RB. Recovery of Chlamydia trachomatis from the endometrium in infertile women with serum antichlamydial antibodies. *Fertil Steril* 1985;44:233–235.

122. Paavonen J, Kiviat N, Brunham RC, et al. Prevalence and manifestations of endometritis among women with cervicitis. *Am J Obstet Gynecol* 1985;152:280–286.

123. Ellis J. Stress proteins as molecular chaperones. In: van Eden W, Young DB, eds. *Stress proteins in medicine.* New York: Marcel Dekkar, 1996:1–26.

124. Kaufmann SH. Heat shock proteins and the immune response. *Immunol Today* 1990;11(4):129–136.

125. Morrison RP, Manning DS, Caldwell HD. Immunology of Chlamydia trachomatis infections. In: Quinn TC, ed. *Sexually transmitted diseases.* New York: Raven Press, 1992:57–84.

126. Witkin SS, Jeremias J, Toth M, et al. Cell-mediated immune response to the recombinant 57-kDa heat-shock protein of Chlamydia trachomatis in women with salpingitis. *J Infect Dis* 1993;167: 1379–1383.
127. Witkin SS, Jeremias J, Toth M, et al. Proliferative response to conserved epitopes of Chlamydia trachomatis and human 60-kilodalton heat-shock proteins by lymphocytes from women with salpingitis. *Am J Obstet Gynecol* 1994;171:455–460.
128. Elias D, Markovits D, Reshef T, et al. Induction and therapy of autoimmune diabetes in the nonobese diabetic (NON/Lt) mouse by a 65-kDa heat shock protein. *Proc Natl Acad Sci U S A* 1990;87: 1576–1580.
129. Hogervorst EJ, Boog CJ, Wagenaar PA, et al. T cell reactivity to an epitope of the mycobacterial 65-kDa heat-shock protein (hsp 65) corresponds with arthritis susceptibility in rats and is regulated by hsp 65-specific cellular responses. *Eur J Immunol* 1991;21:1289–1296.
130. Witkin SS, Jeremias J, Neuer A, et al. Immune recognition of 60 kD heat shock protein: implications for subsequent fertility. *Infect Dis Obstet Gynecol* 1996;4:152–158.
131. Witkin SS. Immune pathogenesis of asymptomatic Chlamydia trachomatis infections in the female genital tract. *Infect Dis Obstet Gynecol* 1995;3:169–74.
132. Batteiger J, MacDonald AB. The role of immunoglobulin in the neutralization of trachoma infectivity. *J Immunol* 1987; 55:1767–1773.
133. Beatty PR, Stephens RS. CD8+ T lymphocyte-mediated lysis of Chlamydia infected L cells using an endogenous antigen pathway. *J Immunol* 1994;153:4588–4595.
134. Rank RG, White HJ. Humoral immunity in the resolution of genital infection in female guinea pigs infected with the agent of guinea pig inclusion conjunctivitis. *Infect Immun* 1979;26:573–579.
135. Starnbach MN, Bevan MJ, Lampe MF. Protective cytotoxic T-lymphocytes are induced during murine infection with Chlamydia trachomatis. *J Immunol* 1994;153:5183–5189.
136. Williams DM, Magee DM, Bonewald LF, et al. A role in vivo for tumor necrosis factor alpha in host defense against Chlamydia trachomatis. *Infect Immun* 1990;58:1572–1576.
137. Zhang Y-X, Stewart S, Joseph T, et al. Protective monoclonal antibodies recognize epitopes located on the major outer membrane protein of Chlamydia trachomatis. *J Immunol* 1987;138:575–581.
138. Beatty WL, Belinger TA, Le DK, et al. Chlamydial persistence mechanism of induction and parallels to a stress-related response. In: Orfila J, Byrne GI, Chernesky MA, et al, eds. *Chlamydial infections.* Bologna, Italy: Societa Editrice Esculapio,1994;415–418.
139. Henry-Suchet J, Askienazy-Elbhar M, Orfila J. Clinical consequences of immune response to CT upper genital tract Infection in women. *Infect Dis Obstet Gynecol* 1996;4:171–175.
140. Campbell LA, Patton DL, Moore DE, et al. Detection of Chlamydia trachomatis deoxyribonucleic acid in women with tubal infertility. *Fertil Steril* 1993;59:45–50.
141. Patton DL, Askienazy M, Henry-Suchet J, et al. Detection of Chlamydia trachomatis in fallopian tube tissue in women with postinfection tubal infertility. *Am J Obstet Gynecol* 1994;171:95–101.
142. Lehtinen M, Paavonen J. Heat shock protein in the immunopathogenesis of Chlamydial pelvic inflammatory disease. In: Orfila J, Byrne GI, Chernesky MA, et al, eds. *Chlamydial infections.* Bologna, Italy: Societa Editrice Esculapio, 1994:599–609.
143. Witkin SS, Sultan KM, Neal GS, et al. Unsuspected Chlamydia trachomatis infection and in vitro fertilization outcome. *Am J Obstet Gynecol* 1994;171:1208–1214.
144. Bensuade O, Morange M. Spontaneous high expression of heat shock proteins in mouse embryonal cells and ectoderm from 8 mouse embryo. *EMBO* J 1983;2:173–177.
145. Mincheva-Nilsson L, Baranov V, Yeung MM, et al. Immunomorphologic studies of human decidua-associated lymphoid cells in normal early pregnancy. *J Immunol* 1994;152:2020–2032.
146. Heybourne K, Fu YX, Nelson A, et al. Recognition of trophoblasts by γδ T cells. *J Immunol* 1994; 153:2918–2926.

3

Pelvic Inflammatory Disease

INTRODUCTION

Pelvic inflammatory disease (PID) is a complex infection that affects millions of women around the world. All women who have not had a hysterectomy and are sexually active are potentially at risk for developing PID. Even women who undergo a procedure requiring instrumentation via the lower genital tract for diagnostic purposes are potentially placed at risk for acquiring PID. Women who have had a hysterectomy and undergo transvaginal aspiration of a pelvic mass are still at risk for developing PID (e.g., aspiration of an ovarian cyst can lead to the formation of an ovarian abscess). In addition, these women are not immune from contracting a sexually transmitted disease (STD) such as *Neisseria gonorrhoeae, Chlamydia trachomatis, Trichomonas vaginalis, Treponema pallidum,* hepatitis B and C, and human papillomavirus (HPV). The urethra, Skene's glands, Bartholin's glands, and the rectum can also be infected. Although the cervix is absent, these sites can serve as possible portals of entry for these organisms and can lead to systemic disease.

This disease, referred to as PID, is actually a spectrum of reproductive tract infections, and can be localized to the cervix, uterus, or fallopian tubes. PID should be viewed as a dynamic progressive infection that can migrate rapidly from the cervix to the uterus to the fallopian tubes and can involve the ovaries. Once the disease has become progressive, it can have devastating consequences on the reproductive tract and the reproductive capabilities of the woman. Unfortunately, the disease is often asymptomatic, and most infected women do not know that they have been infected or that their reproductive capability has been jeopardized. Therein lies the great tragedy of PID. Therefore, all individuals responsible for the care of women (e.g., obstetricians, gynecologists, family practitioners, general internal medicine physicians, emergency room physicians, residents in training, and nurse practitioners) have a significant responsibility in the prevention and proper treatment of PID. These individuals must never assume that a patient is not at risk for contracting a STD and/or developing PID. Regrettably, not all sexually active women presenting to their health care provider will be assessed as at risk for contracting a STD. Another confounding factor is that not all women presenting with a clinical picture suggesting the presence of PID will actually have PID; they will not receive an appropriate evaluation but will most likely be placed on antibiotic therapy unnecessarily. All sexually active women, regardless of age, who possess a cervix, a uterus, fallopian tubes, and ovaries are at risk for contracting a pelvic infection. Health care providers must be aware of the risk factors and subtle presentations associated with infection of the lower and upper genital tract. Physicians and nurse practitioners should have a thorough understanding of the risk factors and should take a thorough history from the patient to determine her degree of risk. Once this has been ascertained, appropriate diagnostic tests can be performed and management can be initiated. The physician should have a thorough knowledge of which antibiotics are appropriate for the treatment of PID.

A second group of women at risk for acquiring PID are those undergoing a transvaginal diagnostic procedure to evaluate the upper genital tract. These women, if their vaginal microflora is altered, can experience upper genital tract invasion by bacteria of the lower genital tract resulting in endometritis and/or salpingitis. If these women have a cervical STD, this organism can be literally pushed into the upper genital tract, resulting in significant infection. The transvaginal procedures in this category include artificial insemination, hysterosalpingography, intrauterine device (IUD) insertion, and fetal reduction.

A third group of women at risk are those with a diagnosis of diverticulosis. These patients are typically older than 35 years. They can develop diverticulitis that can result in the fusion of the inflamed diverticulum to the fallopian tube, ovary, or both organs. This, in turn, results in the formation of a fistula between the two structures permitting transfer of infected material (bacteria-laden feces) to the adnexa resulting in the development of a pyosalpinx, ovarian abscess, or tubo-ovarian complex.

Thus, PID has multiple origins. It can originate from the acquisition of a STD, from the patient's own endogenous vaginal microflora following instrumentation of the upper genital tract via the lower genital tract, or from an adjacent pelvic organ such as an inflamed appendix or diverticulitis. In 1998 it was estimated that the costs of PID and its sequelae were $1.88 billion. The costs were divided into $1.06 billion for treatment of PID, $166 million for the treatment of chronic pelvic pain, $259 million attributable to the management and treatment for ectopic pregnancies, and $360 million of the treatment of infertility caused by PID (1). Thus, most costs attributable to PID are incurred in the initial treatment of PID. Therefore, prevention is the best treatment. Although PID may never be completely eliminated, the incidence can be significantly reduced. Education is probably the most important and most difficult step. Admittedly, this requires a great investment in time, dollars, and the realization that all women are at risk.

Both men and women play key roles in PID that has its origin in STDs; therefore, women must understand how the disease is transmitted and acquired, the factors that place them at risk, and the progressive nature of the disease. Men and women must both assume responsibility for themselves and their sexual practices. Because the male plays a key role in the transmission of STDs, he must assume the responsibility for ensuring that he is not infected or a carrier of an STD. Men who have more than one sexual partner, female or male, can act as a reservoir and a vector of STD transmission because the disease may be asymptomatic. Therefore, men must accept the responsibility of practicing safe sex and be cognizant that their behavior can affect the health of their partners. Likewise, a woman with multiple sexual partners places all those she has sexual contact with in jeopardy. She must recognize the subtle nuances of PID, such as changes in her menstrual pattern, onset of mild pelvic discomfort, and changes associated with sexual intercourse such as pain and postcoital bleeding. Finally, the physician and other caregivers must not overlook subtle signs of infection that are compatible with a diagnosis of PID.

Physicians and nurse practitioners cannot assume, because of a woman's economic status, educational background, position in society, or attire, that she is not at risk for acquiring PID. Therefore, a detailed history must be obtained from each sexually active patient to determine the degree of risk or potential for acquiring PID. This includes all information regarding recent instrumentation or conditions involving other pelvic organs.

EPIDEMIOLOGY

PID is considered one of the most serious and frequent infections in women. The Centers for Disease Control and Prevention (CDC) estimated that in 1998 there were approximately 250,000 physician office visits for PID (2). This is a significant decrease because in 1988 there were approximately 450,000 visits (2) (Fig. 3-1). In 1988, it was estimated that approximately 10% to 15% of

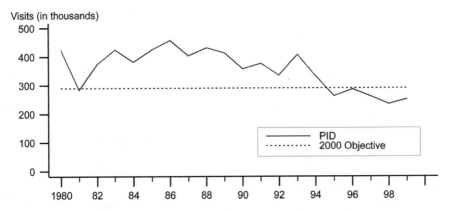

FIG. 3-1. Pelvic inflammatory disease (PID)—initial visits to physicians' offices by women 15 to 44 years of age in the United States from 1980 to 1999. (From *Sexually Transmitted Disease Surveillance, 1999*, U.S. Department of Health and Human Services, Centers for Disease Control, Atlanta, GA and *National Disease and Therapeutic Index*, IMS America, Ltd, with permission.)

reproductive-aged women experienced at least one episode of PID (2). In a recent study of 9,882 sexually active women, 6% (683) reported a history of a STD and 8% (791) reported a history of PID (3). There does appear to be a decrease in the number of cases of PID; however, the question that has not been addressed is whether this decrease is real or if the actual number of cases is underreported because of the current changes in health care. Managed care does create "road blocks" for the patient needing ready access to health care, specifically requiring a referral to see physicians with an interest, the expertise, and experience in recognizing the signs and symptoms of PID. This system makes it difficult and costly for patients to obtain care from specialty physicians. Therefore, has there actually been an increase in the number of asymptomatic and symptomatic cases that is not being identified? There is concern that the current system of health care poses a significant threat to women in the reproductive age group because they are required to see a physician who lacks the training and experience to appropriately recognize the risk factors associated with acquisition of STDs and PID. This is reflected in an increase in the number of infertile women. In addition to errors in diagnosis, there is misuse of antibiotics that can lead not only to the selection of resistant bacteria within the endogenous vaginal microflora but also to incomplete treatment. Another area of concern is the focus on shorter regimens for treating both gonococcal and chlamydial cervical infections. This effort is based on the hope that there will be better compliance with taking prescribed medication. However, available data does not address the results of single-dosing regimens and outcomes with regard to the prevention of subsequent fallopian tube disease and damage. When a woman is diagnosed with cervicitis, there is no way to know whether the disease has progressed to involve the upper genital tract. Therefore, before jumping on the single-dose bandwagon, there should be caution because the result may be an increase in the number of patients experiencing infertility, ectopic pregnancy, and other sequelae of PID. The prevalence of PID will always be significant, regardless of the number of cases estimated, because PID is responsible for approximately 30% of infertility cases and 50% of ectopic pregnancies.

Neisseria gonorrhoeae and *Chlamydia trachomatis* are the most common sexually transmitted bacteria, and are responsible for the largest number of PID cases. The prevalence of *N. gonorrhoeae* has consistently decreased in the United States since 1975, from approximately 425 cases per 100,000 population to 250 cases per 100,000 population in 1998 (Fig. 3-2).

The number of gonorrhea cases decreased significantly in most groups, except among African Americans where there has been a decrease from almost 7,000 cases per 100,000 in 1985 to 4,000 cases per 100,000 in 1998 (Fig. 3-3). However, there was an increase in 1998 over the number of cases in 1996 and 1997. Examining the occurrence of gonorrhea in the United States, it appears that the largest number of cases occurs in the South, Ohio, Illinois, and Missouri (Fig. 3-4).

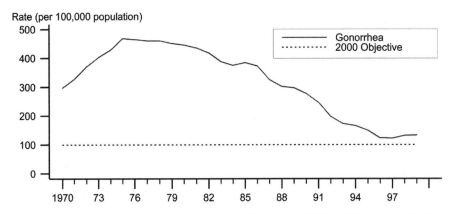

FIG. 3-2. Gonorrhea—reported rates in the United States from 1970 to 1999 and the Healthy People year 2000 objective. (From *Sexually Transmitted Disease Surveillance, 1999*, U.S. Department of Health and Human Services, Centers for Disease Control, Atlanta, GA, with permission.)

Although there was a decrease in the number of *Chlamydia* cases beginning in 1989 through 1996, in 1997 there was an increase that has continued (Fig. 3-5). This increase occurred in all racial and ethnic groups, with the greatest increase seen among African-American and Hispanic women. This increase in the number of *Chlamydia* cases causes concern because the infection tends to be asymptomatic and the subtleness of the clinical presentation is often unrecognized. This results in either no treatment or inappropriate treatment. There was also an increase in relationships between individuals of different races and eth-

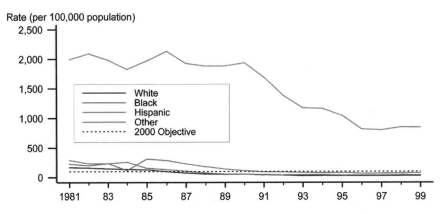

FIG. 3-3. Gonorrhea—rates by race and ethnicity in the United States from 1981 to 1999 and the Healthy People year 2000 objective. "Other" includes Asian/Pacific Islander and American Indian/Alaska native populations. Black, white, and other are non-Hispanic. (From *Sexually Transmitted Disease Surveillance, 1999*, U.S. Department of Health and Human Services, Centers for Disease Control, Atlanta, GA, with permission.)

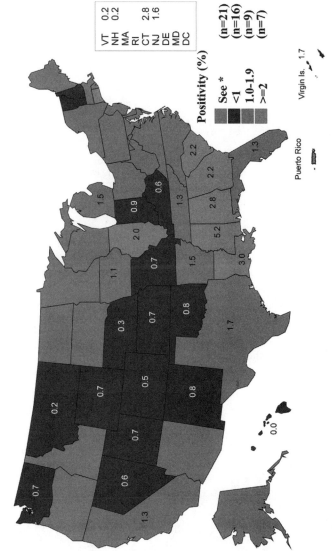

FIG. 3-4. Gonorrhea—positivity among 15- to 24-year-old women tested in family planning clinics by state in 1999. *States reported gonorrhea positivity data on less than 500 women aged 15 to 24 years during 1999 except for New Jersey and Virgin Islands submitting gonorrhea positivity data for July through December only. (From *Sexually Transmitted Disease Surveillance, 1999*, U.S. Department of Health and Human Services, Centers for Disease Control, Atlanta, GA, with permission.)

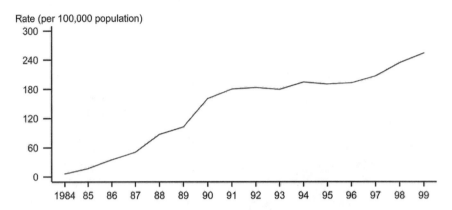

FIG. 3-5. *Chlamydia*—cases reported in the United States from 1984 to 1999. (From *Sexually Transmitted Disease Surveillance, 1999*, U.S. Department of Health and Human Services, Centers for Disease Control, Atlanta, GA, with permission.)

nic origins. An increase in these kinds of relationships has the potential to increase trends in STD transmission. Racial and ethnic boundaries are breaking down, thus allowing for relaxed relationships and the potential of transmission.

Interestingly, the increase in the number of *Chlamydia* cases was not reflected in the number of hospitalizations for acute and chronic PID. Indeed, there was a steady decrease in the number of hospital admissions for PID between 1982 and 1994; however, there was a plateau in the number of PID cases from 1995 to 1997 (Fig. 3-6). Although, on the surface, this appears to be "good news," there should be concern because of the tendency of this disease to be asymptomatic. We may actually be experiencing a false sense of accomplishment because the

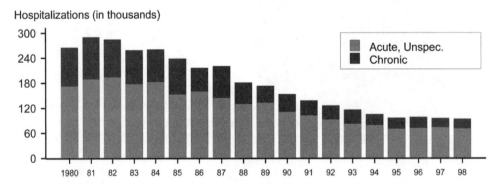

FIG. 3-6. Pelvic inflammatory disease (PID)—hospitalization of women 15 to 44 years of age in the United States from 1980 to 1998. The relative standard error for the estimates of the overall total number of PID cases range from 6% to 9%. (From *National Hospital Discharge Survey*, National Center for Health Statistics, U.S. Department of Health and Human Services, Centers for Disease Control, Atlanta, GA, with permission.)

incidence of chlamydial infection in women is rising (Figs. 3-5, 3-7, and 3-8). Women between the ages of 15 and 35 years may not be evaluated with a focus on the possibility that they might have a chlamydial or gonococcal infection. Although the incidence of chlamydial infection in women is rising, the incidence of gonorrhea appears to be decreasing. The incidence of gonorrhea infection has steadily decreased since 1975 (Fig. 3-2) in all ethnic groups with the most significant decrease among blacks since 1990 (Fig. 3-3). Although the incidence of gonorrhea is decreasing it continues to be a problem throughout the South and West and in Illinois and Missouri (Fig. 3-4). In today's health care environment the emphasis is not on routine screening for STDs because (a) most physicians may not consider the patients in their practice at risk, (b) the health maintenance organization (HMO) may not pay for routine STD screening, and (c) subtle signs and symptoms of STDs are not recognized by the inexperienced physician. The reality is that all individuals participating in sexual intercourse are at risk, and the degree of risk is dependent on whether or not the individual is in a truly monogamous relationship.

Further support that PID may actually be decreasing is reflected in a reduction in the ectopic pregnancy rate (Fig. 3-9). The number of ectopic pregnancies appears to have peaked in 1989. That year the CDC reported approximately 90,000 cases, and in 1997 there were 30,000 cases reported. Although the number of *Chlamydia* cases in women is increasing, the outcome of infection, that is, infertility and ectopic pregnancy rates, are somewhat puzzling. The CDC reports a decline in the incidence of ectopic pregnancy, whereas there appears to be an increase in infertility. Reiterating earlier concerns, this data may be misleading, or perhaps physicians are indeed more thoroughly screening patients, detecting infection earlier and treating it appropriately.

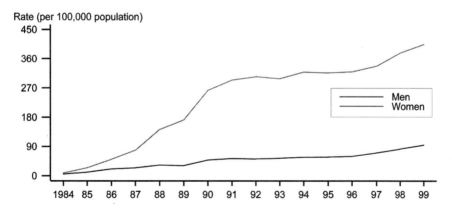

FIG. 3-7. *Chlamydia*—rates by gender in the United States from 1984 to 1999. (From *Sexually Transmitted Disease Surveillance, 1999,* U.S. Department of Health and Human Services, Centers for Disease Control, Atlanta, GA, with permission.)

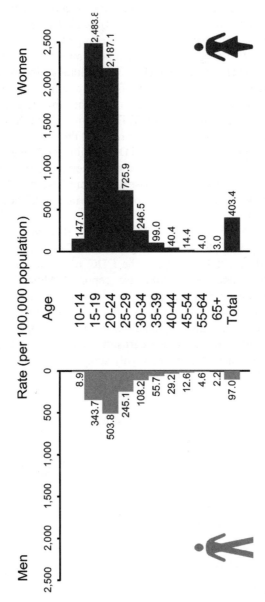

FIG. 3-8. *Chlamydia—age- and gender-specific rates in the United States in 1999. (From Sexually Transmitted Disease Surveillance, 1999,* U.S. Department of Health and Human Services, Centers for Disease Control, Atlanta, GA, with permission.)

Ectopic Pregnancies (in thousands)

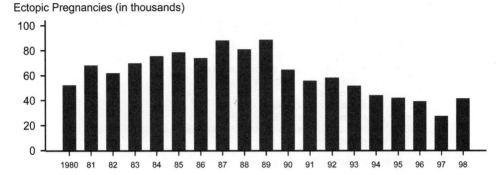

FIG. 3-9. Ectopic pregnancy—hospitalizations of women 15 to 44 years of age in the United States from 1980 to 1998. Some variations in 1981 and 1988 numbers may be due to changes in sampling procedures. The relative standard error for these estimates ranges from 8% to 11%. (From *National Hospital Discharge Survey*, National Center for Health Statistics, U.S. Department of Health and Human Services, Centers for Disease Control, Atlanta, GA, with permission.)

Factors contributing to the potential of women acquiring a STD are complex and often difficult to avoid. The status of the vaginal ecosystem, which frequently is disrupted even though the patient does not realize that there is an abnormality present, can play a significant role in enhancing the risk of infection and development of PID. The degree of cervical ectropion is a significant factor because of the increased surface area of receptive tissue, caused by eversion of the columnar epithelium on the portio of the cervix. Cervical infection is dependent on exposure to an infected partner, the number of exposures, the alteration of the vaginal microflora creating an environment that is favorable to the growth of an infecting organism, the presence of cervical and vaginal inflammation, and the inoculum size. The risk of acquiring a STD is dependent on being exposed to an infected partner and the sexual practice of the patient and the partner. If they are not cohabitating, either individual has multiple partners, and they are not using barrier contraception, the risk for acquiring a STD increases. In addition, the sexual practices are influenced by other behavioral characteristics. For example, if either individual uses illicit drugs, the potential for indiscriminate sexual behavior increases. All these factors should be considered when providing care for women, especially those between 15 and 35 years (Table 3-1).

Individuals most likely to engage in sex with multiple partners are those in the younger age group. The largest number of PID cases occurs in women between the ages of 15 and 25 (4–8). This group is particularly vulnerable because they are more likely to have multiple sexual partners, especially males, and young women tend to have an eversion of their endocervical epithelium on the surface of the portio of their cervix because of the high endogenous estrogen level. Younger women, teenagers in particular, tend to have anovulatory cycles and,

TABLE 3-1. *Risk factors for acquiring PID*

Age of first sexual intercourse, the younger the age the greater the risk
Total number of partners during the patient's lifetime
Number of sexual partners in the last year
Number of sexual partners in the last month
Patient is not cohabitating with current sexual partner
Previous treatment of STD treatment
Previous history of PID
Current sexual partner is not monogamous
Current sexual partner has a STD
Failure to use a barrier method of contraception during sexual intercourse
Use of illicit drugs

PID, pelvic inflammatory disease.

thus, have persistently elevated estrogen levels that produce estrogenized endo-cervical mucus. This mucus facilitates the penetration of bacteria through the endocervix to the uterus allowing the bacteria to colonize and infect the endome-trial tissue (9). This is in contrast to a woman having regular ovulatory cycles who is producing appropriate amounts of estrogen and progesterone. This results in endocervical mucus that is typically thick and tenacious for most of the cycle with estrogenized mucus occurring for a short period during midcycle. The thick, tenacious mucus (progesterone effect) is highly impermeable to bacteria, therefore, hindering but not completely preventing the ascent of bacteria from the lower genital tract and cervix to the upper genital tract.

Contraception plays a significant role in preventing, as well as contributing to, the acquisition of STD and the development of PID. At present, the most effec-tive method of prevention is a barrier method, for example, male and female con-doms, not the diaphragm, associated with a spermicidal agent that has antibac-terial properties (10–13). However, a study by Roddy et al. (14) demonstrated that nonoxynol-9, the most commonly used spermicide, did not protect women against the acquisition of HIV, gonorrhea, or chlamydia. The controversy, espe-cially with regard to nonoxynol-9, will continue regarding the value of spermi-cides as microbicides until intravaginal agents that have demonstrated good *in vitro* and *in vivo* antimicrobial activity with little adverse affect on the vaginal tissue become available. Barrier methods, specifically condoms (both male and female), offer considerable protection against acquisition of STD. The diaphragm also offers a degree of protection as a barrier method, and it is often used in conjunction with a spermicide. However, the diaphragm is not a partic-ularly effective barrier because the vagina is exposed to infectious agents. If the diaphragm is incorrectly positioned, the spermicide is neglected, the diaphragm is removed too soon after sexual intercourse, or it is not fitted correctly, then this is an ineffective method of contraception and prevention against a STD infec-tion. In order for a microbicide to be effective in preventing STD infection, aside from having antimicrobial activity, it must be released from its carrier vehicle over a broad pH range, and it must not induce an inflammatory response in the vagina, or suppress the growth of lactobacilli.

Oral contraceptives have been found to be associated with an increased risk of cervical chlamydial, but not gonococcal, infection (15,16). However, the overall effect of oral contraceptives in reducing the rate of PID is far from settled. There does appear to be an approximately 50% reduction in the incidence of PID among individuals using oral contraceptives (17,18). However, this correlation of a decrease in PID and oral contraceptive use appears to be relative to chlamydial infection but not to gonococcal-associated PID (19,20). The relationship between a protective effect of oral contraceptive use and a reduction in the risk of PID is still unsettled. This theoretical association should not be taken as fact. Patients should be counseled that the use of oral contraceptive pills (OCPs) may decrease, but will not eliminate, the risk of acquiring a STD and, subsequently, PID.

RISK FACTORS

PID is unlike other infections because it can begin as either a unimicrobial or a polymicrobial infection, involving *N. gonorrhoeae* and *C. trachomatis,* and/or it can solely be caused by the endogenous vaginal microflora. Unimicrobial infection, or infection caused by both *N. gonorrhoeae* and *C. trachomatis,* can quickly be joined by the bacteria from the lower genital tract. In moderate to severe PID the bowel, the rectosigmoid colon, rectum, cecum, appendix, and ilium can become inflamed and adherent to the adnexa and the uterus. The inflamed and edematous bowel permits bacteria to migrate through microscopic breaks in the bowel, thereby gaining entrance to the adnexa. This results in abscesses containing bacteria that reflect the bacteria that constitute bowel microflora.

PID also differs from other infections because it consists of a constellation of infected sites like the cervix, uterus, fallopian tubes, and ovaries. Crucial to the diagnosis and treatment of PID is the realization that infection is frequently subtle, and referred to as asymptomatic or "silent" infection. This is erroneous because the disease does have clinical manifestations, although they may be subtle (Table 3-1). Patients with any of the signs or symptoms listed in Table 3-1 should be questioned about recent sexual behavior and screened for *N. gonorrhoeae* and *C. trachomatis.* Patients who develop irregular or breakthrough bleeding, but do not normally experience such irregularities, are often not concerned with the possibility of infection. Other signs such as postcoital bleeding or dyspareunia are often not mentioned to the physician because the patient may not consider it significant.

Although acute and chronic PID can be treated and resolved, the patient who is not diagnosed and treated appropriately early in the disease can often be left with significant lifelong sequelae like chronic pelvic pain or permanently damaged fallopian tubes that can leave her infertile or at risk for ectopic pregnancy. Ultimately, the patient with acute and chronic complex infection, like tubo-ovarian abscesses or intractable pelvic pain, will eventually have a hysterectomy with possible removal of both ovaries and fallopian tubes.

The origin of PID also differs from intraabdominal infections because most infections occur in women between the ages of 15 and 25. In this group of women, the cause is most likely *N. gonorrhoeae, C. trachomatis,* or both; therefore, it is related to their sexual behavior factors. Women older than 25 years of age, especially those older than 35, who contract and develop PID are more likely to be infected with bacteria that are endogenous to the lower genital tract. Unfortunately, factors associated with sexual behavior are not solely related to the patient's own practices but also related to those of her partner as well. For women older than 35, the risk for PID is related to the status of the endogenous vaginal microflora and instrumentation of the upper genital tract via the lower genital tract. In addition, this age group is more likely to have diverticulosis and diverticulitis. As mentioned, there are several factors to consider in assessing the patient's potential risk for acquiring PID (Table 3-1).

The most obvious risk factor is having multiple sexual partners. This includes the patient's male partner having more that one sexual partner and whether or not he is bisexual. If the male partner has multiple female or male sexual partners, this raises the patient's risk of contracting a STD even though she may be monogamous. If he is having sex with multiple partners, this raises the risk of acquiring a STD; therefore, he can transmit the organism or organisms to the patient. Women in truly monogamous relationships have little risk of acquiring a STD. However, as mentioned, if her partner is bisexual, this raises the risk, especially of acquiring human immunodeficiency virus (HIV).

The method of contraception used is related to sexual behavior. When considering a method of contraception, most individuals do not give much thought to the particular method with regard to preventing the acquisition of a STD. Their focus is on prevention of pregnancy. However, the physician or health care provider should thoroughly discuss the risk of STD acquisition and explain that the condom is currently the best method available to prevent contracting a STD. An even better method is the combined use of an oral contraceptive and a condom. Although the diaphragm is a barrier method of contraception, it does not offer the degree of protection needed against transmission or acquisition of a STD because it does not prevent the male from discharging into the vagina. An improperly positioned diaphragm will not prevent urethral discharge and semen from reaching the cervix and endocervical canal.

The use of spermicides, commonly used with a diaphragm, raises concerns. Although there is a suggestion that agents such as nonoxynol-9 have activity against sexually transmitted organisms, spermicides may also have an adverse effect on the endogenous vaginal microflora increasing the likelihood that the vaginal flora is altered. Cook and Rosenberg (13) reported that nonoxynol-9 had an "appreciable protective effect against gonorrhoeae and chlamydial infection." However, a study by Roddy et al. (14) demonstrated that nonoxynol-9 did not protect women against acquisition of HIV, *N. gonorrhoeae,* and *C. trachomatis* in a group of sex workers. The antibacterial properties of nonoxynol-9 have not been well established and require further investigation.

Another form of contraception linked to PID is the IUD. The IUD has a long history of use as a means of birth control until the 1980s when a link was established between the IUD and PID (21–24). A large prospective study of 3,162 women using an IUD were found to have a 3 to 3.5 times higher risk of acquiring PID compared with women who did not use an IUD (24). However, recent analysis has raised concerns over the data published between 1968 and the 1980s. In 1999, Dardano and Burkman (25,26) pointed out that the risks of acquiring PID were associated with both IUD insertion and the acquisition of a STD. A study of 957 women using a copper IUD between 1993 and 1995 revealed no cases of PID within the first 3 months of use (27). In a randomized control study of 930 women divided into two groups, with only one group receiving prophylactic antibiotics, only one case of PID occurred in each group (28).

In 1996, Burkman raised several concerns with the early analysis of IUD use and PID (26). One inherent problem in PID studies is establishing the diagnosis. Jacobson and Westrom (29) highlighted this problem when performing laparoscopies on a group of women with a clinical diagnosis of PID. They found that 1/3 of women with a clinical diagnosis did not actually have PID when examined with the use of laparoscopy. This is a very critical point because patients enrolled in any clinical study of PID will include a significant number of women who do not have an infection. The Women's Health Study of 1,447 women using an IUD and 3,453 controls, the Oxford Planning Association Study of 17,032 women, and the World Health Organization Study all demonstrated that the highest risk of PID was associated with IUD insertion and during the first 20 days postinsertion. The rate of PID at insertion was 9.68/1,000 women years, and after the first 20 days the rate declined to 1.38/1,000 women years (22,30–34). Thus, it appears that the IUD is a safe method of birth control when used in the appropriate patient. The characteristics of an appropriate IUD candidate are listed in Table 3-2.

One study found that the greatest risk of developing PID in association with an IUD is within the first 3 months of use (34). Attempts to reduce the PID risk following IUD insertion have focused on the use of prophylactics administered at the time of insertion. Walsh et al. (35) administered azithromycin to women at

TABLE 3-2. *Criteria for selecting a patient for IUD use*

Must be in a truly monogamous relationship
Must not have had a previous episode of PID
Is not having irregular uterine bleeding
Does not have endocervical mucopus
Has a healthy vaginal microflora (dominated by *Lactobacillus*)
Is not pregnant
Does not have evidence of cervicitis, that is hypertrophy of the endocervical columnar
  epithelium, cervix does not bleed easily, and does not have an inflammatory reaction to a
  Pap smear

IUD, intrauterine device; PID, pelvic inflammatory disease.

the time of IUD insertion and found benefit with regard to preventing subsequent infection. This study was not a particularly well-designed one, however, because of poor controls, but it did address risk with regard to the acquisition of STDs. As noted, patients undergoing any transvaginal invasive procedure to gain entrance to the uterine cavity should be screened for the presence of STDs, bacterial vaginosis (BV), and unimicrobial vaginitis.

There is one area of great concern in relationship to IUD use—use in nulliparous woman. The concern is the potential of infection of the fallopian tubes or salpingitis leading to infertility. Lete et al. (36) reported that the incidence of PID in a group of nulliparous women using an IUD compared with a control group was 1.6% vs 1.1%. These investigators also concluded that being nulliparous was not a contraindication to IUD insertion. This study underscores the need for taking a careful history to determine the patient's degree of risk for potentially contracting a STD, as well as determining the microbiologic status of the lower genital tract.

MICROBIOLOGY

The bacteriology of PID is complex and, initially, may appear to be simple when *N. gonorrhoeae, C. trachomatis,* or both are considered the sole infecting bacteria. However, even when these are the only organisms involved, it is not a simple matter of infection leading to tissue damage. These organisms can trigger a local inflammatory response, initiating release of cytokines that may, in turn, damage the fragile endothelium of the fallopian tubes. Other than acute uncomplicated PID, which is caused by either *N. gonorrhoeae* or *C. trachomatis,* the infection is probably polymicrobial, that is, *N. gonorrhoeae* and *C. trachomatis* (either or both) plus facultative and obligate anaerobes. Nongonococcal, nonchlamydial PID is typically polymicrobial. The confusion over the microbial makeup of PID stems from the nonselective method of obtaining specimens for culture of microorganisms. The microbial cause of endometritis and salpingitis, in the distant past, was determined by obtaining specimens transvaginally, transcervically, or via culdocentesis. The methods are significantly associated with the risk of contamination by bacteria from the vagina. Obtaining specimens via culdocentesis was thought to yield valid specimens, but subsequent studies obtaining specimens from the cul-de-sac via abdominal laparoscopy revealed that the former technique resulted in specimens contaminated by vaginal bacteria (37,38).

Not all PID is related to *N. gonorrhoeae* and *C. trachomatis.* Several studies have failed to recover either of these organisms from patients with acute salpingitis. This led to the theory that either or both of these bacteria initiated infection. Thus, the endogenous bacteria subsequently succeeded in ascending from the lower genital tract through the cervix into the uterus, eventually gaining entrance to and infecting the fallopian tubes (39–41). A second hypothesis assumed that some cases of PID were polymicrobial and initiated without *N.*

gonorrhoeae or *C. trachomatis* (42–44). Several investigators suggested that BV can predispose or facilitate the ascent of *N. gonorrhoeae* or *C. trachomatis* into the upper genital tract (29,45,46). Faro et al. (46) did not find BV to be present in association with acute PID secondary to *N. gonorrhoeae* infection. This study did not find a reduction in *Lactobacillus* or an increase in obligate anaerobic bacteria. There is no doubt that women with an altered vaginal microflora dominated by one or more bacteria can be placed at risk for significant upper genital tract infection. This is especially true if the patient undergoes an invasive procedure such as hysterosalpingography, artificial insemination, *in vitro* fertilization, therapeutic abortion, or surgical completion of a spontaneous abortion. Combinations of bacteria may place the patient at great risk, especially if they have the potential to cause abscesses (e.g., *Escherichia coli* and *Bacteroides fragilis, Prevotella bivia* and *E.coli,* or *P. bivia* and *Enterococcus faecalis*) (47,48).

Although the bacteriology of PID is not completely understood, the physician can be confident in the fact that *N. gonorrhoeae* and *C. trachomatis* are still the leading causes of the spectrum of disease known as PID. However, the physician must be cognizant of the possibility that the endogenous vaginal bacteria, especially the gram-negative facultative and gram-positive obligate anaerobic bacteria, can also be involved in this infection. This is especially possible when the infection has been present for a prolonged period or follows instrumentation of the upper genital tract via the lower genital tract. Therefore, any patient undergoing a procedure that invades the upper genital tract via the lower genital tract must be screened for the presence of *N. gonorrhoeae, C. trachomatis,* and an altered vaginal microflora. This is necessary to prevent the development of PID. Remember, this is an insidious disease. It is frequently undetected in the early stages, eventually resulting in significant tissue destruction, and it can be life threatening. If it continues in an asymptomatic fashion, significant damage to the fallopian tubes can result in placing the patient at risk for an ectopic pregnancy and significant morbidity and mortality. It can also result in the patient being infertile, placing her at risk for the morbidity associated with *in vitro* fertilization.

DIAGNOSIS

The diagnosis of PID depends on understanding that this is a complex disease and may encompass any one part, more than one part, or the entire genital tract. Recognition or detection of cervical infection should not lead the physician to the false sense of security that the disease is limited to the cervix. This may only be the "tip of the iceberg." In actuality, the disease may have progressed to involve the upper genital tract, and, therefore, short-term or inadequate treatment can put the patient at significant risk for serious sequelae.

The symptoms of PID are nonspecific and existent tests are not pathognomonic of this disease. Therefore, there are patients who will be diagnosed with

PID but do not have this infection, and there are individuals with infection that will go undetected. The presentation of PID can be confused with other conditions, and the differential diagnosis is long (Table 3-3). This difficulty in establishing a diagnosis of PID has resulted in the unnecessary administration of antibiotics to individuals suspected of having PID even though they do not have a pelvic infection. As mentioned, Jacobson and Westrom (29) demonstrated, via laparoscopy, that approximately 1/3 of patients with a clinical diagnosis of PID did not have this disease. Twelve percent were found to have other pathologic conditions, and 23% had a normal pelvis.

Clinically, PID is difficult to diagnose, but the diagnosis is frequently made because the patient with lower abdominal or pelvic pain has symptoms and signs that are nonspecific. The pain associated with PID can be described as dull, aching, sharp, intermittent, continuous, and gradual in onset. Both PID associated with gonorrhea and nongonococcal, nonchlamydial, polymicrobial PID are often associated with intense pain. This is in contrast to the pain associated with *C. trachomatis,* which is typically mild. However, infection caused by *C. trachomatis* is often asymptomatic.

The patient with PID, specifically endometritis, can present with intermenstrual bleeding or menorrhagia. This appears to be common with chlamydial PID (47,49). The patient taking OCPs and experiencing irregular uterine bleeding presents the physician with a difficult diagnostic problem. The physician's dilemma is deciding whether the bleeding is secondary to a hormonal imbalance or an infection. The way to solve this problem is to perform a pelvic examination to determine if there is a yellow or greenish discharge, if the discharge is emanating from the endocervix, if there is purulent endocervical mucus, or if there is uterine and adnexal tenderness on motion and palpation of the upper reproductive organs. Thus, the physician should attempt to distinguish between cervicitis and endometritis or to determine if both sites are involved. Cervicitis

TABLE 3-3. *Differential diagnosis of PID*

Appendicitis
Ectopic pregnancy
Torsion of ovarian cyst
Ruptured ovarian cyst
Ovarian cyst
Hemorrhagic ovarian cyst
Peritonitis
Pyelonephritis
Diverticulitis
Meckel's diverticulitis
Colitis
Degenerating myoma
Endometriosis
Ruptured endometrioma
Torsion of hydatid of Morgagni
Paraovarian cyst

PID, pelvic inflammatory disease.

can be diagnosed clinically by the presence of endocervical mucopus, hypertrophy of the endocervical columnar epithelial tissue, and/or the presence of brisk bleeding when the endocervix is gently palpated with a cotton-tipped applicator. Endometritis can be clinically diagnosed by the presence of tenderness on palpation and motion of the uterus and adnexa (50). The endocervical canal can be evaluated by inserting a cotton- or Dacron-tipped applicator into the endocervical canal, rotating it several times then withdrawing it. The tip should be inspected for the presence of mucopus. A specimen should also be obtained and processed for the presence of *N. gonorrhoeae* and *C. trachomatis*. An endometrial biopsy should be performed and the tissue sent for histologic analysis, and part of the specimen should be placed in an anaerobic transport medium. The latter specimen should be cultured for the isolation and identification of *N. gonorrhoeae, C. trachomatis,* and facultative and obligate anaerobic bacteria. The pathologist should be informed that the patient is suspected of having PID; therefore, the presence of plasma cells should be sought. The presence of plasma cells is highly suggestive of and correlates with the presence of endometritis and salpingitis (51–54).

Other reasons for irregular bleeding should be considered such as pregnancy, possible abortion or ectopic pregnancy, endometrial polyps, and uterine fibroids. A pregnancy test should be performed, preferably a quantitative beta-human chorionic gonadotrophin (beta-hCG). Another factor to consider is whether the patient recently experienced a diagnostic or therapeutic procedure that involved passage of instruments through the vagina and endocervical canal into the uterine cavity. These are important considerations in evaluating the patient with irregular uterine bleeding. Therefore, two important diagnostic procedures that can be extremely helpful are a thorough pelvic and bimanual examination. If the patient's bimanual examination suggests that the uterus is enlarged or irregular in contour, a pelvic ultrasound would also be helpful. A saline sonohysterogram should not be performed on a patient who is suspected of having endometritis or salpingitis, however. Doing so will increase the risk of infection and of disseminating an existing infection. If indeed there is an infection and there is significant infectious fluid, performing a sonohysterogram, a hysterosalpingogram, or any procedure in which fluid is injected into the uterus can result in the infected fluid being pushed through the fallopian tubes into the peritoneal cavity. This can result in an intraperitoneal infection and the development of abscesses.

Focusing on the possibility of endometritis or salpingitis in the patient taking OCPs requires the physician to obtain a detailed sexual history. The patient, typically, will not volunteer her sexual history. One important question that must be answered regards the relationship in time between her last menstrual period and sexual intercourse. Intercourse during her menstrual period, or shortly preceding or following her menstrual flow, will increase the possibility of her developing endometritis and salpingitis.

The patient with endometritis can present with irregular or breakthrough bleeding and no other abnormality. This is often misinterpreted as a problem associated with the OCP and the possibility of infection is not considered. Endometritis, unlike postpartum endometritis, can be very subtle and when not considered can lead to the development of an asymptomatic salpingitis. Bimanual examination will often reveal mild tenderness on palpation of the uterus. This should lead the physician to perform an endometrial biopsy. Before performing the biopsy, the vaginal microflora should be assessed to establish whether or not it is altered to avoid introducing obligate anaerobic bacteria as well as *E. coli* and *E. faecalis*, because the combination of *P. bivia* and *E. coli* or *E. faecalis*, as well as *B. fragilis* and *E. coli*, can be abscessogenic.

Disease that has progressed to the fallopian tubes may be asymptomatic or symptomatic. Although the patient with symptomatic salpingitis or PID is not always identified, there are probably many more patients with mild and asymptomatic PID than there are patients with overt symptomatic disease. The CDC criteria for establishing a diagnosis of clinical PID are as follows:

1. Lower abdominal tenderness
2. Adnexal tenderness
3. Cervical motion tenderness

These are considered the minimal criteria and one can easily see that they can be associated with a variety of conditions. These are neither specific nor pathognomonic for PID. Other clinical findings that can strengthen the diagnosis of PID are as follows:

1. Oral temperature greater than 101°F (>38.3°C)
2. Purulent cervical or vaginal discharge
3. Elevated sedimentation rate or C-reactive protein
4. Documented presence of *N. gonorrhoeae* or *C. trachomatis*

The clinical diagnosis is not highly sensitive or specific. In one study of 100 nonpregnant women with acute lower abdominal pain, the preoperative diagnosis was confirmed by laparoscopy in 56% of all patients (55). Twenty-nine of 66 cases of ovarian torsion (44%), 9 of 11 (82%) cases of ovarian cyst, and 12 of 15 (80%) cases of bleeding corpus luteum were confirmed. Among the remaining cases of unsuspected diagnoses were ovarian cysts (24), adhesions (5), bleeding corpus luteum (3), degenerative myomas (3), PID (2), and appendicitis (1). Cibula et al. (56) performed laparoscopy on 141 patients with a clinical diagnosis of PID. Patients underwent laparoscopy within 24 hours of being admitted to the hospital. PID was confirmed in 30% of patients, adhesions in the absence of PID was found in 16% of the patients, and 14% of patients were found to have endometriosis.

Laparoscopic evidence consistent with PID include the presence of hyperemic, edematous fallopian tubes; the presence of pus exiting from the fimbriated ends of the fallopian tubes; and the collection of pus in the posterior cul-de-sac. However, some patients with PID may not develop the signs listed and, therefore, not receive a diagnosis of PID, as with the patient who undergoes laparoscopy

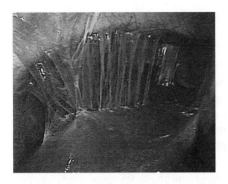

FIG. 3-10. Curtis-Fitz-Hugh syndrome. Notice violin-string adhesions from liver capsules to abdominal wall and note liver in the bottom of the image. (See Color Plate 1 following page 148.)

for acute pain. The pelvis may be normal and no pathology is found, or there may be areas that are mistaken for endometriosis but the patient actually has PID. In this latter situation, unless the areas of suspected endometriosis are classic implants, a biopsy should be taken. This will permit confirmation of endometriosis or negate the clinical diagnosis. Ultrasonographic data supportive of PID are the presence of enlarged fluid-filled fallopian tubes (pyosalpinx); the presence of an enlarged tubo-ovarian complex suggestive of either a symmetrical mass consisting of bowel and adnexa adherent to one another; or the presence of a mass with nonhomogenous fluid that can be multiloculated, suggestive of a tubo-ovarian abscess.

Patients with acute PID can experience disseminated intraabdominal pain secondary to peritonitis. The infected fluid can overlay the entire bowel causing an inflammatory response in the bowel. This can result in adhesion formation and obstruction. Infected fluid can travel up the colonic gutters, reaching the surface of the liver and inferior surface of the diaphragm. This can include an inflammatory response resulting in adhesions and is referred to as the Curtis-Fitz-Hugh syndrome (Fig. 3-10).

Whenever the diagnosis of PID is entertained the patient should be administered antibiotic therapy. Delay in treatment could cost the patient her fertility. There is no reason to be conservative in the approach to a patient suspected of having PID. The patient with acute uncomplicated PID typically responds to antibiotic therapy within 48 to 72 hours, and therapy should be continued for 10 to 14 days in an attempt to curtail the inflammatory response.

TREATMENT

The hallmark of treatment is based on the premise that all patients are infected with *N. gonorrhoeae* and *C. trachomatis*. In addition, the role of the facultative and obligate anaerobic bacteria cannot be discounted. The clinician should assume that there is a complex bacteriologic polymicrobial infection that requires a comprehensive regimen of antimicrobial therapy from the onset, which reduces the risk of damage to the fallopian tubes.

The infectious process involves not only the bacteria and the products they produce and secrete but also the stimulus they provide to the host, specifically the liberation of metabolites that initiate the cytokine cascade in the host. Substance such as tumor necrosis factor α (TNF-α) can have significant adverse effects on the tissue. It is through those bacteria, such as *C. trachomatis,* that an immunologic response is initiated, adhering the release of cytokines, which may be responsible for the tissue damage that results from such infections. In addition, bacteria such as *E. coli* and *E. faecalis* in conjunction with anaerobes counteract synergistically to form abscesses. These abscesses can form within a fallopian tube, in both fallopian tubes and ovaries, in the cul-de-sac, between loops of the bowel, under the liver, between the liver and the diaphragm, and between the spleen and the diaphragm. In fact, an abscess can form anywhere in the peritoneal cavity that infectious fluid can gain access.

Once the diagnosis has been established, the next decision is to determine whether or not the patient is a candidate for outpatient or ambulatory treatment or requires hospitalization and intravenous (IV) administration of antibiotic therapy. If the patient is to be treated in an ambulatory setting, the oral antibiotic regimen chosen should have a broad spectrum of activity and should not be of short duration. The patient should be educated with regard to the seriousness of her infection, the sequelae that can occur, and, therefore, the need to complete the course of therapy. Patients who are candidates for ambulatory treatment should fulfill the following criteria:

1. Cannot be pregnant
2. Must not have nausea or vomiting
3. Must have an oral body temperature less than 101°F
4. Must not have a pelvic mass
5. Must be able to return for reevaluation within 48 to 72 hours
6. Can afford to obtain medication
7. Will be compliant

Pregnant patients who are less that 10 to 12 weeks' gestation can have PID. The gestational sac does not obliterate the uterine cavity before 12 weeks, and the bacteria can infect the basialis layer and gain entrance to the fallopian tubes. Thus, for a patient with a first trimester pregnancy who presents with lower abdominal pain, cervical, uterine, and adnexal tenderness on palpation and motion, the possibility of PID should be considered in addition to a septic abortion.

The patient with nausea who has not vomited is not a candidate for oral antibiotic therapy because all appropriate antibiotics for treating PID will likely worsen her nausea and initiate vomiting. This will discourage her from continuing antibiotic therapy. She will either seek additional help or wait until her condition worsens to return for medical therapy. This is a potentially dangerous situation for the patient especially if her symptoms were mild. A patient with mild symptoms who has an adverse reaction to the antibiotics prescribed will likely discontinue the therapy on her own initiative. This will allow the infection to progress and cause more damage to the fallopian tubes. This reaction to the medication may even dissuade her from returning for her follow-up visit; she may also seek additional help or wait until her condition worsens to return for medical therapy. Delaying antibiotic therapy, even for a short period, can have significant morbidity for the patient.

The presence of a pelvic mass or the suggestion of a mass on pelvic examination, especially if it is symptomatic (suggesting the presence of an inflammatory mass), is a contraindication to outpatient therapy with oral antibiotics. This is because the presence of an inflammatory mass in the pelvis typically means that the lower portion of the small bowel (ileum), the cecum, and the rectosigmoid are usually adherent to the posterior aspect of the uterus and cul-de-sac, thus forming the inflammatory mass. It is usual for the fallopian tubes and ovaries to be involved in the inflammatory mass. This bowel inflammation results in a decrease or absence of peristalsis. Therefore, there is a high probability that any oral medications administered, liquids or solids, will not be tolerated and the patient is likely to vomit. Another possible detriment to achieving success is that the decrease in bowel function may result in decreased absorption of the antibiotics. This will result in decreased serum and tissue levels, thus resulting in decreased efficacy.

The presence of a pelvic mass is not a good prognostic sign if it is an inflammatory mass. This usually indicates that the patient has a pyosalpinx, a tubo-ovarian bowel complex, or a tubo-ovarian abscess. The occurrence of either of these conditions means that the patient may have significant damage to the fallopian tubes and is very likely to be infertile or at risk for ectopic pregnancy.

The antibiotic choices for the ambulatory treatment are several and are based on (a) the spectrum of antibacterial activity needed and (b) whether or not the patient is to be treated solely as an outpatient or is to receive 24 hours of IV therapy followed by oral antibiotics for 14 days.

Treatment regimens for ambulatory treatment of PID are as follows*:

1. Nonpregnant, oral regimens administered for 14 days:
   a. Levofloxacin 500 mg q24h (CDC recommendation)
   b. Ofloxacin 400 mg twice a day for 14 days (CDC recommendation)
   c. Metronidazole (Flagyl) 500 mg three times a day plus Ofloxacin (Floxin) 400 mg twice daily, or Levofloxacin 500 mg once a day for 14 days (CDC recommendation)
   d. Amoxicillin/clavulanic acid (Augmentin) (check dosing available) plus Ofloxacin 400 mg twice daily
   e. Amoxicillin/clavulanic acid plus Doxycycline 100 mg twice daily
2. Short-term parenteral combined with oral therapy (CDC recommendation)*

---

*Centers for Disease Control and Prevention. Sexually transmitted disease treatment guidelines 2002. *MMWR* 2002;51:50–52.

a. Ceftriaxone 250 mg IM in a single dose plus Doxycycline 100 mg orally twice daily for 14 days
b. Cefoxitin 2 g IM in a single dose and Probenecid 1 g orally in a single dose plus Doxycycline 100 mg twice a day for 14 days
c. Can substitute Ceftizoxime, Cefotetan, and Cefoxitin
d. Metronidazole 500 mg orally twice a day for 14 days can be added to any of the above regimens to provide coverage against obligate anaerobic bacteria

A combination of short-term parenteral and oral therapy is indicated for those individuals thought to have significant infection but who have no evidence of a pelvic mass or pelvic peritonitis. These individuals may also have a slight degree of nausea and, therefore, would not tolerate oral antibiotic therapy. If the diagnosis of acute uncomplicated PID is correct, a short course of parenteral antibiotics can result in significant improvement, thereby permitting the administration of comparable oral antibiotics. These individuals do not need to be admitted to the hospital but could treated in a 24- to 36-hour observation area in, or adjacent to, the emergency room. If there is no marked improvement, they should be admitted to the hospital for continued parenteral therapy and further diagnostic testing, like laparoscopy. Once these patients and those treated solely as ambulatory patients are discharged, they should all be reevaluated within 72 hours to determine their response to therapy.

Patients requiring hospitalization are those that:

1. Would be placed on oral therapy but cannot return in 72 hours for reevaluation
2. Have nausea
3. Have fever 101°F or higher
4. Have a pelvic mass
5. Have pelvic peritonitis
6. Have been previously treated for PID

Parenteral treatment regimens for patients requiring hospitalization:

1. Cefotetan 2 g every 12 hours plus Doxycycline 100 mg every 12 hours*
2. Cefoxitin 2 g every 6 hours plus Doxycycline 100 mg every 12 hours*
3. Clindamycin 900 mg every 8 hours plus Gentamicin (see dosing schedule)*
4. Metronidazole 500 mg every 8 hours plus Ofloxacin 400 mg every 12 hours*
5. Ampicillin/sulbactam 3 g every 6 hours plus Doxycycline 100 mg every 12 hours*
6. Piperacillin/tazobactam 3.375 g every 6 hours plus Gentamicin (see dosing schedule)*

*Centers for Disease Control and Prevention. Sexually transmitted disease treatment guidelines 2002. *MMWR* 2002;51:50–52.

7. Piperacillin/tazobactam 3.375 g every 6 hours plus Ofloxacin 400 mg every 12 hours
8. L-ofloxacin 500 mg every 24 hours

Gentamicin can be given either every 8 hours (2 mg/kg of body weight followed by a maintenance dose of 1.5 mg/kg body weight) or once a day (5 mg/kg of body weight). There is no known method to eliminate the risk of ototoxicity or nephrotoxicity; however, administering therapeutic doses and monitoring serum levels can reduce the risk. The serum peak level should be collected 1 hour after the third dose has been completely infused. When a multiple-dosing schedule is used, the peak serum level should be between 4 to 10 μg/mL, and the trough level should be between 1 to 2 μg/mL. When the once-a-day dosing schedule is employed, the serum peak level should be 16 to 24 μg/mL, and the trough level should be less than 1 μg/mL.

Regimens employing L-ofloxacin or metronidazole plus ofloxacin have the advantage that they can be administered parenterally and switched to oral without changing antibiotics, therefore maintaining serum levels. The quinolone provides excellent activity against *N. gonorrhoeae* and *C. trachomatis,* as well as against gram-negative and gram-positive bacteria. L-ofloxacin also has the additional benefit of providing activity against obligate anaerobic bacteria commonly involved in PID. However, if the patient had a pelvic mass or either the suspicion or strong evidence of a pelvic abscess, the combination of metronidazole plus ofloxacin or clindamycin plus ofloxacin would provide increased coverage against obligate anaerobic bacteria, especially *B. fragilis* and the *B. fragilis* group. Gentamicin would have limited value in treating the abscess because this would be an acidic environment, thereby reducing the effectiveness of aminoglycosides. In addition, the abscess contains fragments of nucleic acids that are derived from disrupted cells within the abscess that bind to the aminoglycosides rendering them inactive.

Although the CDC recommends, as alternate treatment regimens, ceftriaxone (250 mg intramuscularly administered once) or cefoxitin (2 g intramuscularly) plus probenecid (1 g orally) plus doxycycline (100 mg orally) twice a day for 14 days, these do not seem appropriate. The assumption is that the patient's PID is acute and minimal and that obligate anaerobes are not a main constituent of the infection. The main bacteria are *N. gonorrhoeae, C. trachomatis,* or both. However, this may not be an assumption that is in the patient's best interest. Data does not address the incidence of infertility following treatment with any of the recommended treatment regimens. Therefore, one of the first principles of therapy is to eradicate the infecting organisms and decrease or prevent the risk of tubal damage. There is no way to determine the duration of the patient's disease. It is assumed that the patient who is seen because of symptomatic PID has only experienced the disease for a short period. This is a faulty assumption because there is no method of determining the extent of the disease. Therefore, when treating PID, the antibiotic regimen that provides the broadest antibacterial activity should be used. It should be explained to the patient that this is a serious disease with significant complications. Therefore, it is imperative that she be compliant with taking the prescribed medications as directed, complete the entire course of medication, and not fail to keep her follow-up appointments. She should also be given a description of the signs and symptoms that might arise should the therapy not be effective. It is imperative that the patient understands that her fertility is in jeopardy and, therefore, that compliance with all aspects of management is essential for success.

REFERENCES

1. Rein DB, Kassler WJ, Irwin KL, et al. Direct medical costs of pelvic inflammatory disease and its sequelae; decreasing but still substantial. *Obstet Gynecol* 2000;95;397–402.
2. Aral SO, Mosher WD, Cates W Jr. Self-reported pelvic inflammatory disease in the United States, 1988. *JAMA* 1991;266:2570–2573.
3. Miller HG, Cain VS, Rogers SM, et al. Correlates of sexually transmitted bacterial infections among U.S. women in 1995. *Fam Plann Perspect* 1999;31:4–9.
4. Forslin L, Falk V, Danielsson D. Changes in the incidence of acute gonococcal and nongonococcal salpingitis. *Br J Vener Dis* 1978;54:247–250.
5. Rees E, Annels EH. Gonococcal salpingitis. *Br J Vener Dis* 1969;45:205–215.
6. McCormack WM, Stumacher RJ, Johnson K, et al. Clinical spectrum of gonococcal infection in women. *Lancet* 1977;1:1182–1185.
7. Arya OP, Mallinson H, Goddard AD. Epidemiological and clinical correlates of chlamydial infection of the cervix. *Br J Vener Dis* 1981;57:118–124.
8. Hobson D, Karayiannis P, Byng RE, et al. Quantitative aspects of chlamydial infection of the cervix. *Br J Vener Dis* 1980;56:156–162.
9. Enhorning G, Huldt L, Melen B. Ability of cervical mucus to act as a barrier against bacteria. *Am J Obstet Gynecol* 1970;108:532–537.
10. Austin H, Louv WC, Alexander WJ. A case-control study of spermicides and gonorrhea. *JAMA* 1984; 251:2822–2824.
11. Quinn RW, O'Reilly KR. Contraceptive practices of women attending the Sexually Transmitted Disease Clinic in Nashville, Tennessee. *Sex Transm Dis* 1985;12:99–102.
12. Louv WC, Austin H, Alexander WJ, et al. A clinical trial of nonoxynol-9 for preventing gonococcal and chlamydial infections. *J Infect Dis* 1988;158:518–523.
13. Cook RL, Rosenberg MJ. Do spermicides containing nonoxynol-9 prevent sexually transmitted infections? A metaanalysis. *Sex Transm Dis* 1998;25:144–150.
14. Roddy RE, Zekeng L, Ryan KA, et al. A controlled trial of nonoxynol 9 film to reduce male-to-female transmission of sexually transmitted diseases. *N Engl J Med* 1998;339:504–510.
15. Harrison HR, Costin M, Meder JB, et al. Cervical *Chlamydia trachomatis* infection in university women: relationship to history, contraception, ectopy, and cervicitis. *Am J Obstet Gynecol* 1985;153: 244–251.
16. Cromer A, Heald FP. Pelvic inflammatory disease associated with *Neisseria gonorrhoeae* and *Chlamydia trachomatis*: clinical correlates. *Sex Transm Dis* 1987;14:125–129.
17. Lee NC, Rubin GL, Grimes DA. Measures of sexual behavior and the risk of pelvic inflammatory disease. *Obstet Gynecol* 1991;77:425–430.
18. Eschenbach DA, Harnisch JP, Holmes KK. Pathogenesis of acute pelvic inflammatory disease: role of contraception and other risk factors. *Am J Obstet Gynecol* 1977;128:838–850.
19. Weström L, Bengtsson LP, Mardh PA. The risk of pelvic inflammatory disease in women using intrauterine contraceptive devices as compared to non-users. *Lancet* 1976;2:221–224.
20. Wolner-Hanssen P, Eschenbach DA, Paavonen J, et al. Decreased risk of symptomatic chlamydial pelvic inflammatory disease associated with oral contraceptive use. *JAMA* 1990;263:54–59.
21. Senanayake P, Krammer DG. Contraception and the etiology of pelvic inflammatory disease: new perspectives. *Am J Obstet Gynecol* 1980;138:852–860.
22. Lee NC, Rubin GL, Ory HW, et al. Type of intrauterine device and the risk of pelvic inflammatory disease. *Obstet Gynecol* 1983;62:1–6.

23. Sparks RA, Purrier BG, Watt PJ, et al. Bacteriological colonisation of uterine cavity: role of tailed intrauterine contraceptive device. *Br Med J* 1981;282:1189–1191.
24. Vessey M, Doll R, Peto R, et al. A long-term follow-up study of women using different methods of contraception—a interim report. *J Biosoc Sci* 1976;8:373–427.
25. Dardano KL, Burkman RT. The intrauterine contraceptive device: an often-forgotten and maligned method of contraception. *Am J Obstet Gynecol* 1999;181:1–5.
26. Burkman RT. Intrauterine devices and pelvic inflammatory disease: evolving perspectives on the data. *Obstet Gynecol Surv* 1996;51(12 Suppl):S35–S41.
27. Skjeldestad FE. How effectively do copper intrauterine devices prevent ectopic pregnancy? *Acta Obstet Gynecol Scand* 1997;76:684–690.
28. Sinei SK, Morrison CS, Sekadde-Kigondu C, et al. Complications of use of intrauterine devices among HIV-1 infected women. *Lancet* 1998;351:1238–1241.
29. Jacobson L, Westrom L. Objectivized diagnosis of acute pelvic inflammatory disease. Diagnostic and prognostic value of routine laparoscopy. *Am J Obstet Gynecol* 1969;105:1088–1098.
30. Burkman RT. Association between intrauterine device and pelvic inflammatory disease. *Obstet Gynecol* 1981;57:269–276.
31. Lee NC, Rubin GL, Borucki R. The intrauterine device and pelvic inflammatory disease revisited: new results from the Women's Health Study. *Obstet Gynecol* 1988;72:1–6.
32. Burkman RT, Lee NC, Ory HW, et al. Response to "The intrauterine device and pelvic inflammatory disease: the Women's Health Study reanalyzed." *J Clin Epidemiol* 1991;44:123–125.
33. Vessey MP, Yeates D, Flavel R, et al. Pelvic inflammatory disease and the intrauterine device: findings in a large cohort study. *Br Med J* 1981;282:855–857.
34. Farley TM, Rosenberg MJ, Rowe JP, et al. Intrauterine devices and pelvic inflammatory disease: an international perspective. *Lancet* 1992;339:785–788.
35. Walsh T, Grimes D, Frezieres R, et al. Randomised controlled trial of prophylactic antibiotics before insertion of intrauterine devices. *Lancet* 1998;351:1005–1008.
36. Lete I, Morales P, de Pablo JL. Use of intrauterine contraceptive devices in nulliparous women: personal experience over a 12-year period. *Eur J Contracep Reprod Health Care* 1998;3:190–193.
37. Sweet RL, Mills J, Hadley KW, et al. Use of laparoscopy to determine the microbiologic etiology of acute salpingitis. *Am J Obstet Gynecol* 1979;134:68–74.
38. Soper DE, Brockwell NJ, Dalton HP. False-positive cultures of the cul-de-sac associated with culdocentesis in patients undergoing elective laparoscopy. *Obstet Gynecol* 1991;77:134–138.
39. Cunningham FG, Hauth JC, Gilstrap LC, et al. The bacterial pathogenesis of acute pelvic inflammatory disease. *Obstet Gynecol* 1978;52:161–164.
40. Chow AW, Malkasian KL, Marshall JR, et al. The bacteriology of acute pelvic inflammatory disease. *Am J Obstet Gynecol* 1975;122:876–879.
41. Monif GR, Welkos SL, Baer H, et al. Cul-de-sac isolates from patients with endometritis-salpingitis-peritonitis and gonococcal endocervicitis. *Am J Obstet Gynecol* 1976;126:158–161.
42. McCormack WM, Nowroozi K, Alpert S, et al. Acute pelvic inflammatory disease: characteristics of patients with gonococcal and nongonococcal infection and evaluation of their response to treatment with aqueous procaine penicillin G and spectinomycin hydrochloride. *Sex Transm Dis* 1977;4:125–131.
43. Eschenbach DA. Epidemiology and diagnosis of acute pelvic inflammatory disease. *Obstet Gynecol* 1980;55(5 Suppl):142S–153S.
44. Sweet RL, Draper DL, Schachter J, et al. Microbiology and pathogenesis of acute salpingitis as determined by laparoscopy: what is appropriate site to sample? *Am J Obstet Gynecol* 1980;138: 985–989.
45. Soper DE, Brockwell NJ, Dalton HP, et al. Observations concerning the microbial etiology of acute salpingitis. *Am J Obstet Gynecol* 1994;170:1008–1017.
46. Faro S, Martens M, Hammill H, et al. Vaginal flora and pelvic inflammatory disease. *Am J Obstet Gynecol* 1993;169:470–474.
47. Paavonen J, Kiviat N, Brunham RC, et al. Prevalence and manifestations of endometritis among women with cervicitis. *Am J Obstet Gynecol* 1985;152:280–286.
48. Paavonen J, Westrom LV. Diagnosis of pelvic inflammatory disease. In: Berger GS, Westrom LV, eds. *Pelvic inflammatory disease.* New York: Raven Press, 1992:48–78.
49. Peterson HB, Galaid EI, Cates W Jr. Pelvic inflammatory disease. *Med Clin North Am* 1990;74: 1603–1615.
50. Peipert JF, Ness RB, Blume J, et al. Pelvic Inflammatory Disease Evaluation and Clinical Health Study Investigators. Clinical predictors of endometritis in women with symptoms and signs of pelvic inflammatory disease. *Am J Obstet Gynecol* 2001;184:856–863.

51. Paavonen J, Teisala K, Heinonen PK, et al. Microbiological and histopathological findings in acute pelvic inflammatory disease. *J Clin Pathol* 1985;38:726–732.
52. Paavonen J, Aine R, Teisala K, et al. Chlamydial endometritis. *J Clin Pathol* 1985;38:726–732.
53. Paavonen J, Aine R, Teisala K, et al. Comparison of endometrial biopsy and peritoneal fluid cytologic testing in the diagnosis of acute pelvic inflammatory disease. *Am J Obstet Gynecol* 1985;151: 645–650.
54. Kiviat NB, Wolner-Hanssen P, Eschenbach DA, et al. Endometrial histopathology in patients with culture-proved upper genital tract infection and laparoscopically diagnosed acute salpingitis. *Am J Surg Pathol* 1990;14:167–175.
55. Cohen SB, Weisz B, Seidman DS, et al. Accuracy of the preoperative diagnosis in 100 emergency laparoscopies performed due to acute abdomen in nonpregnant women. *J Am Assoc Gynecol Laparoscop* 2001;8:92–94.
56. Cibula D, Kozel D, Fucikova Z, et al. Acute exacerbation of recurrent pelvic inflammatory disease. Laparoscopic findings in 141 women with a clinical diagnosis. *J Reprod Med* 2001;46:49–53.

4

Chancroid

INTRODUCTION

Hippocrates recognized a condition in which individuals developed genital ulcers that, in some instances, were associated with the formation of buboes. Hippocrates did not know the cause of this disease. Celsus made additional significant observations and differentiated genital ulcers into two types, those with a dry clean base and those that had a moist and dirty (purulent) base (1). Chancroid was differentiated from syphilis in the mid-1800s, with one report crediting Ricord as the first to differentiate the two diseases (2). In 1852, Brassereau, in France, was credited with establishing chancroid as a separate disease from syphilis. He also observed that infected individuals were able to disseminate the disease to other sites of the body by autoinoculation (3).

The process of autoinoculation was further documented by Ducrey (4,5) who was able to cause infection, in the same patient, by removing an inoculum from an ulcer and introducing it into the skin of the forearm. He described the organism as a short compact streptobacillus with rounded ends. Ducrey was also able to identify the organism in material obtained from a chancre and a bubo, thus confirming the disease was caused by a microorganism. In 1892, Unna (6), studying histologic specimens, was able to stain the organism and describe the gram-negative rods arranged in clumps and chains. In 1920, Teague and Deibert (7) isolated *Haemophilus ducreyi* from approximately 80% of patients with a clinical diagnosis of chancroid.

EPIDEMIOLOGY

Chancroid is most commonly seen in Africa, Asia, and Latin American and may be more common that syphilis (8,9). This disease is more prevalent among the lower socioeconomic classes and is more prominent in males than females (10:1). It also appears that the uncircumcised male is more susceptible than the circumcised male (10,11). At present, the only known route of transmission is via sexual contact. It is not uncommon for the disease to occur in clusters, especially around areas of transient migration such as ports of entry. This is particularly characteristic of individuals returning from tropical areas.

Chancroid is not commonly found in the United States; however, in the late 1980s there was a surge in the incidence of the disease. The Centers for Disease Control and Prevention (CDC) reported that there were 9,515 cases in 1947. This high number of cases continued until 1965. From 1965 through 1984, however, the number of cases averaged approximately 925 per year, with a range of 455 to 1,416 per year. In 1985 there was a surge in the number of cases of chancroid in the United States. The CDC reported a rise to 2,000 cases in 1985, and the prevalence of this disease rose each year thereafter. In 1986 there were 3,000 cases, and in 1987 almost 5,000 cases were reported before the numbers started to decline. In 1988, there were approximately 4,500 cases, and in 1989, 4,250 cases were reported. In 1990, 4,100 cases were reported. This trend continued as the CDC reported approximately 1,800 cases in 1992 and 1,400 in 1993 (12).

The disease is not equally distributed throughout the United States and appears to be more regional. The most U.S. cases were reported in Florida, Georgia, Louisiana, New York, and Texas. The increase in the number of cases from 1986 through 1991 was concentrated in large cities such as Dallas, New Orleans, New York City, Boston, and several cities in Florida (13,14). This increase in number paralleled the increase of primary and secondary syphilis among heterosexual men and women. This increase was also associated with the use of cocaine and the exchange of drugs for sex (15–17).

Sexually transmitted diseases (STDs), such as chancroid, are important risk factors for the heterosexual transmission and acquisition of human immunodeficiency virus (HIV) (18). The mechanism involved in increasing the transmission of HIV is the presence of genital ulcers with an increase in viral shedding at the site of the ulcer (19). The presence of an ulcer also increases susceptibility to HIV by disrupting the epithelial barrier and presenting HIV target cells, macrophages, and CD 4 lymphocytes (20–22).

MICROBIOLOGY

H. ducreyi is the causative agent of chancroid. It is a gram-negative bacillus belonging to the facultative anaerobic group of bacteria. It can be grown on culture media and has a specific requirement for hemin (X factor) (22). Lee (23) demonstrated that *H. ducreyi* has a specific requirement for heme and lacks the enzyme ferrochelatase, which catalyzes the reaction that inserts iron into protoporphyrin IX in the synthesis of heme. The organism's requirement for hemoglobin and heme is specific and when combined with haptoglobin and serum albumin can serve as a suitable source of iron. Sources of iron, such as human transferrin, human lactoferrin, of FeCl₃, however, are not substitutes for hemoglobin or heme when attempting to culture *H. ducreyi* (24).

The organism also appears to have a specific requirement for sodium selenate. In a concentration of 0.1 µg/mL, when added to Mueller-Hinton agar, heme, glutamine, and bovine albumin, sodium selenate stimulated the growth of *H. ducreyi* when grown under microaerophilic, but not ambient, atmospheric conditions (25,26). When Gram stained, the streptobacilli typically appears in a row of chains commonly referred to as a "school of fish." However, the use of the Gram stain to identify *H. ducreyi* from clinical specimens is unreliable. In one study, one out of 19 patients (5.3%) with a clinical diagnosis of chancroid had a positive smear (27).

H. ducreyi is a fastidious bacterium that is difficult to isolate and culture from clinical specimens. There appears to be different nutritional requirements between strains as noted by several investigators (28,29). Several media have been developed for the culture and isolation of *H. ducreyi* with varying degrees of sensitivity. It appears that the following media have the best success rate in culturing *H. ducreyi* (Table 4-1). This media has shown to have a greater than 75% but less than 85% success rate in the culture and isolation of *H. ducreyi* (30). Johnson et al. (31) compared gonococcal based agar plus heart infusion agar supplemented with fetal bovine serum, fresh rabbit blood, Iso Vitale X, and vancomycin with polymerase chain reaction (PCR) in 96 men with genital ulcers for the detection of *H. ducreyi*. This study revealed a 71% sensitivity for culture of *H. ducreyi*.

When obtaining a specimen for the isolation of *H. ducreyi*, it is important to notify the laboratory when the diagnosis is suspected and isolation of the organism will be attempted. Many laboratories do not store the specific medium necessary for the isolation of this organism, and a special transport medium is necessary. The specimen should not be held at room temperature but should be stored at 4°C for no longer than 4 days. In fact, maintaining the specimen at 4°C for 4 days reduced the rate of contamination and increased the positivity rate for isolation of *H. ducreyi* (31). The transport media that yielded the best results were thioglycolate-hemin-based containing either selenium dioxide, glutamine, and albumin or glutamine and albumin (32). Thus, it is imperative that the laboratory be notified when obtaining this type of specimen. The laboratory can offer advice with regard to collection and transport of the specimen as well as prepare to receive and properly process it.

The specimen is best collected from the base of the ulcer and the margins using a swab (33). It is not necessary to preclean the base of the ulcer; however, it seems that cleansing the base with sterile, nonbacterostatic saline would enhance recovery of the organism and is preferred by several investigators

TABLE 4-1. *Media with the highest success rate of growing H. ducreyia*

Mueller-Hinton agar + 5% chocolatized horse blood + 1% Iso Vitale X + vancomycin (3 µg/ml)
Gonococcal agar base + 1% hemoglobin + 5% fetal bovine serum + 1% Iso Vitale X + vancomycin (3 µg/ml)
Gonococcal agar base + 5% Field's extract (Oxoid) + 5% horse blood + vancomycin (3 µg/ml)

[a]Modified from Trees DL, Moorse SA. Chancroid and Haemophilus ducreyi: an update. *Clin Microbiol Rev* 1995;8:357, with permission.

(34–36). Aspirates from buboes are not as successful in retrieving the organism as specimens obtained from ulcers (36).

The distribution of strains and the decision of whether or not reinfection or treatment failure has occurred are important aspects of the management of STDs. Strain typing is also of value in determining if there is a difference in virulence between isolates. Two methods appear to be reliable in identifying specific strains: ribotyping and plasmid analysis. Ribotyping is a method of analyzing specific restriction fragment length polymorphism of ribosomal ribonucleic acid (rRNA) genes, which are highly conserved and present in multiple copies (24). Flood et al. (37) used ribotyping and plasmid analysis to study the outbreak of chancroid in San Francisco between 1989 and 1991. Thirty-two isolates were studied and six different HindIII patterns were identified. Ribotype HindIII-2 was found in four strains and HindIII-11 in one strain from patients who had traveled to Los Angeles, Korea, and El Salvador. This study is in contrast to a study performed on isolates obtained from an outbreak in Orange county in which all strains possessed the 3.2-MDa plasmid and, therefore, were considered to all be of one strain (10).

PATHOGENESIS

The bacteria are typically transmitted during sexual intercourse during the contact of a mucosal surface with a chancre. However, because autoinoculation is possible, infection via nonsexual mucosal contact can occur through a break in the skin. The incubation period is between 4 to 7 days and rarely less than 3 or more than 10 days (38). It is postulated that during sexual intercourse breaks in the vaginal epithelium or epithelial surfaces occur that allow the bacilli to enter the new host. Initially, following the incubation period, a macule or papule develops at the site of inoculation then forms a pustule. After 2 to 3 days, necrosis of the outer layer of the pustule occurs and an ulcer or chancre forms. The ulcer is sharply demarcated with distinct ragged undermined edges, and there is a noticeable absence of induration at the site of the lesion. The base of the ulcer, unlike that of a syphilitic chancre that has a smooth base, has a granular appearance. The ulcer may become covered with a gray to yellow necrotic purulent exudate. Because the chancre is well vascularized, it bleeds easily when scraped. The ulcers of chancroid tend to be very painful. Autoinoculation leads to the formation of multiple lesions, which is common, and often the lesions become confluent forming a large ulceration. Frequently, the lesion becomes secondarily infected, and the edges become shaggy or ragged. A variant of chancroid, "dwarf chancre," is characterized by pustules that do not progress to well-developed ulcerations (39).

Infection in women may be dissimilar to those in men. Chancres that form in the vagina and cervix are typically asymptomatic, whereas those lesions that develop on the vulva are painful. This sets the vulvar chancres apart from those found in conjunction with syphilis. Chancres may develop anywhere there is a

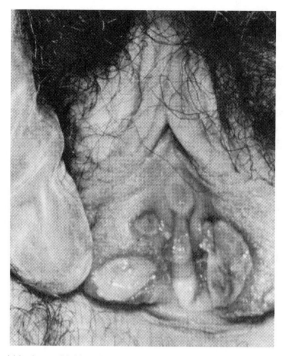

FIG. 4-1. Chancroid lesions of labia minora. (From Kaufman RH, Faro S, Friedrich EG Jr, et al. *Benign diseases of the vulva and vagina,* 4th ed. St. Louis: Mosby, 1994, with permission.) (See Color Plate 2 following page 148.)

break in the tissue that comes in contact with an active chancre. Other common sites are the labia, vestibule, fourchette, and clitoris (Fig. 4-1). Lesions that form on the vaginal epithelium and cervix are usually not associated with pain.

The varied appearance of the chancre may often lead to confusion with other infectious diseases (Table 4-2). The ulcer may be larger than 2 cm; a large ulcer is formed by the coalescence of multiple small ulcers. A follicular ulcer (le chancre mou folliculaire) develops in a hair follicle on the mons or vulva. Because multiple follicles may be involved, this presentation may be confused with a pyogenic infection (40).

The ulcer or chancre of chancroid has three definitive layers (41). The superficial layer is made of necrotic debris consisting of dead cells, fibrin, and neu-

TABLE 4-2. *Differential diagnosis of vulvar ulcers*

Chancroid may be confused with:
 Follicular lesions, folliculitis, or pyoderma
 Dwarf chancroid (formes naines), herpes
 Transient chancroid (chancre mou volant), lymphogranuloma venereum
 Papular chancroid (ulcus molle elevatum), condylomata latum

trophils that have migrated into the area in an effort to eradicate the organisms present in the lesion. The second layer is edematous and contains the proliferation of blood vessels. The bottom layer contains a dense population of inflammatory cells consisting of neutrophils, plasma cells, and fibroblasts. As the lesion ages, lymphoid cells become dominant.

The lymphadenitis associated with genital chancroid is caused by the infiltration of numerous neutrophils and bacteria, which are usually few in number. Lymphadenopathy develops in approximately 50% of patients with chancroid. It is typically unilateral and painful (41–42). Involved lymph nodes can rapidly differentiate into buboes, which spontaneously rupture forming inguinal ulcerations. Suppuration results from the tremendous number of inflammatory cells that migrate into the area producing a pyogenic response. The exact mechanism underlying the development of suppuration has not been determined. The question is how does this process develop in the presence of a relative absence of microorganisms.

Systemic dissemination of *H. ducreyi* has not been demonstrated. Secondary infection of chancroid ulcers may occur with organisms that are endogenous to the vaginal or rectal ecosystems. Bacteria such as members of the Enterobacteriaceae or anaerobes such as *Bacteroides* and *Fusobacterium* can cause sepsis. Gram-negative obligate anaerobic bacteria can cause gangrenous phagedenic ulceration that may result in extensive destruction of the external genitalia (27,43).

CHARACTERISTICS OF THE BACTERIUM

Investigations on the characteristics of the organism have revealed that the bacterium possess extremely fine surface appendages called pili (44). These appendages appear to be similar in all strain studies and have a molecular mass of 24 kDa. Pili receptor sites have not been identified on host cells. Subsequent passage of the organism on culture media did not result in loss of the pili.

H. ducreyi possess lipopolysaccharide but lacks the repeating O-antigens common to the lipopolysaccharide of the Enterobacteriaceae. The lipopolysaccharide of *H. ducreyi* is similar in size and structure to that of other mucosal pathogens and is referred to as a lipooligosaccharide (LOS) (45,46). Intradermal injection of *H. ducreyi* LOS produced skin abscess in rabbits suggesting that LOS may play a role in the pathogenesis of chancroid.

LOS may also play a role in combating the host immune response. The terminal end of LOS Gall—4GlcNAc—can be sialylated similar to the terminal end of gonococcal LOS, converting a serum-sensitive to a serum-resistant organism (47).

DIAGNOSIS

The diagnosis is confirmed by isolating *H. ducreyi* from a lesion. The organism may be noted on the Gram stain of exudate obtained from a scraping of the base of the chancre. However, it is important that no secondary infection be present. The Gram stain will reveal, if *H. ducreyi* is present, gram-negative rods in chains in approximately 35% of the cases (48). The presence of gram-negative bacilli is not sufficient to make a diagnosis of chancroid because the lesion typically becomes secondarily infected. Therefore, it is highly recommended that a specimen be obtained from the lesion to confirm that it is *H. ducreyi*. It is also important to contact the laboratory to inform them that the specimen is forthcoming and *H. ducreyi* is suspected. This will ensure that the specimen is properly prepared and processed appropriately. Because the bacterium is fastidious, it will not survive for a long period if the specimen is maintained on the swab. Therefore, the specimen should be processed immediately. Inoculation of the culture medium at the bedside is the preferred method for isolation of the organism. Aspiration of a lymph node or obtaining purulent material from a suppurative node to isolate the organism is frequently met with negative results because this material usually contains only a scarce population of bacteria. Currently there are no commercially available serologic tests. Experimental techniques involving monoclonal antibodies and deoxyribonucleic acid (DNA) probes are being tested to improve the accuracy of establishing a diagnosis (49,50).

TREATMENT

The CDC recommends the following antibiotics for treatment (51):

Ceftriaxone 250 mg intramuscularly in a single dose
Azithromycin 1 g orally in a single dose
Erythromycin base 500 mg orally QID × 7 days
Ciprofloxacin 500 mg orally BID × 3 days
Ofloxacin 400 mg orally BID × 3 days

Individuals known to have had contact with an infected partner, but who have not manifested a lesion, should be treated with one of the regimens listed. Individuals should be reexamined 7 to 10 days following institution of therapy. Patients with lymphadenopathy may experience resolution but it may be slow, and aspiration of the lymph node may be required. If there appears to be a treatment failure, then the patient must be questioned as to her compliance of therapy. The possibility of a resistant strain, the likelihood of a wrong diagnosis being made, and the possibility of coinfection with the HIV must be entertained. It is also important to review the current effectiveness of the chosen antibiotic. Treatment with sulfonamides, tetracyclines, and penicillins has not been universally effective (12). Fluorinated quinolones, spectinomycin, and cefotaxime have all been demonstrated to be effective against *H. ducreyi* (52–54). Fluorinated quinolones appear to be effective when given to patients who are not positive for HIV (53). Cefotaxime is effective as a three-a-day regimen. *In vitro* activity against *H. ducreyi* has also been reported with other macrolides and third-generation cephalosporins (52). Single-dose treatment for chancroid and longer courses of therapy are required in this population.

In the presence of appropriate antibiotic therapy, sterilization of the ulcer usually occurs in 72 hours. Complete epithelialization of the primary ulcer occurs in 10 days. On rare occasions, slower resolution of the disease, up to 28 days, has been reported (55,56). A temporary enlargement of matted lymph nodes is not indicative of treatment failure unless the ulcer site also shows no improvement. Local therapy with sitz baths with aluminium acetate is useful in providing temporary local relief.

Efficacy of treatment is dependent on whether concurrent HIV infection is present, which increases the probability of failure. This is a likely result when treatment is instituted with single-dose ceftriaxone or fleroxacin (54,57). Initial studies suggest that increasing the duration of treatment to 5 days with fleroxacin 400 mg orally once a day is indicated for the HIV-positive patient with chancroid (58).

Antibiotic resistance has not been a significant problem; however, it is starting to materialize. Erythromycin resistance, minimum inhibitory concentration (MIC) of 4 μg/mL, has been reported from Singapore and Thailand (59,60). Quinolone resistance is not widespread and has not been reported, except for one isolated case from Thailand that was found to be resistant to ciprofloxacin (MIC 2 μg/mL). Resistance to trimethoprim/sulfamethoxazole has a documented increase from 9% in 1988 to 48% in 1991 (60). Strains resistant to trimethoprim/sulfamethoxazole were found to be resistant to trimethoprim as well. Strains resistant to trimethoprim/sulfamethoxazole have been found in the United States, Thailand, and Kenya (61–63). Interestingly, resistance to amoxicillin/clavulanic acid is more common in strains that are beta-lactamase negative than in those that are beta-lactamase positive (61). This data suggests that trimethoprim/sulfamethoxazole, trimethoprim, and amoxicillin/clavulanic acid should not be used to treat chancroid.

REFERENCES

1. Kampmeier RH. The recognition of *Haemophilus ducreyi* as the cause of soft chancre. *Sex Transm Dis* 1982;9:212–213.
2. Schmid GP, Sanders LL Jr, Bount JH, et al. Chancroid in the United States: re-establishment of an old disease. *JAMA* 1987;258:3265–3268.
3. Brassereau PI. *Traite de affections de la peau symptomatiques de la syphilis.* Paris: JB Baillare, 1652.
4. Ducrey A. Il virus dell ulcera venerea. *Gass Int Sci Med* 1889;11:44.
5. Ducrey A. Experimentelle Untersuchungen uber den Ansteckungsstof des weihen Schankers und uber die Bubonen. *Montash Prakt Dermatol* 1889;9:387.
6. Unna PG. Der Streptobacillus. Sex. Des weichen Schenkers. Montash. *Prakt Dermatol* 1892;14:485.
7. Teague O, Deibert O. The value of cultural method in the diagnosis of chancroid. *J Urol* 1920;4:543.
8. Ortiz-Zepeda C, Hernandez-Perez E, Marroquin-Burgos R. Gross and microscopic features in chancroid: a study in 200 new culture proven cases in San Salvador. *Sex Transm Dis* 1994;21:112–117.
9. Piot P, Plummer FA. Genital ulcer adenopathy syndrome. In: Holmes KK, Mardh P-A, Sparling PF, et al., eds. *Sexually transmitted diseases,* 2nd ed. New York: McGraw-Hill, 1990:711–716.
10. Blackmore CA, Limpakarnjanarat K, Rigau-Perez JG, et al. An outbreak of chancroid in Orange County, California: descriptive epidemiology and disease-control measures. *J Infect Dis* 1985;151: 840–844.

11. Hart G. Venereal disease in a war environment: incidence and management. *Med J Aust* 1975;1: 808–810.
12. Sexually transmitted disease surveillance, 1993. Centers for Disease Control and Prevention, US Department of Health and Human Services, Atlanta, GA.
13. Hammond GW, Slutchuk M, Scatliff J, et al. Epidemiologic, clinical, laboratory, and therapeutic features of an urban outbreak of chancroid in North America. *Rev Infect Dis* 1980;2:867–879.
14. Orle KA, Martin DH, Gates CA, et al. Multiplex PCR detection of *Haemophilus ducreyi, Treponema pallidum,* and herpes simplex viruses types 1 and 2 from genital ulcers, abstract C-437. *Abstracts of the 94th Annual Meeting of the American Society of Microbiology.* Washington, DC: 1994:568.
15. Finelli L, Budd J, Spitalny KC. Early syphilis: relationship to sex, drugs, and changes in high-risk behavior from 1987–1990. *Sex Transm Dis* 1993;20:89–95.
16. Martin DH, DiCarlo RP. Recent changes in the epidemiology of genital ulcer disease in the United States: the crack cocaine connection. *Sex Transm Dis* 1994;21(2 Suppl):S76–S80.
17. Roggen EL, DeBreucker S, Van Dyck E, et al. Antigenic diversity in *Haemophilus ducreyi* as shown by Western blot (immunoblot) analysis. *Infect Immun* 1992;60:590–595.
18. Kreiss JK, Coombs R, Plummer F, et al. Isolation of human immunodeficiency virus from genital ulcers in Nairobi prostitutes. *J Infect Dis* 1989;260:380–384.
19. Plummer FA, Wainberg MA, Plourde P, et al. Detection of human immunodeficiency virus type 1 (HIV-1) in genital ulcer exudates of HIV-1 infected men by culture and gene amplification. *J Infect Dis* 1990;161:810–811.
20. Engelkens HJ, ten Kate FJW, Judanarso J, et al. The localization of treponemes and characterization of the inflammatory infiltrate in skin biopsies from patients with primary or secondary syphilis, or early infectious yaws. *Genitourin Med* 1993;69:102–107.
21. Spinola SM, Wild LM, Apicella MA, et al. Experimental human infection with *Haemophilus ducreyi. J Infect Dis* 1994;169:1146–1150.
22. Hammond GW, Lian CJ, Wilt JC, et al. Comparison of specimen collection and laboratory techniques for isolation of *Haemophilus ducreyi. J Clin Microbiol* 1978;7:39–43.
23. Lee BC. Iron sources for *Haemophilus ducreyi. J Med Microbiol* 1991;34:317–322.
24. Trees DL, Moorse SA. Chancroid and *Haemophilus ducreyi*: an update. *Clin Microbiol Rev* 1995;8: 357–375.
25. Vanden Berghe DA. Selenium and the growth of *Haemophilus ducreyi. J Clin Pathol* 1987;40: 1174–1177.
26. Dziuba M, Noble PA, Albritton WL. A study of the nutritional requirements of a selected *Haemophilus ducreyi* strain by impedance and conventional methods. *Curr Microbiol* 1993;27:109.
27. Sturm AW, Stotling GW, Cormane RH, et al. Clinical and microbiological evaluation of 46 episodes of genital ulceration. *Genitourin Med* 1987;63:98–101.
28. MacDonald K, Cameron DW, Inungu G, et al. Comparison of Sheffield media with standard media for the isolation of *Haemophilus ducreyi. Sex Transm Dis* 1989;16:88–90.
29. Morse SA. Chancroid and *Haemophilus ducreyi. Clin Microbiol Rev* 1989;2:137–157.
30. Dangor Y, Miller SD, Koornhof HJ, et al. A simple medium for the primary isolation of *Haemophilus ducreyi. Eur J Clin Microbiol Infect Dis* 1992;11:930–934.
31. Johnson SR, Martin DH, Cammarata C, et al. Alterations in sample preparation increase sensitivity of PCR assay for diagnosis of chancroid. *J Clin Microbiol* 1995;33:1036–1038.
32. Dangor Y, Radebe F, Ballard RC. Transport media for *Haemophilus ducreyi. Sex Transm Dis* 1993;20: 5–9.
33. Taylor DN, Duangmani C, Suvongse C, et al. The role of *Haemophilus ducreyi* in penile ulcers in Bangkok,. Thailand. *Sex Transm Dis* 1984;11:148–151.
34. Crewe-Brown HH, Krige FK, Davel GH, et al. Genital ulceration in males at Ga-Rankuwa Hospital, Pretoria. *S Afr Med J* 1982;62:861–863.
35. Albritton WL, Plummer FA, Sottnek FO, et al. *Haemophilus ducreyi* and *Calymmatobacterium granulomatis.* In Lennette EH, Balows A, Hausler WJ Jr, et al., eds. *Manual of clinical microbiology,* 4th ed. Washington DC: American Society for Microbiology, 1985:869–873.
36. Sottnek FO, Biddle JW, Kraus SJ, et al. Isolation and identification of *Haemophilus ducreyi* in a clinical study. *J Clin Microbiol* 1980;12:170–174.
37. Flood JM, Sarafian SK, Bolan GA, et al. Multistrain outbreak of chancroid in San Francisco, 1989–91. *J Infect Dis* 1993;167:1106–1111.
38. Ronald AR, Plummer FA. Chancroid and *Haemophilus ducreyi. Ann Int Med* 1985;102:705–707.
39. Gaisin A, Heaton CL. Chancroid: alias soft chancre. *Int J Dermatol* 1975;14:188–190.
40. Chapel TA, Brown WJ, Jefferies C, et al. How reliable is the morphological diagnosis of penile ulcerations? *Sex Transm Dis* 1977;4:150–152.

41. D'Costa LJ, Bowmer I, Nsanze H, et al. Advances in the diagnosis and management of chancroid. *Sex Transm Dis* 1986;13(3 Suppl):189–191.
42. Plummer FA, D'Costa LJ, Nsanze H, et al. Clinical and microbiological studies of genital ulcers in Kenyan women. *Sex Transm Dis* 1985;12:193–197.
43. Ronald AR, Albritton WL. Chancroid and *Haemophilus ducreyi.* In: Holmes KK, Mardh PA, Sparling PF, et al., eds. *Sexually transmitted diseases.* New York: McGraw-Hill, 1984;385–393.
44. Spinola SM, Castellazzo A, Shero M, et al. Characterization of pili expressed by *Haemophilus ducreyi. Microb Pathog* 1990;9:417–426.
45. Mandrell RE, Griffiss JM, Macher BA. Lipopooligosaccharides (LOS) of *Neisseria gonorrhoeae* and *Neisseria meningitidis* have components that are immunochemically similar to precursors of blood group antigens: carbohydrate sequence specificity of the mouse monoclonal antibodies that recognize crossreacting antigens on LOS and human erythrocytes. *J Exp Med* 1988;168:107–126.
46. Melaugh W, Phillips NJ, Campagnari AA, et al. Structure of the major lipo-oligosaccharide from the *Haemophilus ducreyi* strain 35000 and evidence for additional glycoforms. *Biochemistry* 1994;33: 13070–13078.
47. Melaugh W, Phillips NJ, Campagnari AA, et al. Partial characterization of the major lipo-oligosaccharide from a strain of *Haemophilus ducreyi,* the causative agent of chancroid, a genital ulcer disease. *J Biol Chem* 1992;267:13434–13439.
48. Choudhary BP, Kumari S, Bhatia R, et al. Bacteriological study of chancroid. *Indian J Med Res* 1982; 76:379–385.
49. Sheldon WH, Heyman A. Studies on chancroid: I. Observations on the histology with an evaluation of biopsy as a diagnostic procedure. *Am J Pathol* 1946;22:415.
50. Karim QN, Finn GY, Easmon CS, et al. Rapid detection of *Haemophilus ducreyi* in clinical and experimental infections using monoclonal antibody: a preliminary evaluation. *Genitourin Med* 1989; 65:361–365.
51. Parsons LM, Shayegani M, Waring AL, et al. DNA probes for the identification of *Haemophilus ducreyi. J Clin Microbiol* 1989;27:1441–1445.
52. Centers for Disease Control and Prevention. Sexually transmitted disease treatment guidelines, 2002. *MMWR* 2002;51:11-12.
53. Fransen L, Nsanze H, Ndinya-Achola JO, et al. A comparison of single dose spectinomycin with five days of trimethoprim-sulfamethoxazole for the treatment of chancroid. *Sex Transm Dis* 1987;14: 98–101.
54. Plummer FA, Maggwa N, D'Costa LJ, et al. Cefotaxime treatment of *Haemophilus ducreyi* infection in Kenya. *Sex Transm Dis* 1984;11:304–307.
55. MacDonald KS, Cameron DW, D'Costa LJ, et al. Evaluation of fleroxacin (RO 23-6240) as single oral dose therapy of culture proven chancroid in Nairobi, Kenya. *Antimicrob Agents Chemother* 1989; 33:612–614.
56. Dangor Y, Ballard RC, Miller SD, et al. Treatment of chancroid. *Antimicrob Agents Chemother* 1990; 34:1308–1311.
57. Ballard RC, Duncan MO, Fehler HG, et al. Treating chancroid: summary of studies in Southern Africa. *Genitourin Med* 1989;65:54–57.
58. Asin J. Chancroid: a report of 1402 cases. *Am J Syph Gon Vener Dis* 1952;36:483.
59. Tyndall MW, Malisa M, Plummer FA, et al. Ceftriaxone no longer predictably cures chancroid in Kenya. *J Infect Dis* 1993;167:469–471.
60. Tyndall MW, Plourde PJ, Agoki E, et al. Fleroxacin in the treatment of chancroid: an open study in men seropositive or seronegative for the human immunodeficiency virus type 1. *Am J Med* 1993;94: 855–885.
61. Slootmans L, Vanden Berghe DA, Van Dyck E, et al. Susceptibility pf 40 *Haemophilus ducreyi* strains to 34 antimicrobial products. *Antimicrob Agents Chemother* 1983;24:564–567.
62. Van Dyck E, Bogaerts J, Smet H, et al. Emergence of *Haemophilus ducreyi* resistance to trimethoprim-sulfamethoxazole in Rwanda. *Antimicrob Agents Chemother* 1994;38:1647–1648.
63. Plourde PJ, D'Costa LJ, Agoki E, et al. A randomized, double-blind study of the efficacy of fleroxacin versus trimethoprim-sulfamethoxazole in men with culture-proven chancroid. *J Infect Dis* 1992; 165:949–952.

5

Granuloma Inguinale

Granuloma inguinale (GI), a chronic progressive disease, was first described by McLeod in 1882. The disease typically involves the genital region and is considered a sexually transmitted disease (STD). Donovan, in 1905, demonstrated the presence of an organism in tissue specimens obtained from patients with active disease, and the infection was referred to as Donovania granulomatis (1).

Because the organism has not been grown on artificial media, its biochemical and microbiologic characteristics are not fully known. Recently, the organism was named *Calymmatobacterium granulomatis*. In tissue specimens, the organism typically appears within phagocytic mononuclear cells and forms complexes called "Donovan bodies" (2) (Fig. 5-1).

EPIDEMIOLOGY

In 1991, the Centers for Disease Control and Prevention (CDC) reported 29 cases of GI in the United States (3). In 1984, 20 cases were reported in the state of Texas (4). The disease, however, is primarily found in West New Guinea, among aborigines in Australia, in India, in the Caribbean, and in Africa, as well as in subtropical areas (5). Genital ulcerative diseases (GUDs), such as granuloma inguinale and lymphogranuloma venereum, are common in tropical and subtropical regions but uncommon in developed countries. However, other GUDs, such as herpes, are not uncommon in developing countries and are recognized as a cofactor for heterosexual transmission of human immunodeficiency virus (HIV). Men with GUD serve as an important vector in the transmission of HIV in the general population, particularly to women (6).

The route of transmission has not been completely elucidated; however, there is strong evidence that indicates the primary route of transmission is via sexual contact. In many cases, active lesions cannot be detected, but, in approximately 12% to 52% of cases, infection is known to be present within a marital or long-term sexual relationship (7). Homosexuals with anal lesions tend to pass the disease to their partners, who often develop the lesion on their penises (8,9).

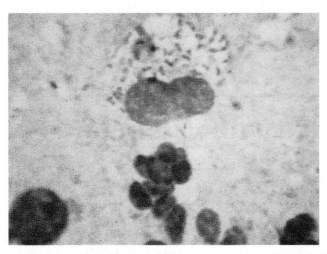

FIG. 5-1. Donovan bodies contained within vacuoles of a mononuclear cell. Note the bipolar staining, which is typical of *Calymmatobacterium granuloma*. (See Color Plate 3 following page 148.)

Autoinoculation also occurs and is easily accomplished by manually transferring the organism from an active lesion to a distant site. Thus, a new lesion arises after touching an active lesion and then scratching at a distant site with the same hand. Dissemination of the disease has been reported to involve the oropharynx, liver, thorax, and skeletal system (10–13). A unique characteristic of the disease is that it does not appear to be highly contagious and requires repeated exposure to cause infection. In New Guinea there is a concentration of cases among children, ages 1 to 4, and in individuals older than 15 years. It is hypothesized that the disease is concentrated in children because they acquire the infection by sitting on the laps of infected individuals (14).

In 1996, a study was conducted in Durban, South Africa to determine if there is an increasing prevalence of GI in women. In the clinical records of 123 women diagnosed with GI, 52 (42%) were pregnant. The only detectable difference between pregnant and nonpregnant women was an increase in rectal and pelvic lesions in the latter group. Thirty-six (69%) delivered vaginally and 16 were delivered by cesarean section. There was no evidence of congenital GI, and maternal GI had no influence on the pregnancy outcome. Although GI is increasing in pregnancy, this did not enhance dissemination (15).

MICROBIOLOGY

Calymmatobacterium granuloma is an encapsulated gram-negative bacterium. The organism is phagocytized by histocytic cells or, occasionally, by polymorphonuclear leukocytes or plasma cells. The bacterium remains within these intracellular vacuoles throughout its life cycle. The bacterium reproduces within these vacuoles, producing 20 to 30 bacteria per vacuole. An infected cell will usually hold several bacteria-containing vacuoles. Once the host cell has been exhausted of its nutrients and bacterial reproduction has been completed, the vacuole lyses and the cell ruptures liberating the bacteria (16).

PATHOGENESIS

Initially an inflammatory nodule develops at the site of inoculation. The lesion progressively enlarges and undergoes central necrosis to form a beefy, granulomatous ulcer (Fig. 5-2). The ulcer, via autoinoculation, gives rise to new lesions that may coalesce with adjacent lesions to form large granulomatous masses (Fig. 5-3) The ulcer is usually painless, unless it becomes secondarily infected and develops a border of granulation tissue with a red base. Progressive lesions develop along the route of lymphatic drainage; however, these lesions are not true buboes. Although they do not typically involve lymph nodes, they are subcutaneous lesions. Keloids develop when ulcers healed by fibrosis lack pigmentation. Fibrosis and lymphatic obstruction results from the enlarging ulcers that may cause gross distortion of tissue, such as vulvar elephantiasis. On occasion, the lymph nodes draining the affected area become infected and develop into a bubo. The presence of a bubo may raise the possibility of other STDs, such as

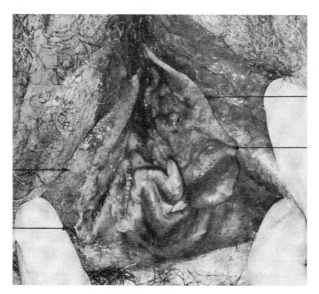

FIG. 5-2. Granuloma inguinale large granular, raised ulceration involving extensive areas of the vulva. This lesion has been mistaken for carcinoma of the vulva. (From Kaufman RH, Faro S. *Benign diseases of the vulva and vagina,* 4th ed. St. Louis: Mosby, 1994:62, Figure 5.9 on page 71, with permission.) (See Color Plate 4 following page 148.)

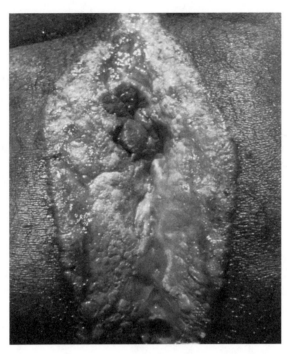

FIG. 5-3. Granuloma inguinale large ulceration involving an extensive area in the perianal region. This lesion, most likely, arose by autoinoculation of adjacent areas and coalescence of these lesions. The base is beefy red and friable. (From Lambert HP, Farrar WE. *Infectious disease illustrated. An integrated text and color atlas.* Philadelphia: WB Saunders and London, New York: Gower Medical Publishing, 1982:23, Figure 9.54, with permission.) (See Color Plate 5 following page 148.)

lymphogranuloma venereum. Hematogenous dissemination of the disease has been recorded but is rare. When GI is discovered in extragenital sites, a primary genital infection is usually present.

DIAGNOSIS

The laboratory confirmation of GI requires the identification of Donovan bodies in a biopsy specimen obtained from a lesion. A Wright or Giemsa stain of the material from the ulcer may identify Donovan bodies (17). The organism, Donovan bodies, stains blue or black within vacuoles of large mononuclear cells (Fig. 5-1).

The laboratory should be consulted before obtaining the specimen. By alerting the pathologist that the patient may have GI, he or she will be prepared to receive and process the specimen. This will result in specific direction for obtaining and transporting the specimen appropriately. Traditionally the specimen is crushed on a glass slide, allowed to air dry, and stained with Giemsa or Wright stain.

Detection of Donovan bodies has also been reported with Papanicolaou smears. Typically, there is a noticeable inflammatory cell infiltrate, predominantly neutrophils, epithelioid histocytes, and Donovan bodies with vacuoles contained in the histocytes (18,19).

THERAPY

Primary therapy is the administration of tetracycline 500 mg orally four times a day for 21 days. Patients who are allergic to tetracycline or who are pregnant may be treated with erythromycin 500 mg four times a day for 21 days (20). However, erythromycin has not been totally effective, and, therefore, subsequent or combination therapy may be necessary. This raises a significant problem for the obstetrician because there is a reluctance to use antibiotics such as chloramphenicol, cotrimoxazole, gentamicin, or streptomycin.

Chloramphenicol, although not contraindicated in pregnancy, must be used with great care and should not be used if a premature birth is anticipated or the patient is near term. This is because the use of chloramphenicol in preterm and newborn infants is associated with the "gray baby" syndrome. This syndrome results from the administration of excess dosages of chloramphenicol that the immature liver is unable to clear. Circulatory collapse results, and it is associated with a 50% mortality rate (21,22). The syndrome is characterized by abdominal distention, vomiting, pallor, cyanosis, and circulatory collapse. The cyanosis results in these infants appearing gray or ashened, thus the term gray baby syndrome. Because chloramphenicol does cross the placenta, the dose should not exceed the recommended 500 mg every 8 hours. If the drug must be used in late pregnancy, during labor, or during lactation, signs of toxicity in the infant must be monitored. Treatment may require nothing more than discontinuing antibiotic exposure to the infant. Both exchange transfusion and charcoal-column hemoperfusion have been used successfully (23–27).

Trimethoprim/sulfamethoxazole and trimethoprim may also be used in pregnancy but should be avoided in the first trimester. Both of these agents have been shown to be teratogenic when administered to pregnant animals in high doses. Because trimethoprim is a folic acid antagonist, it should be avoided in the first trimester. However, in one study the drug was administered to 10 pregnant patients during the first 16 weeks of their pregnancy and no fetal malformations were observed (28). Sulfonamides compete with bilirubin for albumin binding sites; therefore, it is recommended that these antibiotics have limited use in pregnant women. The sulfonamides are usually restricted to those individuals who are not expected to deliver either while taking this medication or shortly after completing a course of therapy. Use of sulfonamides may increase the free serum bilirubin levels resulting in jaundice or even kernicterus. Subsequently, it has been demonstrated that sulfadoxine/pyrimethamine (Fansidar) and sulfamethoxazole/trimethoprim (Cotrimoxazole) can be used in pregnancy (29,30).

Gentamicin readily crosses the placenta, and the mean peak level in the umbilical vein is 30% to 40% of that in the maternal serum (31). The actual degree of ototoxicity in the fetus, as a result of maternal gentamicin use, is not known. However, aminoglycoside therapy should be used in pregnancy only when there is no suitable alternative.

Therefore, in the pregnant patient, it is extremely important to establish the correct diagnosis. Successful treatment may require the use of antibiotics, which may be associated with significant risk for toxicity to the fetus.

Recent studies have begun to seek antibiotics that reduce toxicity, are efficacious, and are safe in pregnancy. Ceftriaxone, 1 g intramuscularly, was administered daily to eight women and four men, for a total of 7 to 26 g. Four patients responded to 7 to 10 g, whereas the remainder responded to an additional course of ceftriaxone (32).

Azithromycin, 1 g orally, was administered once a week for 4 weeks to seven patients. Four patients had complete resolution and three were improved. Four patients received 500 mg of azithromycin daily for 7 days with one patient reporting complete resolution and three patients showed improvement. Seventeen additional patients received azithromycin and responded favorably (33). Ceftriaxone and azithromycin offer a possibility for treatment of donovanosis that can be used in both the nonpregnant and pregnant patient.

Antibiotics such as chloramphenicol, gentamicin, and cotrimoxazole have also shown effectiveness (Table 5-1) but are associated with significant potential toxicity. Ampicillin has not been shown to be as effective as other agents and requires a prolonged course (34). Therefore, ampicillin should not be used in pregnant patients. Successful therapy will produce a positive response in approximately 1 week and healing of the lesions within 4 to 6 weeks. Inadequate therapy may result in abscess formation, even if it appears that the ulcerations are healing. Therefore, it is important that therapy be continued until all lesions have healed and there is no evidence of active disease. Patients who develop scarring and fibrosis, causing significant discomfort, will require surgical intervention.

TABLE 5-1. *CDC recommendations for antibiotic treatment of Granuloma inguinale*[a]

Doxycycline 100 mg orally twice a day for at least 3 weeks.
Trimethoprim-sulfamethoxazole one double strength (800 mg/160 mg) tablet orally twice a day for at least 3 weeks.
Alternative choices:
Ciprofloxacin 750 mg orally four times a day for at least 3 weeks.
Erythromycin base 500 mg orally four times a day for at least 3 weeks.
Azithromycin 1 g orally once a week for at least 3 weeks.
If no improvement is seen within the first 3 to 4 days, begin an aminoglycoside, e.g., gentamicin 1 mg/kg of body weight every 8 hours.

CDC, Centers for Disease Control and Prevention.
[a]From Centers for Disease Control and Prevention. Sexually transmitted diseases guidelines, 2002. *MMWR* 2002;51:16-18, with permission.

TABLE 5-2. *Screen patients positive for a sexually transmitted disease*

1. Specimens for culture:
    Endocervix: *Neisseria gonorrhoeae*
                      Chlamydia trachomatis
    Vagina and rectum: *Streptococcus agalactiae*
2. Serologic test:
    Syphilis
    HIV
    Hepatitis (if positive, test for Hepatitis C and D)
3. Evaluate the vaginal ecosystem for:
    Bacterial vaginosis
    Trichomonas vaginalis

The differential diagnosis of vulvar ulcerations must include both sexually and nonsexually transmitted diseases. It is important to accurately diagnose the cause of a GUD because of the differences in treatment. In a study conducted in Atlanta, Georgia, herpes simplex was cultured more frequently than *Haemophilus ducreyi* in patients who presented with signs or symptoms suggestive of chancroid (35). The patient should be counseled about the possibility of contracting acquired immunodeficiency syndrome (AIDS), because patients with ulcerative diseases are at a significant risk for acquiring the disease. Any patient diagnosed with a specific STD should always be screened for a battery of STDs (Table 5-2). Biopsy specimens should also be processed for histologic examination, because carcinoma of the vulva has also been associated with GI (36).

REFERENCES

1. Hart G. Donovanosis. In: Holmes KK, Mardh RA, Sparling PF, et al., eds. *Sexually transmitted diseases.* New York: McGraw-Hill, 1984;393.
2. Chandra M, Jain AK. Fine structure of *Calymmatobacterium granulomatis* with particular reference to the surface structure. *Indian J Med Res* 1991;93:225–231.
3. Centers for Disease Control and Prevention—Summary of notifiable diseases, United States 1991. *MMWR* 1991;40:3.
4. Rosen, Tschen JA, Ramsdell W, et al. Granuloma inguinale. *J Am Acad Dermatol* 1984;11:433–437.
5. Mitchell KM, Roberts AN, Williams VM, et al. Donovanosis in Western Australia. *Genitourin Med* 1986;62:191–195.
6. O'Farrell N. Global eradication of donovanosis an opportunity for limiting the spread of HIV-1 infection. *Genitourin Med* 1995;71:27–31.
7. Bhagwandeen BS, Nakik KG. Granuloma venereum (granuloma inguinale) in Zambia. *East Afr Med J* 1977;54:637–642.
8. Hart G. Chancroid, donovanosis, lymphogranuloma venereum. Atlanta, GA: U.S. Department of Health, Education and Welfare, Centers for Disease Control, 1975:75–83.
9. Marmell M. Donovanosis of the anus in the male. An epidemiologic consideration. *Br J Vener Dis* 1958;34:213.
10. Kirkpatrick DJ. Donovanosis (granuloma inguinale) a rare cause of osteolytic bone lesions. *Clin Radiol* 1970;21:101–105.
11. Sehgal UN, Prasad AL. Donovanosis. Current concepts. *Int J Dermatol* 1986;25:8–16.
12. Kampmeier RH. Granuloma inguinale. *Sex Transm Dis* 1984;11:318–321.
13. Zigas V. Medicine from the past. Donovanosis project in Goilala (1951–1954). *Papua New Guinea Med J* 1971;14:148.

14. Dodson RF, Fritz GS, Hubler WR Jr, et al. Donovanosis. A morphologic study. *J Invest Dermatol* 1974;62:611–614.
15. Hoosen AA, Mphatsoe M, Kharsany AB, et al. Granuloma inguinale in association with pregnancy and HIV infection. *Int J Gynecol Obstet* 1996;53:133–138.
16. DeBoer A. Cytologic identification of Donovan bodies in granuloma inguinale. *Acta Cytol* 1984;28: 126.
17. Hoosen AA, Draper G, Moodley J. Granuloma inguinale of the cervix a carcinoma look-alike. *Genitourin Med* 1990;5:380.
18. Leiman G, Markowitz S, Margolius KA. Cytologic detection of cervical granuloma inguinale. *Diagn Cytopathol* 1986;2:138–143.
19. Robinson HM, Cohen MM. Treatment of granuloma inguinale with erythromycin. *J Invest Dermatol* 1953;20:407.
20. Sutherland JM. Fatal cardiovascular collapse of infants receiving large amounts of chloramphenicol. *Am J Dis Child* 1959;97:761.
21. Burns LE, Hodgman JE, Cass AB. Fatal circulatory collapse in premature infants receiving chloramphenicol. *New Engl J Med* 1959;261:1318.
22. Kessler DL, Smith AL, Woodrum DE. Chloramphenicol toxicity in a neonate treated with exchange transfusion. *J Pediatr* 1980;96:140.
23. Stevens DC, Kleiman MB, Lietman PS, et al. Exchange transfusion in acute chloramphenicol toxicity. *J Pediatr* 1981;99:651.
24. Mauer SM, Chavers BM, Kjellstrand CM. Treatment of an infant with severe chloramphenicol intoxication using charcoal column hemoperfusion. *J Pediatr* 1980;96:136.
25. Freundlich M, Cynamon H, Tamer A, et al. Management of chloramphenicol intoxication in infancy by charcoal hemoperfusion. *J Pediatr* 1983;103:4985.
26. Centers for Disease Control. Adverse reactions to Fansidar and update recommendations for its use in the prevention of malaria. *MMWR* 1985;33:713.
27. Leading article. Pyrimethamine combinations in pregnancy. *Lancet* 1983;2:1005–1007.
28. Yoshioka H, Monma T, Matsuda S. Placental transfer of gentamicin. *J Pediatr* 1972;80:121.
29. Merianos A, Gilles M, Chauah J. Ceftriaxone in the treatment of chronic donovanosis in central Australia. *Genitourin Med* 1996;70:84–89.
30. Bowden FJ, Mein J, Plunkett C, Bastian I. Pilot study of azithromycin in the treatment of genital donovanosis. *Genitourin Med* 1996;72:17–19.
31. Breschi LC, Goldman G, Shapiro SR. Granuloma inguinale in Viet Nam. Successful therapy with ampicillin and lincomycin. *J Am Vener Dis Assoc* 1975;1:118.
32. Salzman RS, Kraus SF, Miller RG, et al. Chancroidal ulcers that are not chancroid. Cause and epidemiology. *Arch Dermatol* 1984;120:636–639.
33. Sengupta BS. Vulvar carcinoma in premenopausal Jamaican women. *Int J Gynecol Obstet* 1980;17: 526.
34. Thew MA, Swift JT, Heaton CL. Ampicillin in the treatment of granuloma inguinale. *JAMA* 1969;210:866–867.
35. Chen CY, Mertz KJ, Spinda SM, et al. Comparison of enzyme immunoassays for antibodies to Haemophilus ducreyi in a community outbreak of chancroid in the United States. *Jour Infect Dis* 1997;175:1390–1395.
36. Sengupta BS. Vulval cancer following or co-existing with chronic granulomatous diseases of vulva. An analysis of its natural history, clinical manifestation and treatment. *Trop Doc* 1981;11:110–114.

6

Vaginal Microflora

INTRODUCTION

The vaginal ecosystem (VE) is a dynamic and complex biocommunity consisting of several distinct but interactive components. Some of the constituents function independently of one another, others act synergistically, and still others act antagonistically. One of the more complex components of the VE is the endogenous vaginal microflora, which consists of gram-positive and gram-negative aerobic, facultative, and obligate anaerobic bacteria (Table 6-1). The synergistic and antagonistic action between the endogenous vaginal microflora, in conjunction with other components of the VE, results in a balanced ecologic system commonly referred to as a healthy vaginal ecosystem (HVE). Any factor or condition that results in a shift in this balance or equilibrium results in an imbalance in the VE and an alteration in the vaginal microflora. In a balanced VE, the dominant bacterium is *Lactobacillus* (Fig. 6-1). Specifically, it is a *Lactobacillus* species, such as *Lactobacillus acidophilus, Lactobacillus casei, Lactobacillus crispatus,* and *Lactobacillus gasseri,* that produces a variety of organic acids including lactic acid, hydrogen peroxide (H_2O_2), and bacteriocin (1–4). The latter is a protein that inhibits the growth of other bacteria, including other species of *Lactobacillus*. The importance of maintaining a HVE is reflected not only in the maintenance of a healthy vagina but also in the general well being of either the obstetric or gynecologic patient. A disrupted or unhealthy VE can lead to localized conditions such as bacterial vaginosis (BV), an altered vaginal microflora (AVM) (e.g., colonization by *Streptococcus agalactiae* or *Escherichia coli*), vulvovaginal candidiasis (VVC), and upper genital tract infection leading to chorioamnionitis and/or postpartum endometritis in the pregnant patient and posthysterectomy pelvic infection (5–9).

There has been a tremendous effort put forth to report clinical observations of alterations in the vaginal microflora. Many investigators attempted to associate a relationship between an AVM and infections of the lower and upper genital tract. However, there is considerable confusion over some of these suggested relationships, mainly those centered on BV. The present discussion focuses on specific conditions of the AVM and their relationship to infections of the upper

TABLE 6-1. *Endogenous bacteria of the lower genital tract*

Facultative anaerobes	
Gram-positive	Gram-negative
Lactobacillus	Escherichia coli
Corynebacterium	Enterobacter aerogenes
Diphtheroids	Enterobacter agglomerans
Enterococcus faecalis	Enterobacter cloacae
α-hemolytic streptococci	Klebsiella pneumoniae
Staphylococcus aureus	Morganella morganii
Staphylococcus epidermidis	Proteus mirabilis
	Proteus vulgaris

Obligate anaerobes	
Gram-positive	Gram-negative
Eubacterium	Bacteroides fragilis
Peptococcus niger	Fusobacterium necrophorum
Peptostreptococcus anaerobius	Fusobacterium nucleatum
	Mobiluncus curticei
	Prevotella biviua
	Prevotella melaninogenica
	Veillonella

and lower genital tract. The intent of this chapter is to assist the reader in using current information to diagnose and manage various alterations in the vaginal microflora, and to ultimately restore the VE to a healthy state. Because sexually transmitted diseases (STDs) typically occur as infections originating in the lower genital tract and can be present with conditions such as an AVM, this discussion

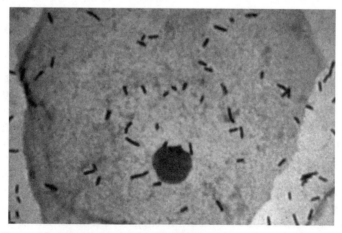

FIG. 6-1. Gram stain representation of a healthy vaginal ecosystem. Note: the squamous epithelia cell is well estrogenized, and the dominant bacterium is large gram-positive rods. There is a noticeable absence of other bacteria and white blood cells. (See Color Plate 6 following page 148.)

is included to enable physicians to thoroughly evaluate the lower genital tract and to understand that these conditions can coexist. It is important to understand the microbial physiology of the lower genital tract because alterations in the VE may mimic or mask concomitant infections, especially STDs.

MICROBIOLOGY OF THE VAGINA

The endogenous vaginal microflora is unique because in a healthy state it can assist the host defenses in warding off infection, such as STDs, postoperative infections, and chorioamnionitis. The concept of a VE is not unique, because other ecosystems occur at other sites in and on the body (e.g., skin, rectum, oral cavity, and large and small bowel). In addition to the bacterial array of genera and species present in the vagina that make up the endogenous vaginal microflora, from 8% to 68% of asymptomatic women are colonized by yeast; *Candida albicans* is the dominant genus and species (10,11). Although these reports describe a broad range of rates, the investigations conducted with good mycologic techniques yield isolation rates with asymptomatic women of 7.8%, 14.9%, and 25.9% (10,12). A well-designed study comparing the isolation rates of yeast from asymptomatic women with HVEs is needed to determine the rate of colonization. It would also be helpful to follow these women for 12 months to determine the number that develops symptomatic VVC. Although *Lactobacillus* plays a key role in maintaining a HVE, not all species have a beneficial effect. The key species of *Lactobacillus* that assist in maintaining a HVE (*L. acidophilus, L. crispatus, L. casei,* and *L. gasseri*) produce a variety of organic acids, including lactic acid, H_2O_2, and bacteriocin (13–15). Because *Lactobacillus* not only appears to be the dominant bacterium in a HVE but also plays a key role in maintaining the healthy state of the patient, factors that influence the growth of *Lactobacillus* ultimately determine the status of the VE.

Lactic acid, as well as other organic acids produced by *Lactobacillus,* plays an essential role in maintaining the pH at less than 4.5, which is unfavorable to the growth of many bacteria, especially the endogenous vaginal pathogenic microorganism (Table 6-2). Although *Lactobacillus* prefers a pH higher than 4.5 to achieve optimal growth, just as the other endogenous bacteria do, it has evolved and adapted to grow at lower pH levels (pH $\geq$ 3.5 to $\leq$ 4), although at much slower growth rates (Fig. 6-1). Thus, by controlling the hydrogen ion concentration in the environment, it can negatively affect growth of the pathogenic bacteria that are commonly found to inhabit the vagina. The ability to produce H_2O_2 is another mechanism that allows *Lactobacillus* to maintain dominance over the obligate anaerobic bacteria that lack the enzyme catalase (16,17). Hydrogen peroxide producing lactobacilli are dominant in the vagina of women with a HVE but not in women with bacterial vaginitis or vaginosis (1). The microflora that constitutes BV is mainly made of obligate anaerobic bacteria that lack catalase. However, the obligate anaerobic bacteria are not the sole organisms present. The facultative anaerobic bacteria, like *E. coli,* are also present although in lower numbers, as are gram-positive bacteria such as streptococci and enterococci.

TABLE 6-2. *Bacterial growth in response to pH of the environment*

pH ≤ 4

   Lactobacillus grows but at a slow rate.
   Other bacteria, especially the pathogenic bacteria, do not grow. If they do grow, their growth
   is not significant but does allow the organism to survive.

pH > 4 ≤ 4.5

   Competition begins between all bacteria present in the vagina, especially the facultative
   gram-negative bacteria and gram-positive bacteria, such as *Enterococcus faecalis* and
   Streptococcus agalactiae. The growth of these organisms, and especially *Gardnerella
   vaginalis,* results in a decrease in the hydrogen ion and oxygen concentrations, thus
   creating a more alkaline and anaerobic environment. The continued growth of *G.
   vaginalis* eventually results in the depletion of oxygen.

pH ≥ 5

   Lactobacillus begins losing its ability to compete with other bacteria when the pH is >4.5.
   When the pH is >5, the lactobacilli do not compete with other bacteria present, and their
   concentration decreases to <10^3 bacteria/mL of vaginal fluid. *G. vaginalis* and the
   obligate anaerobic bacteria gain dominance, and the concentration per bacterial species
   is ≥10^6 bacteria/mL of vaginal fluid. The gram-negative facultative bacteria are present,
   but their concentration is less than that of the obligate anaerobes and greater than the
   lactobacilli.

This is an important concept because treatment of BV can result in a shift toward allowing one or more of the nonobligate anaerobic bacteria to become dominant. Thus, treatment of BV can result in the patient developing *E. coli, Enterococcus,* or group B streptococcus (GBS) vaginitis. Therefore, in women with little or no hydrogen peroxide producing lactobacilli, the noncatalase-producing bacteria can easily overgrow the lactobacilli, thus establishing an AVM. Klebanoff postulated that vaginal bacteria capable of producing H_2O_2 directly or through the H_2O_2 peroxidase-halide system inhibited the growth of the pathogenic bacteria (2). The third defensive factor produced by the lactobacilli is bacteriocin, a low molecular weight protein that inhibits the growth of many bacteria especially other lactobacilli, *Gardnerella vaginalis, E. coli, Prevotella bivia,* and *Peptostreptococcus.*

All three of these mechanisms appear to function in an antagonistic manner enabling *Lactobacillus* to maintain dominance and, in turn, establish a HVE. In patients who have a HVE, *Lactobacillus* is present in a concentration of 10^6 or more bacteria/mL of vaginal fluid, whereas the pathogenic bacteria are present in a concentration of 10^3 or less bacteria/mL of vaginal fluid. The maintenance of this ratio of lactobacilli to other bacteria (greater than or equal to 1000:1) is extremely important because if the balance is altered, a change in vaginal flora can occur and any one or more of the bacteria can assume dominance. Disruption of the equilibrium of the VE can lead to the development of BV or dominance by other bacteria, such as *E. coli* or *S. agalactiae.* Dominance by *S. agalactiae* can result in a variety of significant infections. For example, any of the following conditions could occur in the pregnant patient: septic abortion, premature rupture of amniotic membranes, chorioamnionitis, and postpartum endometritis. In the patient with chronic illness, *S. agalactiae* can cause significant morbidity and mortality (18). The patient whose vaginal microflora is dominated by *S. agalactiae* can be either asymptomatic, as is commonly seen in the obstetric and gynecologic patient, or symptomatic complaining of vaginal "soreness" or burning or swelling of the labia and increased discharge. Evaluation of the vagina of a patient whose vaginal microflora is dominated by *S. agalactiae* can be confirmed by a vaginal pH 5 or greater, a negative whiff test, and the observation of cocci as well as the absence of both large bacillary forms and clue cells when the vaginal discharge is examined microscopically. If a variety of bacteria gain dominance the patient can develop BV. In situations in which combinations of bacteria become dominant, the healthy patient can be placed in "harm's way," especially if she is the recipient of an invasive gynecologic procedure, such as transvaginal and transcervical artificial insemination, hysterosalpingography, or hysterectomy. Combinations such as *P. bivia* and *Enterococcus faecalis,* and *P. bivia* and *E. coli* are abscessogenic (19). Therefore, if these bacteria become dominant, are each present in a concentration of 10^6 or greater, and gain entrance to the upper genital tract, there is the potential for serious infection to occur. Physicians must be aware of the two contributing factors that they can encounter when performing invasive procedures of the upper genital tract via transgressing the vagina and cervix. The potential for introducing a large inoculum into the upper genital tract is significant considering the large number of bacteria present when an AVM exists. Another factor to consider is the trauma induced in the upper genital tract. Thus, the ratio of *Lactobacillus* to pathogenic bacteria ($\geq$ 1000:1) becomes reversed (1:$\geq$ 1000) (lactobacilli/pathogenic bacteria). Therefore, there is a significant increase in the inoculum size of the pathogenic bacteria. In conditions in which the inoculum size of virulent bacteria is 10^6 CFU/mL or greater, if the bacteria gain entrance to the upper genital tract, the threat of infection becomes significant. It is extremely important for all physicians who render care to women, especially those who perform invasive procedures of the upper genital tract via the vagina and cervix, to be very cognizant of the characteristics that constitute both a healthy and a disrupted VE.

The characteristics of a HVE are (Fig. 6-1) as follows:

A white to slate-gray discharge
The absence of vaginal odor
The consistency of the discharge may be liquid to pasty
The pH is 3.8 to 4.2
The presence of estrogenized squamous epithelial cells
The gross architecture of the squamous epithelial cells can be easily seen microscopically
White blood cells (WBCs) are rarely seen microscopically, usually less than 4/hpf
Large bacilli are the dominant bacterial morphotype, presumably *Lactobacillus*

A pH between 4.2 and 4.5 may indicate that the balance of the VE is being threatened, and the balanced environment is tenuous at best where a shift to imbalance can easily occur. In a situation where the vaginal pH is more than 4 but less than or equal to 4.5, microscopic analysis may reveal a noticeable scarcity of bacillary forms (lactobacilli), as well as the absence of other bacteria, or the presence of one or more bacterial morphotype. Determining the vaginal pH and performing a microscopic examination of the vaginal discharge is extremely important when evaluating patients complaining of vaginal discomfort. This evaluation is not difficult to do, does not require sophisticated equipment, is inexpensive to perform, and is not time-consuming. The finding of a pH less than 5 does not, in itself, establish that the VE is in a healthy state. The patient with a pH 4.5 or less may have a heavy colonization of yeast. Patients may also have a vaginal pH 4.5 or higher but have a vaginal flora dominated by *E. coli, S. agalactiae,* or another bacterium. These patients also have a negative potassium hydroxide (KOH) (whiff) test. The microscopic analysis performed under these circumstances may assist in ruling out the presence of vaginal candidiasis or trichomoniasis. One may also observe the early development of BV with a flora dominated by *G. vaginalis.* This can be inferred by noting the presence of clue cells, aggregates of free-floating gram-negative bacteria, and the absence of a morphologically diverse population of individual gram-negative and gram-positive bacteria floating freely in the vaginal fluid. Recognizing the presence of an abnormality that is not an infectious condition but rather a disrupted state of the vaginal microflora and differentiating between BV and a unibacterial AVM, like *E. coli* or GBS, may be very helpful in restoring the VM and ecosystem to a healthy state. This can reduce the indiscriminate use of antibiotics that can facilitate driving the already disrupted vaginal flora to further disruption.

THE ALTERED VAGINAL MICROFLORA

The concept of an AVM provides insight into the microbial pathophysiology leading to pelvic infections but does not explain how the alterations in the VE occur. Many pelvic infections give the allusion that they developed spontaneously. Postoperative pelvic infection can develop following major and minor invasive procedures conducted under sterile conditions. This is often both frustrating and perplexing to the physician because a review of the case does not provide an answer as to why or how the infection developed. There is also the belief that the patient became infected because of a break in sterile technique, which is often erroneous. These infections are usually mild but can be very serious, resulting in significant morbidity to the patient. The overwhelming majority of postoperative pelvic infections are derived from the patient's own vaginal microflora. Many, if not most, of these patients receive prophylactic antibiotics, and yet 5% to 20% will develop infection. If the patient has an associated STD (like *Neisseria gonorrhoeae* or *Chlamydia trachomatis*), the presence of leukorrhea, increased vascularity, and cytokine response will increase the potential for more virulent bacteria to gain a foothold in initiating a soft tissue pelvic infection. Available data have demonstrated that alterations in the vaginal microflora can lead to acquisition and transmission of human immunodeficiency virus (HIV) and other STDs (20). Women with BV exposed to HIV-infected sexual partners are more likely to acquire the virus then women without BV (21–23). Conditions that give rise to an AVM and cervicitis have been associated with increased shedding of HIV in the female genital tract (24). Bacteria such as *Peptostreptococcus asaccharolyticus* and *P. bivia* were shown to stimulate HIV expression in monocytoid cells (25). These same investigators found that *Bacteroides ureolyticus, Peptostreptococcus anaerobius,* and *L. acidophilus* did not stimulate or enhance HIV expression.

Therefore, the physician must be very aware of the status of the VE and pay particular attention to the vaginal microflora. Determining the vaginal pH and microscopically examining the vaginal discharge can ascertain the general characteristics of the vaginal microflora. Many have advocated using molecular techniques to determine what is and what is not in the vagina with regard to organisms. Highly specific tests such as the polymerase chain reaction (PCR) assays can detect fragments of pathogenic bacteria deoxyribonucleic acid (DNA); however, this would not necessarily be the bacterium responsible for the infections. The results of such assays are not immediately known and are costly. A rapid office test to evaluate vaginal discharge called the Fem Exam is available. This is a colorimetric test that uses a card the size of a credit card. There are two wells on the card, one for determining pH and the other for the presence of amines (whiff tests). However, using this card can often lead physicians astray. A patient may have a vaginal pH greater than 5 with a negative amine test. If a wet mount is not done the physician will not know the nature of the alteration in the vaginal microflora. Suppose the patient has a pH less than 5 and a negative amine test but is symptomatic? Microscopic examination of the discharge is still necessary. A third scenario could be that the patient's vaginal pH is greater than 5 and amines are positive. If nothing further is done, like a wet mount, an inflammatory condition may go unnoticed, and the patient will not be evaluated for possible STD. Therefore, at the present time, there is no rapid test (like determining pH and examining the vaginal discharge microscopically) that can take the place of performing the classic evaluation of vaginal discharge.

Although office evaluations using pH paper, a whiff test, and the microscope are not as sensitive or as specific as PCR analysis, they are rapid (taking less than 5 minutes) and inexpensive and the necessary information is quickly ascertained. Simple office tests such as determining the vaginal pH and microscopic analysis of the vaginal discharge will yield significant information such as the acidity of the vagina and the bacterial makeup of the endogenous microflora. A pH 5 or greater immediately informs the physician that there is a high probability that the vaginal microflora is altered. Microscopic examination can reveal either the presence of one dominant bacterium or the presence of more than one morphologic bacterium. In addition, microscopic examination of the vaginal discharge can reveal the presence of inflammation, that is, the presence of WBCs indicating the possible existence of infection. Specimens obtained from the vagina should be taken when the microscopic analysis reveals the absence of *Lactobacillus* and BV, as well as the presence of a single dominant morphotype such as cocci. If there is a purulent discharge the examiner should look for *Trichomonas vaginalis,* perhaps even culture for it, and culture the endocervix for *N. gonorrhoeae* and *C. trachomatis.* It does not benefit the physician or the patient to obtain vaginal microbiology only to receive information such as normal vaginal flora or lactobacilli present. There is also no benefit in performing vaginal cultures for patients with BV.

Figure 6-2 depicts a sample scheme in the evaluation of a patient suspected of having vaginitis or an AVM. If there are a significant number of WBCs present in the vaginal discharge (WBCs greater than 5 cells/hpf) and no vaginal pathogens present (e.g., trichomonads), then the patient should be evaluated for cervicitis. The endocervical discharge should be examined for the presence of mucopus, and the endocervical canal should be sampled for the detection of *N. gonorrhoeae* and *C. trachomatis.*

AVM is a general term describing a disruption in the vaginal flora in which *Lactobacillus* has lost dominance. It should not be confused with the term BV. It can encompass BV but is not restricted to it; therefore, the two are synonymous but not equal. The evolution from a healthy vaginal microflora to an AVM can result in either BV or a bacterial vaginitis dominated by GBS, *E. coli,* or any bacterium including *Lactobacillus. Lactobacillus,* although not a virulent organism, can cause significant infection in both healthy patients and those patients with chronic illness. Cox et al. (26) reported *Lactobacillus* chorioamnionitis and bacteremia, as well as vertical transmission resulting in neonatal bacteremia in healthy pregnant women. *Lactobacillus* has also been the etiologic agent causing dental disease, infective endocarditis, urinary tract infections, chorioamnionitis, endometritis meningitis, intraabdominal abscess, liver abscess, splenic abscess, and bacteremia (27–31). It is not understood how this evolution from a *Lactobacillus*-dominant flora to a microflora dominated by one or more other bacteria occurs. In the evolution of BV it appears that *G. vaginalis,* or perhaps another bacterium, is able to overcome the suppressive effect of *Lactobacillus* initiating a shift in the microflora even though the initiating event is not known. However, once the balance is tipped and favors the growth of *G. vaginalis* a cascade of events occurs, resulting in a rise in pH with a simultaneous decrease in the oxygen concentration. There is a period when *G. vaginalis* assumes dominance and lactobacilli growth continues to decline reaching very low levels (10^3 or less bacteria/mL of vaginal fluid). If for some reason the cascade of events is inhibited, the vaginal microflora can achieve a state in which *G. vaginalis* maintains dominance but this probably rarely occurs. The continued growth of *G. vaginalis* results in a pH greater than 5, and the eventual estab-

---

FIG. 6-2. Algorithm for the evaluation and management of altered vaginal microflora. ˙Culture vagina [e.g., *Escherichia coli* or group B streptococcus (GBS) dominance]. ¨Culture vagina and cervix for STD.

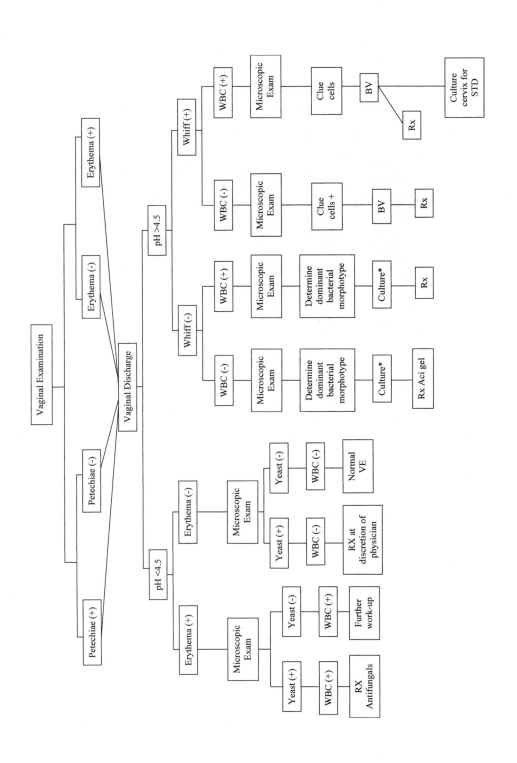

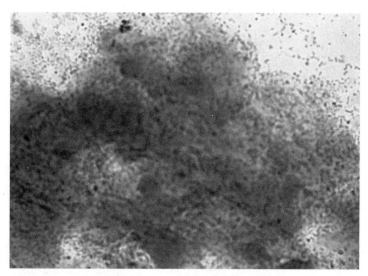

FIG 6-3. Gram stain of vaginal discharge: clue cells. Note: the squamous epithelial cells are obliterated by densely adhering gram-negative rods (*Gardnerella vaginalis*). There are numerous individual free-floating bacteria in the vaginal discharge. There is a noticeable absence of white blood cells. (See Color Plate 7 following page 148.)

lishment of an anaerobic environment. This permits the growth of various obligate anaerobic bacteria (Fig. 6-3).

There are eight different biotypes of *G. vaginalis,* and some are resistant to the bacteriocin produced by *Lactobacillus* (32–35). It is possible that if the growth of a resistant *G. vaginalis* strain gains a foothold it can overcome the suppressive effects of bacteriocin produced by the endogenous strains of *Lactobacillus. G. vaginalis* produces catalase, is not affected by the H_2O_2 that is produced by *Lactobacillus,* and can compete well for nutrients. *G. vaginalis* can outgrow *Lactobacillus* and gain dominance. This is a possible mechanism for transition from a healthy vaginal microflora to one that is dominated by pathogenic bacteria.

Obstetric and gynecologic patients are at risk for a variety of infections if their vaginal microflora becomes altered and dominated by one or more pathogenic bacteria. The obstetric patient with an AVM is at risk for premature labor, premature rupture of amniotic membranes, septic abortion, cystitis, pyelonephritis, and postpartum endometritis. Any one of these infections can potentially place the patient in septic shock and significantly increase the seriousness of the infection that can result in death. The issue concerning the relationship between BV and premature labor and delivery has not been decided. There have been two randomized double-blinded studies comparing metronidazole with placebo for the treatment of BV in pregnancy to determine if the prematurity rate can be reduced. Unfortunately, these studies did not show a significant reduction in the prematurity rate for the treated patients compared with the untreated group (36,37).

BACTERIAL VAGINOSIS

BV has received a great deal of attention over the last 10 years, but it is still somewhat of an enigma because the microbiology of this AVM is not very well understood. The discussions concerning the terminology are important, but their relationship to the clinical significance of BV is not particularly relevant. This is because the terminology does not influence either the understanding or treatment of BV. Discussions concerning the nomenclature of this condition (i.e., should it be BV, vaginal bacteriosis, or simply referred to as an AVM) have not produced any clarification in our understanding of the microbiology of the lower genital tract. There is a significant lack of information regarding the microbial physiology of the vaginal microbiology and how it relates to infectious diseases and to the healthy state of the genital tract. The one fact that all can agree on is that this condition, BV, is an altered state of the vaginal microflora and it is characterized by an overgrowth of bacteria dominated by mainly obligate anaerobic bacteria.

BV can be clinically characterized by (a) well-estrogenized squamous epithelial cells, (b) adherent bacteria densely covering many of the squamous epithelial cells, (c) lack of *Lactobacillus* dominance, (d) the dominance of a variety of bacterial genera and species, (e) obligate anaerobic bacteria that outnumber facultative bacteria, (f) a preponderance of bacteria that are pathogenic and extremely virulent, (g) a fish-like odor emanating from the vagina, and (h) a noticeable absence of WBCs (Fig. 6-3). Thus, BV is not an infection; it is an alteration in the endogenous microflora of the VE. BV does not insight an inflammatory response, hence the absence of WBCs. However, the bacteria that constitute BV can cause infection given the appropriate environment. Therefore, it must be recognized that patients with BV are potentially at risk for developing infection if (a) immunosuppressed, (b) an inoculum is introduced into an area of the body not commonly exposed to a significant number of bacteria, and (c) subjected to trauma (surgery) that creates an environment conducive to the growth of bacteria.

Statistically, BV has been associated with many infectious conditions involving the female genital tract. However, the strongest association has been the development of postoperative pelvic infection following obstetric and gynecologic surgery. There also appears to be a significant association between BV and the risk of acquiring a STD, including HIV (38,39); however, the relationship between BV and pelvic inflammatory disease (PID) needs further clarification. There have been several studies linking BV and PID, but one study did not find a relationship between BV and acute gonococcal PID (40–43). In addition, the association between BV and preterm labor remains controversial. Two randomized double-blind studies, one published in 1997 and the other in 2000, failed to show any association between the treatment of BV with metronidazole and a reduction in preterm labor (36,37). However, these studies did not attempt to determine if there was a cause and effect relationship between BV and preterm labor. Instead, these studies focused on treatment.

MICROBIOLOGY OF BV

BV, like all alterations in the vaginal microflora, evolves from a healthy vaginal microflora. The initiating factors that cause changes in the VE and influence the growth of the microbial component are unknown. When dominant *Lactobacillus* is antagonistic toward *Gardnerella,* and when the latter bacterium is stimulated to grow, it causes a change in the pH of the vaginal environment and a decrease in the oxygen concentration. Although *Lactobacillus* prefers a pH of 5 or greater, it apparently is not a good competitor and its growth is inhibited (Fig. 6-4) by the growth of *Gardnerella.* The continued growth of *Gardnerella* results in the vaginal pH rising to greater than 5 and the environment becoming anaerobic by depleting oxygen. Because these conditions favor the growth of obligate anaerobes, they become the dominant microbes in the VE. Interestingly, the facultative anaerobic bacteria switch metabolism from aerobic to anaerobic and continue to grow. This creates a complex microbial environment. It can be hypothesized that the facultative anaerobes, even though they are present in smaller numbers, may very well be the initiators of infection. This is likely caused by their ability to reproduce more rapidly than obligate anaerobes. Once gaining entrance to a site destined to become infected, they create an anaerobic environment permitting growth of the obligate anaerobes, thus giving rise to polymicrobial infections. This hypothesis is supported by analyzing the postpartum endometritis that develops within 24 to 48 hours of delivery. Postpartum endometritis tends to be unimicrobial mainly because of GBS *and E. coli,* whereas an infection that manifests for more than 48 hours is polymicrobial and involves facultative and obligate anaerobes. Therefore, once an abnormal vaginal microbiology or AVM is established, it is difficult to restore the endogenous

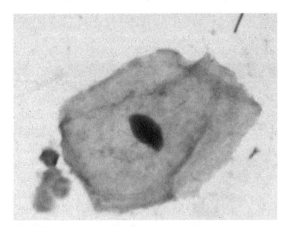

FIG. 6-4. Gram stain of vaginal discharge following treatment of a patient with bacterial vaginosis. Note the following: (a) clue cells are absent, (b) a well-estrogenized squamous epithelial cell without adherent bacteria is present, (c) two white blood cells are present, and (d) the dominant bacteria are large gram-positive bacilli consistent with *Lactobacillus.* (See Color Plate 8 following page 148.)

vaginal microflora to a *Lactobacillus*-dominant microflora. Many studies examining treatment regimens, mainly metronidazole and clindamycin, note that neither has been very successful. This is likely because most physicians approach an AVM as an infection when it is often not an infection.

PREVENTION AND TREATMENT

The best defense against BV or any AVM is prevention, and this begins with screening. Women presenting for any gynecologic problem or annual examination should have an evaluation of the VE. The VE can be viewed as a window not only to the vaginal health but also to the general health of the patient. This is not unlike examining the oral cavity and gums for signs of periodontal disease. Recognizing early signs of the vaginal flora shifting from a *Lactobacillus*-dominant flora to an altered state affects both the vaginal health and, potentially, the general health of the patient. For example, obstetric and gynecologic patients are at a greater risk for postoperative infection and acquisition of STDs. This is especially important if the patient is scheduled to have a procedure involving the upper genital tract via the lower genital tract.

Treatment is focused on the use of clindamycin vaginal cream or ovules, metronidazole vaginal gel, or oral metronidazole. However, treatment with oral and intravaginal preparations has not been especially rewarding. The restoration of a healthy vaginal microflora or "cure" rate was approximately 68.1% in patients treated with clindamycin ovules for 3 days compared with 66.7% in patients treated with 7 days of oral metronidazole 500 mg given twice daily (43). Intravaginal metronidazole has not proven any more efficacious than clindamycin cream or oral metronidazole (43).

Treatment of BV should be directed at restoring the VE to a healthy state not at the eradication of a bacterium or bacteria. The relatively poor response to current therapy is compounded by the failure to reexamine the patient following a course of therapy to determine if the pH level has returned to less than 4.5 and if the lactobacilli have assumed the position of dominance (Fig. 6-1). Currently, there is no treatment that is truly satisfactory.

If pH is a significant factor, and currently available microbiologic data strongly indicates that the hydrogen ion concentration does affect the growth of bacteria in the vagina, then treatment regimens should include mechanisms or agents to alter the pH. Because BV and other AVM are not infections, one cannot achieve a cure. As mentioned, when treating these conditions, one does not try to eradicate a bacterium or bacteria, as is the goal in treatment of a true infection. Treatment of an AVM will have an impact on the total microflora of the vagina. Studies have shown that patients treated for AVM with various antibiotics did not significantly alter the *Lactobacillus* content of the vagina over the short term.

Patients should be reevaluated following completion of therapy; that is, the vaginal pH and microscopic analysis of the vaginal discharge should be conducted. The goal is to restore the pH between 3.8 and 4.2, and the dominant bacterial morphotype should be large bacillary forms. Squamous cells should be well estrogenized, no bacteria should be adherent to the squamous epithelial cells, and there should be no or few (5 cells/hpf or less) WBCs present (Fig. 6-1). Following treatment, the pH may be 5 or greater, but the bacteriology has shifted, *Lactobacillus* did not achieve dominance, and there may be a scarcity of bacteria (Fig. 6-4). To determine the dominant bacterium, a culture must be done.

SUMMARY

The purpose of discussing the vaginal microflora is to emphasize that an AVM is more likely to occur in women who are sexually active. An AVM in a sexually active woman can be a clue to the presence of a STD. The presence of WBCs in the vaginal discharge should encourage the physician to seek causes of inflammation because cervical infection is likely to be present. Obtaining a detailed sexual history can assist in determining the patient's level of risk for being exposed to a STD and the likelihood that the patient may indeed be infected.

REFERENCES

1. Eschenbach DA, Davick PR, Williams BL, et al. Prevalence of hydrogen peroxide-producing *Lactobacillus* species in normal women and women with bacterial vaginosis. *J Clin Microbiol* 1989;27: 251–256.
2. Klebanoff SJ, Hillier SL, Eschenbach DA, et al. Control of the microbial flora of the vagina by H_2O_2-generating lactobacilli. *J Infect Dis* 1991;164:94–100.
3. Skarin A, Sylwan J. Vaginal lactobacilli inhibiting growth of *Gardnerella vaginalis, Mobiluncus* and other bacterial species cultured from vaginal content of women with bacterial vaginosis. *Acta Path Microb Immuno Scand Sect B* 1986;94:399–403.
4. Aroutcheva A, Simoes JA, Faro S. Antimicrobial protein produced by vaginal *Lactobacillus* species, recovery and purification. *Infect Dis Obstet Gynecol* 2000;8:202(abst).
5. Korn AP, Bolan G, Padian N, et al. Plasma cell endometritis in women with symptomatic bacterial vaginosis. *Obstet Gynecol* 1995;85:387–390.
6. Silver HM, Sperling RS, St. Clair PJ, et al. Evidence relating bacterial vaginosis to intra-amniotic infection. *Am J Obstet Gynecol* 1989;161:808–812.
7. Watts DH, Eschenbach DA, Kenny GE. Early postpartum endometritis: the role of bacteria, genital mycoplasma, and *Chlamydia trachomatis*. *Obstet Gynecol* 1989;73:52–60.
8. Soper DE, Bump RC, Hurt WG. Bacterial vaginosis and trichomoniasis vaginitis are risk factors for cuff cellulitis after abdominal hysterectomy. *Am J Obstet Gynecol* 1990;163:1016–1023.
9. Lin L, Song J, Kimber N, et al. The role of bacterial vaginosis in infection after major gynecologic surgery. *Infect Dis Obstet Gynecol* 1999;7:169–174.
10. Timonen S, Salo OP, Meyer B, et al. Vaginal mycosis. *Acta Obstet Gynaecol Scand* 1966;45:232–247.
11. Daus AD, Hafez ES. *Candida albicans* in women. *Nurs Res* 1975;24:430–433.
12. Oriel JD, Partridge BM, Denny MJ, et al. Genital yeast infections. *Br Med J* 1972;4:761–764.
13. Redondo-Lopez V, Cook RL, Sobel JD. Emerging role of lactobacilli in the control and maintenance of the vaginal bacterial microflora. *Rev Inf Dis* 1990;12:856–872.
14. Mardh PA, Soltesz LV. In vitro interactions between lactobacilli and other microorganisms occurring in the vaginal flora. *Scand J Infect Dis* 1983;40:47–51.
15. Mehta AM, Patel KA, Dave PJ. Purification and properties of the inhibitory protein isolated from *Lactobacillus acidophilus* AC1. *Microbios* 1983;38:73–81.
16. Hillier SH, Krohn MA, Klebanoff SJ, et al. The relationship of hydrogen peroxide-producing lactobacilli to bacterial vaginosis and genital microflora in pregnant women. *Obstet Gynecol* 1992;79: 369–373.
17. Whittenburg R. Hydrogen peroxide formation and catalase activity in the lactic acid bacteria. *J Gen Microbiol* 1964;35:13–26.

18. Tyrrell GJ, Senzilet LD, Spika JS, et al. Invasive disease due to group B streptococcal infection in adults: results from a Canadian, population-based, active laboratory surveillance study—1996. Sentinel Health Unit Surveillance System Site Coordinators. *J Infect Dis* 2000;182:168–173.

19. Husni RN, Gordon SM, Washington JA, et al. *Lactobacillus* bacteremia and endocarditis: review of 45 cases. *Clin Infect Dis* 1997;25:1048–1055.

20. van De Wijgert JH, Mason PR, Gwanzura L, et al. Intravaginal practices, vaginal flora disturbances, and acquisition of sexually transmitted diseases in Zimbabwean women. *J Infect Dis* 2000;181: 587–594.

21. Taha TE, Hoover DR, Dallabetta GA, et al. Bacterial vaginosis and disturbances of vaginal flora: association with increased acquisition of HIV. *AIDS* 1998;12:699–706.

22. Sewankambo N, Gray RH, Wawer MJ, et al. HIV-1 infection associated with abnormal vaginal flora morphology and bacterial vaginosis. *Lancet* 1997;350:546–550.

23. Cohen CR, Duerr A, Pruithithada N, et al. Bacterial vaginosis and HIV seroprevalence among female commercial sex workers in Chiang Mai, Thailand. *AIDS* 1995;9:1093–1097.

24. Mostad SB, Kreiss JK. Shedding of HIV-1 in the genital tract. *AIDS* 1996;10:1305–1315.

25. Hashemi FB, Ghassemi M, Faro S, et al. Induction of human immunodeficiency virus type 1 expression by anaerobes associated with bacterial vaginosis. *J Infect Dis* 2000;181:1574–1580.

26. Cox SM, Phillips LE, Mercer LJ, et al. Lactobacillemia of amniotic fluid origin. *Obstet Gynecol* 1986;68:134–135.

27. Dickgiesser U, Weiss N, Fritsche D. *Lactobacillus gasseri* as the cause of septic urinary infection. *Infection* 1984;12:14–16.

28. Digamon-Beltran M, Feigman T, Klein SA, et al. Lactobacillemia in pregnancy. *South Med J* 1985; 78:1138–1139.

29. Sherman ME, Albrecht M, DeGirolami PC, et al. An unusual case of splenic abscess and sepsis in an immunocompromised host. *Am J Clin Pathol* 1987;88:659–662.

30. Andriessen MP, Mulder JG, Sleijfer DT. Lactobacillus septicemia an unusual complication during the treatment of metastatic choriocarcinoma. *Gynecol Oncol* 1991;40:87–89.

31. Ingianni A, Petruzzelli S, Morandotti G, et al. Genotypic differentiation of *Gardnerella vaginalis* by amplified ribosomal DNA restriction analysis (ARDRA). *FEMS Immunol Med Microbiol* 1997;18: 61–66.

32. Piot P, Van Dyck E, Peeters M, et al. Biotypes of *Gardnerella vaginalis*. *J Clin Microbiol* 1984;20: 677–679.

33. Nath K, Choi DJ, Devlin D. The characterization of *Gardnerella vaginalis* DNA using non-radioactive DNA probes. *Res Microbiol* 1991;142:573–583.

34. Cohen CR, Duerr A, Pruithithada N, et al. Bacterial vaginosis and HIV seroprevalence among female commercial sex workers in Chiang Mai, Thailand. *AIDS* 1995;9:1093–1097.

35. McLean NW, McGroarty JA. Growth inhibition of metronidazole-susceptible and metronidazole-resistant strains of *Gardnerella vaginalis* by lactobacilli in vitro. *Appl Environ Microbiol* 1996;62: 1089–1092.

36. McDonald HM, O'Loughlin JA, Vigneswaran R, et al. Impact of metronidazole therapy on preterm birth in women with bacterial vaginosis flora (*Gardnerella vaginalis*): a randomised, placebo-controlled trial. *Br J Obstet Gynaecol* 1997;104:1391–1397.

37. Carey JC, Klebanoff MA, Hauth JC, et al. Metronidazole to prevent preterm delivery in pregnant women with asymptomatic bacterial vaginosis. NICHHD Network of Maternal-Fetal Medicine Units. *N Engl J Med* 2000;342:534–540.

38. Martin HL, Richardson BA, Nyange PM, et al. Vaginal lactobacilli, microbial flora, and risk of human immunodeficiency virus type I and sexually transmitted disease acquisition. *J Infect Dis* 1999; 180:1863–1868.

39. Behets FM, Williams Y, Brathwaite A, et al. Management of vaginal discharge in women treated at a Jamaican sexually transmitted disease clinic: use of diagnostic algorithms versus laboratory testing. *Clin Infect Dis* 1995;21:1450–1455.

40. Faro S, Martens M, Maccato M, et al. Vaginal flora and pelvic inflammatory disease. *Am J Obstet Gynecol* 1993;169:470–474.

41. Barbone F, Austin W, Louv WC, et al. A follow-up study of methods of contraception, sexual activity, and rates of trichomoniasis, candidiasis, and bacterial vaginosis. *Am J Obstet Gynecol* 1990;163: 510–514.

42. Berger BJ, Kolton S, Zenilman JM, et al. Bacterial vaginosis in lesbians: a sexually transmitted disease. *Clin Infect Dis* 1995;21:1402–1405.

43. Paavonen J, Mangioni C, Martin MA, et al. Vaginal clindamycin and oral metronidazole for bacterial vaginosis: a randomized trial. *Obstet Gynecol* 2000;96:256–260.

7

Trichomonas

INTRODUCTION

Donne, in 1836, was the first investigator to describe the protozoan *Trichomonas vaginalis*. Hohne, in 1936, demonstrated a relationship between the presence of *T. vaginalis* and the development of symptoms localized to the vagina. Hohne also described the association of trichomoniasis with an increase in vaginal discharge. Trussell and Plass (1), in 1940, were able to fulfill Koch's postulates by inoculating vaginas of healthy volunteers with pure cultures of *T. vaginalis* and establishing acute symptomatic vaginitis. In 1947, Trussell (2) published a monograph on *T. vaginalis* describing the extent of this infection in the lower genital tract. Subsequent to the work of Trussell, *T. vaginalis* has been the subject of intense study because of the related infectious complications associated with vaginal trichomoniasis. Although effective antimicrobial therapy (metronidazole) was developed and continues to be effective, urogenital trichomoniasis continues to be one of the world's most prevalent sexually transmitted diseases (STD). This, in part, is because of patients developing persistent and chronic infection, an allergy to metronidazole, and the emergence of *T. vaginalis* strains resistant to metronidazole. Trichomonads that parasitize humans are unique in that each species occupies a specific anatomic site in the host. Each species has evolved a distinctive structure, function, and relationship to the host. Pregnancy, for example, appears to favor the growth of *T. vaginalis* and is associated with an increase in symptoms. However, the reason for the increase in symptomatic trichomonas infection in the pregnant patient has not yet been elucidated. Thus, *T. vaginalis,* although recognized for many decades, continues to be surrounded by many perplexing problems such as the life cycle of the organism, including the pathophysiology of symptomatic and asymptomatic infection. One area that is not fully understood is the interaction of *T. vaginalis* with other microbes in regard to the basis of the infectious process, as well as the protozoan's possible relationship to other serious pelvic infections [e.g., pelvic inflammatory disease (PID), infertility, premature labor, premature rupture of amniotic membranes, and postoperative pelvic cellulitis]. Although vaginitis is probably the most common problem that patients seek medical treatment for, the incidence of trichomoniasis has decreased in the United States and Scandinavia since 1976 (3).

MICROBIOLOGY

There are five known species, all members of the order Trichomonadida and the family Trichomonadidae. The species are *Trichomonas tenax, T. vaginalis, Trichomonas fecalis, Pentatrichomonas,* and *Dientamoebafragilis.* The latter two organisms actually belong to the subfamily Dientamoebae of the family Monocercomonadidae (4). The present discussion focuses on the most common species encountered in the obstetric and gynecologic patient, *T. vaginalis.*

The morphology of the urogenital trichomonad is dependent on the physiologic condition of the anatomic site that is infected. The pH, temperature, oxygen concentration and ionic concentrations of the microenvironment, and the vaginal ecosystem are all important in determining the structural configuration of the organism. It is important to understand that the vaginal ecosystem exists in a delicate dynamic equilibrium. This microecosystem is very complex and is not regulated by the host or the metabolic products released into the environment. The interaction between microbes, as well as the host, plays a role in either the maintenance or disruption of this ecosystem. In addition to the endogenous microflora, there are exogenous factors such as microorganisms and chemical and sexual activity that also play a role in determining the state of this microecosystem.

Typically, *T. vaginalis* has four anteriorly located flagella, which can easily be seen when examining the organism isolated from culture or from vaginal discharge (Fig. 7-1). The nucleus is located in the anterior portion of the cell. An

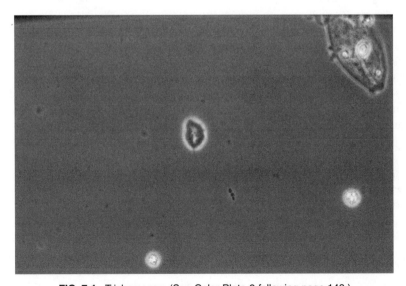

FIG. 7-1. Trichomonas. (See Color Plate 9 following page 148.)

undulating membrane extends from the anterior portion of the protozoan and is attached to the body for a distance equal to ½ to ⅔ of the organism's body length.

Eight serotypes of *T. vaginalis* have been identified (5). Although strains possess both unshared and shared antigens, these antigens are not associated with pathogenicity (6,7). Because *T. vaginalis* is a parasite of mucosal surfaces, IgA is of considerable importance. IgA does not function to initiate complement-mediated cytotoxicity. Therefore, it would not be expected that this antibody would exhibit a lethal effect on this organism. Sufficient studies in this area have not been conducted to determine the effect of IgA on trichomonads. Direct killing of *T. vaginalis* has been accomplished by polymorphonuclear neutrophils (8). The process is dependent on the oxygen concentration and activation of a complement but not a specific antibody. It has been demonstrated that activation of the alternate pathway stimulates production of C3b. The C3b fragment binds to the parasite, which in turn allows the polymorphonuclear leukocytes to bind to the C3b sites via their receptors (9,10). Although the presence of trichomonads in the vagina can stimulate antibody production, it does not confer immunity to the individual. This is readily seen in clinical practice, because it is common to find patients who have recurrent infection.

T. vaginalis, when present in the human host, must exist in a relationship with the endogenous vaginal microflora and establish a new ecosystem that ensures the protozoan's survival. It is generally accepted that 25% to 50% of women with trichomoniasis are asymptomatic. Therefore, the protozoan must develop a synergistic or, perhaps, commensal relationship when in the asymptomatic state and its number must be kept below a threshold that will initiate symptomatic infection. When the latter state is achieved or created, the trichomonads have entered an antagonistic relationship with other inhabitants of the vaginal ecosystem. Bacteria are the dominant microbial inhabitants of the vaginal ecosystem, with lactobacilli being the dominant bacterium. In a healthy vaginal ecosystem, the nonpathogenic bacteria exist in a harmonious state with one another, and they are antagonistic to the pathogenic bacteria. These relationships allow the nonpathogenic bacteria to dominate and suppress the growth of the pathogenic bacteria. It is this physiologic state that prevents the potentially pathogenic bacteria from adhering to the epithelial cells, along with a healthy functioning localized immunologic system, thus preventing initiation and the eventual establishment of an infectious process. Although the pathogens are always present in the vaginal ecosystem, their numbers are kept low and their growth suppressed; thus they are neither able to produce toxins in a significant concentration nor able to alter the environment of the ecosystem to favor their growth and inhibit the growth of lactobacilli.

Successful colonization of the lower genital tract by protozoans, such as *T. vaginalis,* and bacteria is dependent on several conditions being present within the ecosystem. Most microorganisms prefer an environmental temperature of 37°C but will tolerate a range of temperatures that permit them to maintain dominance. Some microorganisms have the ability to adapt to marked variations in temperature by producing structures that are resistant to extremes in temperatures, such as spores or capsules. The temperature of the vagina does not vary greatly when a patient is healthy but can vary when the patient develops an increase in body temperature. However, there have not been any studies regarding possible changes in the microflora when there are significant changes in temperature.

In a healthy state, *Lactobacillus acidophilus,* or other species of lactobacilli produce lactic acid, hydrogen peroxide, and bacteriocin or lactocin (a protein that inhibits the growth of bacteria). *L. acidophilus* maintains dominance and the stability of the vaginal ecosystem by secreting lactic acid, which maintains the pH of the environment between 3.8 and 4.2. This acid concentration is not favorable to either the growth of the pathogenic bacteria or *T. vaginalis.* The production of hydrogen peroxide is toxic to anaerobic bacteria because these organisms lack catalase and, therefore, cannot break down hydrogen peroxide. Bacteriocin inhibited the growth of bacteria that constitutes the bacterial vaginosis (BV) flora, as well as other bacteria. Growth of bacteria such as *Gardnerella vaginalis* causes the pH to rise and the oxygen concentration to decrease. This change in environmental conditions favors the growth of *T. vaginalis.*

Glycogen is the principal carbohydrate in the vaginal ecosystem. When the glycogen concentration is elevated, the hydrogen ion concentration becomes elevated via the production of organic acids, and the pH tends to be less than 4.5. This situation favors the growth of aerobic organisms as well as yeast. This represents an example of a host factor that assists in maintaining the equilibrium of a healthy vaginal ecosystem, which, in turn, has a direct effect on the composition of the endogenous microflora.

Typically, the microflora of the vaginal ecosystem is characterized by a dominance of gram-positive aerobic bacteria, especially *L. acidophilus.* The secondary bacteria are streptococci of the viridans group and diphtheroids. A variety of bacteria may also be isolated from the lower genital tract during either the healthy or unhealthy state. The difference between the two states is reflected, in the latter state, by the increase in the numbers of pathogenic bacteria that make up the vaginal flora. In the unhealthy or disrupted state, no one bacterium assumes dominance, rather many different bacteria become dominant (Table 7-1).

Another factor that is host dependent is the presence of estrogen in the vaginal environment. Estrogen appears to play a role in whether or not *T. vaginalis* exists in a mobile, flagellated, or spheroid form. The flagellated mobile form is found both in women who have an acute infection and in pregnant women. The spheroid form is more likely to be associated with premenarchal girls and postmenopausal women (11). Sharma et al. (12) reported a case of a postmenopausal woman allergic to metronidazole who was cured of vaginal trichomoniasis following discontinuation of estrogen therapy.

In 1968, Jirovec and Petru (13) published a grading scale that was adapted from one developed by Schroder (14). This grading system continues to be used

TABLE 7-1. *Dominant bacteria of an unhealthy vaginal ecosystem*

Gardnerella vaginalis
Escherichia coli
Streptococcus agalactiae
Enterococcus faecalis
Prevotella biviua
Prevotella melaninogenicus
Bacteroides fragilis
Peptostreptococcus anaerobius
Eubacterium
Bifidobacterium
Clostridium
Mycoplasma hominis

today to evaluate vaginal discharge for the management of vaginitis (Table 7-2). A Grade II vaginal discharge is characteristic of BV, and a Grade V discharge is characteristic of trichomoniasis (11–18).

There may be confusion when the microscopic examination of the vaginal discharge reveals the presence of clue cells, a variety of bacterial morphotypes, and many white blood cells (WBCs). This can be interpreted as a Grade III discharge that resembles BV, but the presence of WBCs indicates that the patient has two simultaneous conditions. Thus, it is likely that a STD or inflammatory condition of the lower genital tract is present. However, a clinical finding of WBCs in the vaginal discharge should lead the physician to seek other causes and investigate the possibility of cervical infection, as well as upper genital tract involvement.

Several investigators have studied the relationship between *T. vaginalis* and the endogenous flora of the vaginal ecosystem. In one study comparing 104 women with trichomoniasis to 232 women without evidence of trichomoniasis, no differences were identified in isolation rates of *Mycoplasma, Ureaplasma, Lactobacillus, Candida, Streptococcus agalactiae,* or *Enterobacter faecalis* (19). In another study when the numbers of lactobacilli were altered, changes in the

TABLE 7-2. *Grading system for characterizing vaginal discharge*

Grade	Characteristics
0	Premenarchal, healthy, no lactobacilli, other bacteria rare
I	Premenopausal, healthy, many estrogenized squamous epithelial cells present, many lactobacilli, WBC rare
II	Unhealthy, many estrogenized squamous epithelial cells, clue cells present, many different bacterial morphotypes are present including gram-positive and gram-negative bacteria, WBC rare
III	Purulent discharge, characteristics are similar to Grade II
IV	Gonococcal discharge, intracellular gram-negative diplococci can be found
V	*Trichomonas vaginalis* vaginitis
VI	Yeast vaginitis

WBC, white blood cell.

isolation of *T. vaginalis* resulted. When the population of *Lactobacillus* was significantly decreased and *T. vaginalis* was present, there was a slight increase in the number of anaerobe species (20). Hawes et al. (21) reported that in a study of 182 women over a 2-year period a decrease in hydrogen peroxide producing lactobacilli was associated with an increase in vaginitis. However, vaginal trichomoniasis was associated with a new sexual partner and not influenced by the status of the vaginal hydrogen-peroxide producing lactobacilli. In a study of 1,562 premenarchal children, determined by cytologic analysis of vaginal epithelium, 3% to 8% were found to have vaginal trichomoniasis (22). Thus, the presence or absence of lactobacilli docs not appear to place the individual at a greater risk for acquiring trichomoniasis.

In vitro studies have shown that there may be synergy as well as antagonism between the endogenous bacteria of the lower genital tract and *T. vaginalis.* Bacteria such as *Micrococcus, Staphylococcus aureus,* and *E. faecalis* appear to act synergistically with *T. vaginalis. Proteus vulgaris* and *Pseudomonas aeruginosa* appear to be antagonistic when grown in the same environment with *T. vaginalis* (23,24). When high concentrations of *T. vaginalis* are mixed with lactobacilli, the bacteria do not survive; however, when high concentrations of lactobacilli are used, the bacteria do survive (25).

Currently available data demonstrates that microorganisms, such as *Escherichia coli* and *Mycoplasma hominis,* have the ability to attach to the protozoan and be carried into the fallopian tubes, as well as into the peritoneal cavity. *M. hominis* and *Ureaplasma urealyticum* have been found within membranous vesicles inside the protozoan (26,27). The protozoan has been isolated from the peritoneal cavity by the aspiration of peritoneal fluid via laparoscopy from women with PID (28). These studies will have significant impact if proven accurate because *T. vaginalis* will have to be considered a significant pathogen with the potential to cause, or at least contribute to, soft tissue pelvic infection. In addition, this organism may also serve as another cause of the so-called silent or asymptomatic PID.

EPIDEMIOLOGY

T. vaginalis is a fastidious organism and is dependent on its host for survival. There is no known cyst stage. Herein lies the difficulty in understanding how this organism is able to survive during periods of environmental stress. The absence of a cyst or spore stage would prevent the trichomonads from surviving exposure during periods of desiccation, high temperature, or unfavorable hydrogen ion concentrations. However, when the organism is outside the confines of the host, it can survive if the humidity of the environment is high, thereby preventing desiccation. The protozoan has been isolated from baths; poorly chlorinated water, such as that found whirlpools and hot tubs; and from swimming pools (29,30). Interestingly, studies have revealed that *T. vaginalis* has survived in vaginal exudates at 100°C for up to 48 hours (30). The organism has also survived up to 3 hours in urine and up to 6 hours in ejaculated semen (31). The protozoan has also been found to survive in water on washcloths at a temperature of 350°C (13,32). Approximately one third of washcloths found to be contaminated with *T. vaginalis* contained viable organisms after 2 to 3 hours, and 10% had viable protozoans up to 24 hours after being contaminated (32). In one study, 37% of women with vaginal trichomoniasis were found to leave urine on toilet seats after voiding, and 36% of the samples contained viable trichomonads. Toilet seats seeded with vaginal exudates containing viable trichomonads were found to have viable organisms for up to 45 minutes (33,34).

Although there is evidence that suggests that *T. vaginalis* can be transmitted via nonsexual contact, this has not been demonstrated. Therefore, it is generally agreed that acquisition is primarily, and almost exclusively, through sexual intercourse (35–37). Transmission of the protozoan may occur via sexual contact, excluding sexual intercourse. Acquisition of *T. vaginalis* has been reported to occur between a lesbian couple. A recent report demonstrated that transmission occurred between the couple via mutual masturbation. This couple was reported to be in a monogamous relationship and did not have sex with males. They did not use sexual instruments (e.g., penetrating instruments) (38).

Transmission to newborn infants may occur as the infant passes through the birth canal. There have been three cases of pneumonia in infants from which *T. vaginalis* was recovered from the respiratory tract and no other pathogen–bacterial, viral, or yeast–or other protozoan could be detected (39,40). The risk of contracting trichomoniasis is directly related to the number of sexual partners that the individual is directly or indirectly exposed to. This, in turn, is related to the number of individuals in the pool of contacts that are infected with *T. vaginalis*. The age group at greatest risk for acquiring trichomoniasis is the same as the group that is at risk for contracting gonorrhea and chlamydial infection. This is between 20 and 30 years of age, which is the age at which there is the greatest likelihood of heterogenous sexual activity. However, unlike gonorrhea, which tends to decrease in frequency as the at-risk population ages, the frequency of trichomoniasis infection tends to increase in women 30 to 40 years of age (13,26).

The greatest risk factors for acquiring trichomoniasis are race, use of contraceptives other than condoms, and a past history of a STD. Several studies have shown that African American women are at greater risk for having trichomoniasis than Hispanics or Caucasians. This also appears to be true for acquiring gonorrhea (13,26). Earlier studies suggested that oral contraceptive use was associated with a decrease in trichomoniasis compared with an intrauterine device or individuals that do not use contraception. Patients not using contraceptives were twice as likely to acquire trichomoniasis as those using contraceptive pills (41,42).

There has been concern that the male may serve as an asymptomatic carrier and, therefore, is an important vector and reservoir for transmission to their sexual partners. It has been hypothesized that the male may be symptomatic, not infected with T. vaginalis, but found to have nongonococcal, nonchlamydial ure-thritis or prostatitis (43–45). In one study, *T. vaginalis* was isolated from 50 of 447 males being evaluated in a STD clinic (46). The organism was isolated from 9 (17%) of 52 males who had sexual contact with women known to have vagi-nal trichomoniasis. 27 of the 52 infected males had symptoms of urethritis. The males usually became symptomatic within 24 hours following contact with an infected partner. A pure trichomonal infection in the male produces a clear to slightly purulent urethral discharge.

PATIENT EVALUATION

The patient with symptomatic vaginal trichomoniasis usually presents with a malodorous vaginal discharge. Occasionally itching, soreness, or dyspareunia will be associated with vaginal trichomoniasis. Typically, the discharge is dirty gray to green in color, may or may not be frothy, and is usually liquid. Petechial hemorrhages are present on the cervix in 25% of the cases. The diagnosis can be established in approximately 75% of the cases by carefully examining the vagi-nal discharge microscopically. The vaginal pH is 5 or greater when the patient has trichomoniasis. Therefore, if the patient's vaginal discharge is dirty gray, yel-low, or green, the pH should be determined, and if 5 or greater, microscopic eval-uation of the discharge should be performed. This can easily be accomplished by obtaining an aliquot of the discharge from the fornix or lateral wall of the vagina with a cotton-tipped applicator. The applicator should be immersed in 2 mL of normal saline, swirled vigorously, and removed from the saline; then a glass slide is touched with the applicator to dislodge one to two drops of diluted vagi-nal discharge. A glass coverslip is placed over the specimen and examined microscopically under 40× magnification. Trichomonads can be easily identified by noting their elliptical shape, swimming motion, and beating flagella. Careful focus with the fine adjustment will reveal the presence of their four anterior fla-gella. It is the whipping, back-and-forth motion of the flagella that give the pro-tozoans their characteristic swimming movements. The trichomonads are larger than a WBC but smaller than mature squamous epithelial cells. It is important to note the presence of any other abnormality present in the vaginal discharge, such as clue cells suggesting the presence of BV.

Individuals who have a vaginal discharge characterized by the presence of many WBCs, the absence of clue cells, or the absence of yeast or pseudohyphae should be considered suspicious for the presence of trichomoniasis. In these instances, the pH should be determined. If the pH is 5 or greater and the micro-scopic evaluation does not reveal a pathogen, then a specimen should be obtained for the inoculation of Diamond's medium for the growth of *T. vaginalis*. The culture medium should be examined daily for the presence of trichomonads.

The method employed to establish a diagnosis of trichomoniasis has been of concern because there is no rapid method that has both a high degree of sensi-tivity and specificity. (Sensitivity is defined as the percentage of culture-positive specimens identified as positive by microscopy or other tests. Specificity is defined as the percentage of culture-negative specimens identified as negative by microscopy or other tests.) Using the characteristics of discharge is neither sensitive nor specific because 50% who do not have a discharge resembling that associated with trichomoniasis are not infected (47,48). Microscopic examination of the vaginal discharge (wet prep) is the most commonly employed method for establishing a diagnosis of trichomoniasis. The specificity and sensitivity of the wet prep compared with culture has been reported to range from 96% to 100% and 38% to 82%, respectively (49,50). Robertson et al. (51) did not confirm the high specificity with microscopy as reported by others. They compared wet prep with a centrifuge specimen examined under phase contrast microscopy to culture and could not confirm 10 of 44 specimens that had been identified as positive by microscopic examination of a wet prep. In an attempt to enhance the accuracy of establishing the correct diagnosis, the Gram stain has been employed. Cree (52) detected *T. vaginalis* in Gram-stained specimens of vaginal exudate in 66% of 249 individuals with culture-proven infection. The false-positive rate in this study was only 7%. Sorbrepena (53) reported successful identification of *T. vaginalis* by Gram stain in twice the number of individuals as was identified by microscopic examination of unstained vaginal discharge (wet prep).

Trichomonads are frequently reported by the cytopathologist when reading Papanicolaou (Pap) smears. In one study comparing Pap smear with culture and wet prep microscopy, the Pap smear was found to be inferior. In this study, 126 infections were diagnosed by Pap smear but could not be confirmed by other methods (54). Perl (55) studied 1,199 patients and found 666 positive for trichomoniasis on Pap smear. However, of the positives, 37% could not be confirmed.

New methodology is constantly sought to improve the reliability of establishing the diagnosis. Several new, so-called rapid tests are available and being developed, but none are truly rapid and all are more costly. The only meaningful test that has clinical application is one that can produce results in 5 to 10 minutes and is not expensive. If test results cannot be available during the time the patient is being evaluated, then the test is not particularly useful. In addition, these tests will most likely require the presence of someone other than the physician and the nurse to perform, and Clinical Laboratory Improvements Amendment (CLIA) certification will be required, therefore, making the test impractical. If the specimen has to be sent out for processing, the cost will increase because of all that will be involved to send and process the specimen and to report the result to the physician and the patient. Finally, another telephone call will have to be made to prescribe medication for the patient.

Driving the development of the new test is that many investigators are of the opinion that (a) many physicians do not take the time to examine vaginal discharge thoroughly, (b) many physicians are inexperienced in evaluating vaginal discharge, and (c) use of the wet prep to diagnose trichomoniasis is not extremely sensitive and specific. One group of investigators found that examining the vaginal discharge microscopically (wet prep) at the time the Pap smear is obtained may be beneficial in the management of the patient and reduce the need for repeat Pap smears. They found that an inflammatory Pap smear was associated with BV ($p < 0.0001$), excess WBCs ($p < 0.0001$), trichomoniasis ($p < 0.0001$), abnormal wet preps in general ($p < 0.0001$), and positive cervical cultures for *Neisseria gonorrhoeae* and *Chlamydia trachomatis* ($p < 0.001$) (56).

There is considerable concern over the patient who fails to respond to treatment and may have a strain that is resistant to metronidazole. First, the patient must be educated as to the means of *T. vaginalis* acquisition, which is primarily via sexual contact. Second, treatment must be administered to the patient and her sexual partner(s). If the patient has multiple sexual partners, her behavior must be modified. The patient should insist that her contacts wear a condom during the act of sexual intercourse. Third, the patient should be reevaluated following completion of treatment to document that the trichomonads have been eradicated and that the vaginal ecosystem has been restored to a healthy state.

Management of the sexual partner is as important as the management of the patient. Both partners must complete a full course of therapy. It is best that they take metronidazole over the same period, to prevent cross infection. However, this will not ensure that the organism is eradicated in both individuals. If the male develops a trichomoniasis of the prostate he may require a longer treatment regimen. *T. vaginalis* was first described in expressed prostatic fluid obtained from husbands of infected women in 1936 (57). Isolation of trichomonads from men who have had sexual intercourse with women infected with vaginal trichomoniasis ranges from 9% to 100% (58,59). Of the males diagnosed with urethritis who have not responded to several courses of antibiotics, 85% were subsequently found to harbor *T. vaginalis* (60,61). One difficulty with these early studies is that the patients were not evaluated for the presence of *N. gonorrhoeae, C, trachomatis, M. hominis, U. urealyticum,* or herpes simplex.

It may be that the significance of *T. vaginalis* infection in males resides in the fact that infection tends to be latent. Several studies have demonstrated the presence of *T. vaginalis* in symptomatic husbands and sexual partners of infected women (13,62,63). In one investigation, 30 husbands of infected women were cultured; 60% of the husbands were found to be positive for *T. vaginalis,* and 61% of these infected males were asymptomatic (64). The percentage of male sexual contacts of infected women who subsequently develop symptomatic urethritis and are found to be positive for *T. vaginalis* ranges from 16% to 83% (65).

The fact that partners may be treated simultaneously does not ensure that the trichomonads will all be killed simultaneously nor that adequate levels of metronidazole will be achieved in the prostate gland. This is an important consideration because if the trichomonads have invaded the prostate gland, eradication becomes more difficult. A second consideration is that infection in the male may involve other sites, such as the epididymitis, posthitis (infection of the foreskin), balanitis (inflammation of the glans penis), and may cause draining sinuses of the median raphe (33,40,66–71). *T. vaginalis* has also been found in association with penal ulcers (44,70). In a classic study performed by Weston and Nicol (64), in 1963, males were examined 2 days after exposure to infected females, and the organism was recovered from 70% of the males. Increasing the interval between exposure and examination correlated with a decrease in the recovery rate of the protozoan. After an interval of 14 days only 30% of the exposed males were found to be positive for *T. vaginalis*. Thirty days after exposure, only 23% of the males remained positive and subsequent examination failed to recover trichomonads.

Trichomoniasis infection in males can be summarized as follows: (a) symptomatic infection is common; (b) males exposed to infected females should be considered colonized, whether asymptomatic or symptomatic; (c) symptomatic male infection is typically diagnosed as urethritis and these individuals have a purulent discharge; and (d) prostatitis is rare. The women's health physician should remember that all women with documented vaginal trichomoniasis should be considered a vector for the transmission of *T. vaginalis*. Finally, when treating a women for trichomoniasis, it is imperative that her sexual partner be treated, whether he or she is symptomatic or not.

TREATMENT

The only approved antitrichomonal agent approved in the United States is metronidazole, which was approved for use in 1963. Metronidazole was synthesized from Streptomyces (72). The antibiotic known as metronidazole (Flagyl) was approved in France in 1980. The delay in the United States was because of concern over the presence of the nitro group, which made the drug similar to chloramphenicol. There were also reports of leukopenia associated with metronidazole use (73). Other nitroimidazoles available outside the United States are nimorazole (Naxogin), tinidazole (Fasign), omidazole, scenidazole, camidazole, and misonidazole (74,75). Two new forms of the drug are available that are associated with less gastrointestinal side effects, Flagyl 375 mg capsule and Flagyl ER. (A 750 mg tablet that has been incorporated into a matrix that allows for the drug to be released slowly or over an extended period.) This new formulation, extended release (ER), allows for once-a-day dosing.

Metronidazole is almost completely absorbed by the gastrointestinal tract when taken orally, and approximately 95% of the drug is bioavailable. Peak serum levels are achieved in 1 to 3 hours following an oral dose. However, if taken after consuming a meal, absorption is delayed and peak serum levels may not be reached for 3 hours (76,77). Metronidazole is metabolized by the liver into at least five different metabolites (78). Approximately 20% to 30% of the daily dose is excreted in the urine and feces. Studies have demonstrated small amounts of mutagenic derivatives and an acetamide in the urine of patients receiving the drug (79). When metronidazole is administered vaginally, as a cream or suppository, absorption does occur with peak levels of 0.2 μg/mL within 12 to 24 hours following a 500-mg dose. Absorption is greater when the antimicrobial agent is in a cream versus a suppository (80). Common side effects are listed in Table 7-3. Patients who are taking metronidazole should be advised not to consume alcohol containing liquid because they may suffer abdominal pain (a reaction similar to the one experienced when alcohol is consumed by patients taking disulfiram) (81). Metronidazole should be administered with care to patients taking anticonvulsants and warfarin because it can enhance the action of these medications (82).

The standard regimens for the treatment of trichomoniasis are either 2 g administered as a single dose, 250 mg three times daily, or 500 mg twice daily for 7 days. Two new dosage forms are available: 375 mg taken twice daily and 750 mg ER (Flagyl ER) given once daily for 7 days. The 2-g single oral dose regimen is favored by some physicians because it can be taken once and, therefore, compliance is greater. However, there is a considerable amount of gastrointestinal discomfort. In cases in which trichomoniasis is diagnosed accidentally (e.g., by Pap smear) and the patient is asymptomatic, treatment should not be instituted without confirming the diagnosis. If left untreated, the patient will ultimately serve as a vector for transmission of *T. vaginalis*. In addition, she will eventually experience acute exacerbations of acute infection and may develop an abnormal Pap smear (83). It is important that males are treated when they are exposed to a known infected partner. If the exposed male is left untreated, approximately 24% of his subsequent partners will become infected (84). Failures caused by resistant strains of *T. vaginalis* are sensitive to less than 1 µg/mL up to 16 µg/mL (85–87). However, sensitivity testing is dependent on whether the organism has been tested under aerobic or anaerobic conditions. Various concentrations have been found to be effective. However, there is general agreement that under normal anaerobic conditions most strains are susceptible to metronidazole at a concentration of 3 µg/mL or less and under aerobic conditions 25 µg/mL or less (88).

Although the organism has remained relatively sensitive to metronidazole, resistance to that drug has been reported (89). Other investigators have found resistant strains but were able to treat patients successfully by increasing the dose

TABLE 7-3. *Adverse reactions to metronidazole*

Nausea
Vomiting
Gastric pain
Metallic taste
Headache
Dizziness
Peripheral neuropathy
Seizures
Ataxia
Disulfiram-like reaction

of metronidazole (90–93). Patients who appear to have intractable or resistant trichomoniasis should be managed by first having the organism isolated and sensitivity to metronidazole determined. Isolates that have an aerobic minimum inhibitory concentration (MIC) greater than 50 but less than 200 μg/mL will be moderately sensitive, whereas those isolates with a MIC greater than 200 μg/mL will be resistant (91). Thus, a patient with a moderately to highly resistant strain will require a total daily dose of metronidazole from 2 to 3.5 g a day for 7 to 14 days. Treatment can be administered by combining oral and vaginal administration of metronidazole. In cases in which high doses of oral metronidazole cannot be tolerated, the drug can be given intravenously. High doses of metronidazole (more than 2 g/day) can induce nausea, vomiting, gastrointestinal discomfort, headache, and peripheral neuropathy, which usually appears within 72 hours of beginning the administration of metronidazole.

Treatment of trichomoniasis during pregnancy poses significant potential problems. Trichomoniasis is associated with septic abortion, preterm labor, premature rupture of amniotic membranes, chorioamnionitis, and postpartum endometritis. Metronidazole does cross the placenta but has not been shown to produce teratogenic effects in the fetus (94). However, the concern for potentially adverse effects on the fetus continues to exist among obstetricians. Therefore, there is a reluctance to administer the drug to pregnant women, especially in the first trimester. A meta-analysis was performed on all references of congenital malformations associated with metronidazole use in pregnancy from 1966 to 1996. Only four studies fulfilled the inclusion criteria (95–99). A recent review of the literature on metronidazole use in pregnancy revealed that there has been no association between the drug and teratogenic effects in the fetus regardless of which trimester the fetus was exposed to metronidazole (100). In view of the fact that there is no suitable alternative, metronidazole should be administered for the treatment of trichomoniasis. An alternative treatment modality that has been tested, but is not satisfactory, is clotrimazole. Cure rates of 41% to 81% have been reported when 100-mg vaginal suppositories are administered daily for 7 days (101–103).

Transmission of *T. vaginalis* to the newborn has been reported (104). The effect of neonatal infection is not well understood, and, therefore, treatment is not recommended unless infection is symptomatic or persists beyond 6 weeks. However, this may be an instance when polymerase chain reaction (PCR) detection of *Trichomonas* has a role. Taking the position that one should not treat a known infection unless it is apparently symptomatic does not appear to be prudent. Because the organism can invade the lower urinary tract, it may be mistaken for a bacterial infection. If it is not detected, the symptoms may also be misconstrued for some other condition leading to inappropriate testing and treatments. I would recommend that infants, born to women with known trichomoniasis at the time of delivery, be evaluated with the most sensitive test available to detect the presence of trichomonads and treated appropriately.

Metronidazole does gain entrance to breast milk, and, therefore, a breast-feeding infant can acquire metronidazole from the mother. It has been documented that a single 2-g dose administered to the mother will result in a concentration of 25 mg/L of breast milk (105).

Metronidazole is fairly well tolerated by most patients; however, true allergy is rare but does occur. Allergy to metronidazole is characterized by urticaria, pruritus, rash, vasodilation, flushing, and bronchospasm (106). Although hypersensitivity reactions typically occur shortly after exposure to the allergen (within 60 minutes), the allergic reaction to metronidazole may occur after 24 hours. The severity of the reaction may vary from mild to true anaphylaxis, hypotension, cardiac arrhythmias, syncope, seizures, loss of consciousness, shock, and death.

Because there is no alternative to metronidazole for the treatment of trichomoniasis, patients who have not responded to lesser treatment regimens should be desensitized to metronidazole. Desensitization should be carried out in a setting where the patient's vital signs can be continuously monitored and there can be an immediate response to any adverse event that may occur during the desensitization process (Table 7-4). An anesthesiologist should be alerted and available during the patient's desensitization and up to 24 hours after metronidazole has been administered.

Pearlman et al. (106) reported on two women with documented allergy to metronidazole who underwent desensitization. These investigators tested each patient to determine if they were truly allergic to metronidazole by applying 0.2 mm of 0.75% metronidazole vaginal gel to the vaginal epithelium. A positive result was documented by the presence of a wheal at the test site. They then proceeded to desensitize the patient by administering increasing incremental doses of metronidazole (Table 7-5). These investigators were successful in desensitizing the patients and eradicating their infection. Faro successfully desensitized a patient who was allergic to metronidazole by modifying the protocol of Pearlman et al. The patient was an African-American woman who had symptomatic trichomoniasis of the lower genitourinary tract for 4 years. The patient's allergic reaction to metronidazole was characterized by the development of a rash and shortness of breath 24 hours after taking metronidazole. This occurred on two separate occasions, and both times she was treated with antihistamines and

TABLE 7-4. *Items necessary for desensitization to metronidazole*

Automated blood pressure recorder
Continuous monitoring of oxygen saturation
Continuous cardiac monitoring
Intravenous fluids
Epinephrine
Oxygen
Metaproterenol
Hydrocortisone
Diphenhydramine
Aminophylline
Cimetidine
Resuscitation equipment

TABLE 7-5. *Protocol for desensitization to metronidazole[a]*

Dose	Fluid infused
5 µg	1 mL
15 µg	1mL
50 µg	1 mL
150 µg	3 mL
500 µg	1 mL
1.5 mg	3 mL
5 mg	1 mL
15 mg	3 mL
30 mg	6 mL
60 mg	2 mL
125 mg	25 mL
Oral dose administered at 1-hour intervals	
250 mg	1 tablet
500 mg	1 tablet
2 g	4 tablets

[a]Modified from Pearlman MD, Yasher C, Ernst S, et al. An incremental dosing protocol for women with severe vaginal trichomoniasis and adverse reactions to metronidazole. *Am J Obstet Gynecol* 1996;174:934–936, with permission.

steroids, which successfully interrupted the reaction. Because the patient had a strong history for allergy to metronidazole, a test to the agent was not performed before instituting desensitization. Faro modified the recommended protocol by not administering metronidazole, but instead completed the process by infusing the following doses: 250 mg, 500 mg, 500 mg, and 500 mg intravenously every 8 hours. The patient was discharged from the hospital 24 hours after the last dose. This was then followed by Flagyl 375 mg orally twice a day for 10 days. The patient was contacted daily to determine if any adverse reaction had occurred. The patient was reevaluated at the completion of therapy, and in 3 weeks complete resolution of her symptoms had occurred; the organism could not be detected by either microscopic examination or by culture.

PATHOGENESIS

Trichomonads are commonly found in the vagina during acute symptomatic infection but may also be found in Skene's and Bartholin's glands, as well as in the bladder. Trichomonads have been found to cause lower urinary tract infection in approximately 10% to 20% of women with vaginal trichomoniasis (107). *T. vaginalis* can be recovered in clean voided urine specimens from the urethra in approximately 50% of women with vaginal trichomoniasis and have a concomitant urethral discharge with dysuria (108). Thus, the organism has been postulated as a possible source of PID. Strength for this position has been derived from data provided by scanning electron microscopy (108). When treating an infected woman, it is important to consider that the organism can reside in sites other than the vagina. This is especially true when consideration is given to use of intravaginal preparations to treat symptomatic or asymptomatic infection. Typical signs and symptoms of PID are not associated with trichomoniasis of the upper genital tract; lower abdominal pain is found in 2% to 15% of patients (109–112). Other than isolation of the trichomonads, physical findings that are specific for trichomoniasis-associated PID do not exist. A frothy or foamy vaginal discharge is found in only 15% to 25% of patients, the color of the discharge may vary from gray to yellow, and the discharge may or may not be malodorous. Petechial hemorrhages of the vaginal epithelium and portio of the cervix occur in approximately 25% of infected patients (113).

The infection is responsive to hormonal changes of the host. The disease appears to become latent during the follicular phase and ovulation. The organism tends to favor a less acidic environment and prefers to inhabit the endocervical canal where it is likely to establish an asymptomatic infection. Therefore, patients who present with a purulent vaginal discharge or a dirty gray discharge with a significant number of WBCs but no identifiable pathogen on microscopic examination of the vaginal discharge should have (a) a specimen of the vaginal discharge cultured in Diamond's medium for the isolation of *T. vaginalis* and (b) a specimen obtained from the endocervical canal to examine microscopically and to inoculate Diamond's medium. During the luteal phase and menstruation, the organism again seeks an existence in the vagina. *T. vaginalis* penetrates the surface epithelium of the vagina and lies intracellularly, as well as intercellularly (114). The organism may cause surface necrosis of the epithelium, abscess, and erosion of the epithelium of the vagina. These tissue reactions are accompanied by a polymorphonuclear leukocyte infiltration. Macrophages, lymphocytes, and plasma cells are also found to accompany the polymorphonuclear leukocytes. *T. vaginalis* may cause an intraepithelial edema that reflects a picture similar to that seen with the human papilloma virus infection, that is, koilocytosis (115,116). However, the perinuclear edema seen with trichomoniasis produces a clear halo, which is not as wide as that seen with koilocytosis and tends to be glandular.

Chronic infection of the cervix and the endocervix may be accompanied by hyperplasia of the endocervical epithelium, parabasal cell hyperplasia of the squamous epithelium, and parabasal cell hyperplasia of the squamous epithelium. In addition, squamous cell metaplasia of the cervix may also occur. The organism commonly invades the endocervical clefts causing inflammation that can initiate closures of these clefts, forming small abscesses. These areas become chronically infected with trichomonads that can survive in these isolated regions because they are nourished by serum and the pH remains neutral. This change in pH favors the growth of the trichomonads and anaerobic bacteria as well as *E. coli, E. faecalis,* and so forth. Combinations of bacteria such as *Prevotella bivia* and *E. coli* or *E. faecalis* are abscessogenic (117). The organisms, *T. vaginalis* and bacteria, can be liberated when a Pap smear is obtained, via trauma such as either sexual activity, or any mechanical abrasion that can disrupt the surface epithelium. When conditions throughout the lower genital tract are not favorable for the wide distribution of *T. vaginalis,* its possible presence should be suspected when a patient's Pap smear repeatedly returns with a diagnosis of inflammation. If a thorough examination of the lower genital tract, including evaluation of the vaginal ecosystem, reveals no abnormality then a localized cervical infection should be considered. Evaluation of the endocervical discharge can be accomplished by (a) wiping away all excess discharge from the portio of the cervix, (b) gently inserting a cotton-tipped swab into the endocervical canal, (c) removing the swab and placing 2 to 3 mL of normal saline then agitating the swab, (d) placing one to two drops of the diluted discharge on a glass slide then placing a coverslip over the specimen, and (e) microscopically examining under 40× magnification. The endocervix should be cultured for *N. gonorrhoeae, C. trachomatis, M. hominis,* and *U. urealyticum.*

T. vaginalis is often found in association with other sexually transmitted organisms. The two most common are the human papillomavirus and *C. trachomatis.* Other infectious agents that have been reported in association with trichomoniasis are *Candida, Actinomyces,* herpes, and adenovirus. Studies have suggested that the trichomonads are capable of ingesting *C. trachomatis* (118,119). This may have significant implications, if proven true, for it may serve as a mechanism for simultaneously transmitting two infections. It is also important to be alert to the fact that trichomoniasis may serve as an indicator for the presence of other sexually transmitted organisms. Trichomoniasis has been found to be associated with symptoms and signs of urethritis. The prevalence of *N. gonorrhoeae* and *C. trachomatis* was similar in patients with and without trichomoniasis (120). Male patients with trichomoniasis but not another STD were often symptomatic having urethral discharge and inflammation. (120). Women infected with *T. vaginalis* were more likely to be positive for other sexually transmitted organisms. For example, 31% of women with *T. vaginalis* were also infected with *N. gonorrhoeae* versus 11% without concomitant trichomoniasis; 18% were coinfected with *C. trachomatis* versus 15% without trichomoniasis; 87% were also positive for *Mycoplasma*; 75% had BV compared with 47% with BV but without trichomoniasis; 44% had a mucopurulent cervicitis with trichomoniasis compared with 31% with mucopurulent cervicitis alone (121).

REFERENCES

1. Trussell RE, Plass ED. The pathogenicity and physiology of a pure culture of *Trichomonas vaginalis.* Am J Obstet Gynecol 1940;40:833.
2. Trussell RE. *Trichomonas vaginalis and trichomoniasis.* Springfield, IL: Charles C. Thomas, 1947.
3. Kent HL. *Epidemiology of vaginitis. Am J Obstet Gynecol* 1991;165:1168–1176.
4. Honiberg BM. Taxonomy and nomenclature. In: Honigberg BM, ed. *Trichomonads parasitic in humans.* New York: Springer Verlag, 1990:3–35.
5. Kott H, Adler S. A serological study of *Trichomonas* species parasitic in man. *Trans R Soc Trop Med Hyg* 1961;55:333–344.
6. Su-Lin K-E, Honigberg BM. Antigenic analysis of *Trichomonas vaginalis* strains by quantitative fluorescent antibody methods. *Z Parasitenkd* 1983;69(2):161–181.
7. Su-Lin K-E, Honigberg BM. Antigenic analysis of *Trichomonas vaginalis. J Protozool* 1976;23: 18A.
8. Rein MF, Sullivan JA, Mandell GL. Trichomonacidal activity of human polymorphonuclear neutrophils: killing by disruption and fragmentation. *J Infect Dis* 1980;142:575–585.
9. Gillin FD, Sher A. Activation of the alternate complement pathway by *Trichomonas vaginalis. Infect Immun* 1981;34:268–273.

10. Holbrook TW, Boackle RJ, Vesely J, et al. *Trichomonas vaginalis*: alternative pathway activation of complement. *Trans R Soc Trop Med Hyg* 1982;76:473–475.
11. Soszka S, Kazanowska W, Kuczynska K, et al. *Trichomonas vaginalis* at different life stages of women. *Wiad Parazytol* 1990;36(5–6):211–217.
12. Sharma R, Pickerin T, McCormick WM. Trichomoniasis in a postmenopausal women cured after discontinuation of a salutary effect on *Trichomonas vaginalis*. *Sex Transm Dis* 1997;24:543–545.
13. Jirovec O, Petru M. *Trichomonas vaginalis* and trichomoniasis. *Adv Parasitol* 1968;6:117–188.
14. Schroder R. Zur Pathogenese und Klinik des vaginalen Fluoirs. *Zentralbl Gynakol* 1921;45: 1350–1361.
15. Goldacre MJ, Watt B, Loudon N, et al. Vaginal microbial flora in normal young women. *Br Med J* 1979;1:1450–1453.
16. Spiegel CA, Amsel R, Eschenbach D, et al. Anaerobic bacteria in nonspecific vaginitis. *N Engl J Med* 1980;303:601–607.
17. Blackwell AL, Fox AR, Phillips I, et al. Anaerobic vaginosis (non-specific vaginitis): clinical, microbiological, and therapeutic findings. *Lancet* 1983;2:1379–1382.
18. Taylor E, Blackwell AL, Barlow D, et al. *Gardnerella vaginalis,* anaerobes, and vaginal discharge. *Lancet* 1982;1:1376–1379.
19. Mason PR, MacCallum MJ, Poynter B. Association of *Trichomonas vaginalis* with other microorganisms. *Lancet* 1982;1:1067.
20. Levinson ME, Trestman I, Quach R, et al. Quantitative bacteriology of the vaginal flora in vaginitis. *Am J Obstet Gynecol* 1979;133:139–144.
21. Hawes S, Hillier SL, Benedetti J, et al. Hydrogen peroxide-producing lactobacilli and acquisition of vaginal infections. *J Infect Dis* 1996;174:1058–1063.
22. Stefanovic J. Trichomoniasis in girls during the period of hormonal inactivity. *Bratisl Lek Listy* 1990; 91:780–782.
23. Robinson SC, Mirchandam G. Observations on vaginal trichomoniasis. IV. Significance on vaginal flora under various conditions. *Am J Obstet Gynecol* 1965;91:1005–1012.
24. Szreter H. Influence of microorganisms on the survival rate of *Trichomonas vaginalis* in physiologic salt solution. *Wiad Parazytol* 1979;25:409–415.
25. Soszka S, Kuczynsha K. Effect of *T. vaginalis* on the physiological flora. *Wiad Parazytol* 1977;23: 519–523.
26. Rein MF, Muller M. *Trichomonas vaginalis.* In: Holmes KK, Mardh PA, Sparling PF, et al., eds. *Sexually transmitted diseases.* New York: McGraw-Hill, 1984:525–535.
27. Santler R, Thurner J, Poitschek C. Trichomoniasis. *Z Hautkr* 1976;51:757–761.
28. Keith L, Berger GS, Edelman A, et al. On the causation of pelvic inflammatory disease. *Am J Obstet Gynecol* 1984;149:215–224.
29. Kozlowska D, Wichrowska B. The effect of chlorine and its compounds used for disinfection of water on *Trichomonas vaginalis*. *Awiad Parazytol* 1976;22:433–435.
30. Whittington MJ. The survival of *Trichomonas vaginalis* at temperatures below 370C. *J Hyg* 1951; 22:400–409.
31. Gallai Z, Sylvestre L. The present status of urogenital trichomoniasis: a general review of the literature. *Appl Ther* 1966;8:773–778.
32. Burch TA, Rees CW, Reardon LV. Epidemiological studies on human trichomoniasis. *Am J Trop Med* 1959;8:312–318.
33. Kessel JF, Thompson CF. Survival of *Trichomonas vaginalis* in vaginal discharge. *Proc Soc Exp Biol Med* 1950;74:755–758.
34. Whittington JM. Epidemiology of infections with *Trichomonas vaginalis* in the light of improved diagnostic methods. *Br J Vener Dis* 1957;33:80–91.
35. Krieger JN. Urologic aspects of trichomoniasis. *Invest Urol* 1981;18:411–417.
36. Catterall RD, Nicol CS. Is trichomonal infection a veneral disease? *Br Med J* 1960;1:1177–1179.
37. Catterall RD. Trichomonal infections of the genital tract. *Med Clin North Am* 1972;56:1203–1209.
38. Kellock D, O'Mahony CP. Sexually acquired metronidazole resistant trichomoniasis in a lesbian couple. *Genitourin Med* 1996;72:60–61.
39. Hiemstra I, Van Bel F, Berger HM. Can *Trichomonas vaginalis* cause pneumonia in newborn babies? *Br Med J* 1984;289:355–356.
40. McLaren LC, Davis LE, Healy GR, et al. Isolation of *Trichomonas vaginalis* from the respiratory tract of infants with respiratory disease. *Pediatrics* 1983;71:888–890.
41. Bramley M, Kinghorn G. Do oral contraceptives inhibit *Trichomonas vaginalis*? *Sex Transm Dis* 1979;6:261–263.
42. Birnbaum H, Kraussold E. Incidence of the *Blastomyces* and trichomonad infections during the use of hormonal and intrauterine contraception. *Zentralbl Gynakol* 1975;97:1636–1640.

43. Gardner WA Jr, Culberson DE, Bennett DB. *Trichomonas vaginalis* in the prostate gland. *Arch Pathol Lab Med* 1986;110:430–432.
44. Kuberski T. *Trichomonas vaginalis* associated with nongonococcal urethritis and prostatitis. *Sex Transm Dis* 1980;7:135–136.
45. Mardh PA, Colleen S. Search for uro-genital tract infections in patients with symptoms of prostatitis. Studies on aerobic and strictly anaerobic bacteria, mycoplasmas, fungi, trichomonads and viruses. *Scand J Urol Nephrol* 1975;9:8–16.
46. Meares EM Jr. Prostatitis syndromes: new perspectives about old woes. *J Urol* 1980;123:141–147.
47. Fouts AC, Kraus SJ. *Trichomonas vaginalis*: re-evaluation of its clinical presentation and laboratory diagnosis. *J Infect Dis* 1980;141:137–143.
48. McLellan R, Spence MR, Brockman M, et al. The clinical diagnosis of trichomoniasis. *Obstet Gynecol* 1982;60:30–34.
49. Martin RD, Kaufman RH, Burns M. *Trichomonas vaginalis*: a statistical evaluation of diagnostic methods. *Am J Obstet Gynecol* 1963;87:1024–1027.
50. McCann JS. Comparison of direct microscopy and culture in the diagnosis of trichomoniasis. *Br J Vener Dis* 1974;50:450–452.
51. Robertson DH, Lumsden WH, Fraser KF, et al. Simultaneous isolation of *Trichomonas vaginalis* and collection of vaginal exudates. *Br J Vener Dis* 1969;45:42–43.
52. Cree GE. *Trichomonas vaginalis* in Gram-stained smears. *Br J Vener Dis* 1968;44:226–227.
53. Sorbrepena RL. Identification of *Trichomonas vaginalis* in Gram-stained smears. *Lab Med* 1980;11:558–560.
54. Mason PR, Super H, Fripp PJ. Comparison of four techniques for the routine diagnosis of *Trichomonas vaginalis* infection. *J Clin Pathol*1976;29:154–157.
55. Perl G. Errors in the diagnosis of *Trichomonas vaginalis* infections as observed among 1199 patients. *Obstet Gynecol* 1972;39:7–9.
56. Eltabbakh GH, Eltabbakh GD, Broekhuizer FF, et al. Value of wet mount and cervical culture at the time of cervical cytology in asymptomatic women. *Obstet Gynecol* 1995;85:499–503.
57. Drummond AC. Trichomonas infestation of the prostate gland. *Am J Surg* 1936;31:98–103.
58. Sylvestre L, Belanger M, Gallai Z. Urogenital trichomoniasis in the male: review of the literature and report on treatment of 37 patients by a new nitroimidazole derivative (Flagyl). *Can Med Assoc J* 1960;83:2295–2299.
59. Kawamura N. Trichomoniasis of the prostate. *Jpn J Clin Urol* 1973;27:335–344.
60. Gallai Z, Sylvestre L. The present status of urogenital trichomoniasis: a general review of the literature. *Appl Ther* 1966;8:773–778.
61. Fullilove RE Jr. *Trichomonas vaginalis* in men. *J Med Soc NJ* 1983;80:94–96.
62. Willcox RR. Epidemiological aspects of human trichomoniasis. *Br J Vener Dis* 1960;36:167–174.
63. Jennison RF. Incidence of *Trichomonas vaginalis* in marital partners. *Br J Vener Dis* 1960 36:163–166.
64. Weston TE, Nicol CS. Natural history of trichomonal infection in males. *Br J Vener Dis* 1963;39:251–257.
65. Counts WE, Silva-Inzunza B, Tallman B. Genitourinary complications of non-gonococcal urethritis and trichomoniasis in males. *Urol Int* 1959;9:189–208.
66. Kuberski T. *Trichomonas vaginalis* associated with non-gonococcal urethritis and prostatitis. *Sex Transm Dis* 1980;7:135–136.
67. Catterall RD. Diagnosis and treatment of trichomonal urethritis in men. *Br J Med J* 1960;2:113–115.
68. Wilson A, Ackers JP. Urine culture for the detection of *Trichomonas vaginalis* in men. *Br J Vener Dis* 1980;56:46–48.
69. Watt L, Jennison RF. Incidence of *Trichomonas vaginalis* infection of the median raphae of the penis. *Br J Vener Dis* 1960;36:163–166.
70. Soendjojo A, Pindha S. *Trichomonas vaginalis* infection of the median raphe of the penis. *Sex Transm Dis* 1981;8:255–257.
71. Sowmini CN, Vijayalakshmi K, Chellamuthiah C, et al. Infections of the median raphe of the penis: report of 3 cases. *Br J Vener Dis* 1973;49:469–474.
72. Maeda K, Osato T, Umexawa H. A new antibiotic: Azomycin. *J Antibiot* 1953;6A:182.
73. Anonymous. Flagyl, a systemic trichomonacide. *Med Lett* 1963;5:33–34.
74. Miller MW, Howes HL, English AR. Tinidazole, a potent new antiprotozoal agent. *Antimicrob Agents Chemother* 1969;9:257–260.
75. Muller M. Action of clinically utilized 5-nitroimidazoles on microorganisms. *Scand J Infect Dis* 1981;26:31–41.
76. Houghton GW, Smith J, Thorne PS, et al. The pharmacokinetics of oral and intravenous metronidazole in man. *J Antimicrob Chemother* 1979;5:621–623.

77. Levison ME. Microbiological agar diffusion assay for metronidazole concentration in serum. *Antimicrobial Agents Chemother* 1974;5:466–468.
78. Stambaugh JE, Feo LG, Manthei RW. The isolation and identification of the urinary oxidative metabolites of metronidazole in man. *J Pharmacol Exp Ther* 1968;161:373–381.
79. Stambaugh JE, Feo LG, Manthei RW. Isolation and identification of the major urinary metabolite of metronidazole. *Life Sci* 1967;6:1811–1819.
80. Alper MM, Barwin BN, McLean WM, et al. Systemic absorption of metronidazole by the vaginal route. *Obstet Gynecol* 1985;65:781–784.
81. Winter D, Stanescu C, Sauvard S. The effect of metronidazole on the toxicity of ethanol. *Biochem Pharmacol* 1969;18:1246–1248.
82. O'Reilly RA. Stereospecific interaction of warfarin and metronidazole. *Fed Proc* 1975;34:259.
83. Koss IG, Wolinksa WH. *Trichomonas vaginalis* cervicitis and its relationship to cervical cancer. *Cancer* 1959;12:1171–1193.
84. Watt L, Jennison RF. Incidence of *Trichomonas vaginalis* in marital partners. *Br J Vener Dis* 1960; 36:163–170.
85. Korner B, Jensen HK. Sensitivity of *Trichomonas vaginalis* to metronidazole, tinidazole, and nifuratel in vitro. *Br J Vener Dis* 1976;52:404–408.
86. McFadzean JA, Pugh IM, Squires SL, et al. Further observations on strain sensitivity of *Trichomonas vaginalis* to metronidazole. *Br J Vener Dis* 1969;45:161–162.
87. Nielsen R. *Trichomonas vaginalis.* II. Laboratory investigations in trichomonas. *Br J Vener Dis* 1973;49:531–535.
88. Ralph ED, Darwish R, Austin TW, et al. Susceptibility of *Trichomonas vaginalis* strains to metronidazole: response to treatment. *Sex Transm Dis* 1983;10:119–122.
89. Robinson SC. *Trichomonal vaginitis* resistant to metronidazole. *Can Med Assoc J* 1992;86:665.
90. Pereyra AJ, Lansing JD. Urogenital trichomoniasis: treatment with metronidazole in 2,002 incarcerated women. *Obstet Gynecol* 1964;24:499–508.
91. Lossick JG, Muller M, Gorrell TE. In vitro drug susceptibility and doses of metronidazole required for cure in cases if refractory vaginal trichomoniasis. *J Infect Dis* 1986;153:948–955.
92. Forsgren A, Forssman L. Metronidazole-resistant *Trichomonas vaginalis. Br J Vener Dis* 1979;55: 351–353.
93. Kulda J, Vojtechovska M, Tachezy J, et al. Metronidazole resistance of *Trichomonas vaginalis* as a cause of treatment failure in trichomoniasis—a case report. *Br J Vener Dis* 1982;58:394–399.
94. Amon K, Amon I, Muller H. Maternal-fetal passage of metronidazole. In: Hejzlar M, Semonsky M, Masak S, eds. *Advances in antimicrobial antineoplastic chemotherapy,* vol 1. Baltimore: University Park Press, 1972:113–115.
95. Caro-Paton T, Carvajal A, Martin de Diego I, et al. Is metronidazole teratogenic? A meta-analysis. *Br J Clin Pharmacol* 1997;44:179–182.
96. Morgan IFK. Metronidazole treatment in pregnancy. In: Collier PI, ed. *Metronidazole, proceedings.* Geneva, Switzerland and London: Royal Society of Medicine, International Congress and Symposium Series, the Royal Society of Medicine, 1979.
97. Rosa FW, Baum C, Shaw M. Pregnancy outcomes after first-trimester vaginitis drug therapy. *Obstet Gynecol* 1987;69:751–755.
98. Piper JM, Mitchel EF Jr., Ray WA. Prenatal use of metronidazole and birth defects: no association. *Obstet Gynecol* 1993;82:348–352.
99. Heinonen OP, Slone D, Shapiro S. *Birth defects and drugs in pregnancy.* Littleton, MA: Publishing Sciences Group, 1977:296–302.
100. Struthers BJ. Metronidazole appears not to be a human teratogen: review of the literature. *Infect Dis Obstet Gynecol* 1997;5:326–535.
101. Schnell JD. The incidence of vaginal *Candida* and *Trichomonas* infections and treatment of *Trichomonas vaginitis* with clotrimazole. *Postgrad Med* 1974;50(Suppl 1):79–81.
102. Legal HP. The treatment of trichomonas and *Candida vaginitis* with clotrimazole vaginal tablets. *Postgrad Med* 1974;50(Suppl 1):81–83.
103. Lohmeyer H. Treatment of candidiasis and trichomoniasis of the female genital tract. *Postgrad Med* 1974;50(Suppl 1):78–79.
104. Trusell RE, Wilson ME, Longwell FH, et al. Vaginal trichomoniasis: complement fixation, puerperal morbidity, and early infection of newborn infants. *Am J Obstet Gynecol* 1992;44:292–300.
105. Erickson SH, Oppenheim GL, Smith GH. Metronidazole in breast milk. *Obstet Gynecol* 1981;57: 48–50.
106. Pearlman MD, Yasher C, Ernst S, et al. An incremental dosing protocol for women with severe vaginal trichomoniasis and adverse reactions to metronidazole. *Am J Obstet Gynecol* 1996;174:934–936.
107. Mason PR. Trichomoniasis. New ideas on an old disease. *S Afr Med J* 1980;58:857–859.

108. Wallin JE, Thompson SE, Zaidi A, et al. Urethritis in women attending an STD clinic. *Br J Vener Dis* 1981:57:50–54.
109. Mardh PA, Westrom L. Tubal and cervical cultures in acute salpingitis with special reference to *Mycoplasma hominis* and T-strain mycoplasmas. *Br J Vener Dis* 1970;78:269.
110. Keith LG, Berger GS, Edelman DA, et al. On the causation of pelvic inflammatory disease. *Am J Obstet Gynecol* 1984;149:215–224.
111. Honigberg BM. Trichomonads of importance in human medicine. In: Kreier JP, ed. *Parasitic protozoa.* New York: Academic Press, 1978:276–280.
112. Wisdom AR, Dunlap EMC. Trichomoniasis: study of the disease and its treatment in women and men. *Br J Vener Dis* 1965;41:909–916.
113. Rein MF, Muller M. *Trichomonas vaginalis.* In: Holmes KK, Mardh PA, Weisner PH, eds. *Sexually transmitted disease.* New York: McGraw-Hill, 1984:525–536.
114. Frost JK. *Trichomonas vaginalis* and cervical epithelial changes. *Ann N Y Acad Sci* 1962;97: 792–799.
115. Hypes RA, Ladwig PP. Leukocytic clusters on epithelial cells in cervicovaginal smears: a presumptive test for *Trichomonas infection. Am J Clin Pathol* 1956;26:94–97.
116. Kolstad P. The colposcopic picture of *Trichomonas vaginitis. Acta Obstet Gynecol Scand* 1964;43: 388–398.
117. Martens MG, Faro S, Phillips LE, et al. Female genital tract abscess formation in the rat: use of pathogens including enterococci. *J Reprod Med* 1993;38:280–286.
118. Gardner WA Jr., Culberson DE, Benett BD. *Trichomonas vaginalis* in the prostate gland. *Arch Pathol Lab Med* 1986;110:430–432.
119. Naib ZM. Stepping up the search for vaginal pathogens. Symposium. *Contem Obstet Gynecol* 1984; Oct/Dec:139–149, 194–215.
120. Krieger JN, Jenny C, Verdon M, et al. Clinical manifestations of trichomoniasis in men. *Ann Intern Med* 1993;118:844–849.
121. Wolner-Hanssen P, Krieger JN, Stevens CE, et al. Clinical manifestations of vaginal trichomoniasis. *JAMA* 1989;261:571–576.

8

Vulvovaginal Candidiasis

INTRODUCTION

Vulvovaginal candidiasis (VVC) is an ancient disease, but it was not recognized as a microbial disease until 1849. Wilkinson (1) first described the organism from microscopic observations of material obtained from a genital lesion. In the 1930s, two groups of investigators, led by Plass and Hesseltine, linked the fungus to the clinical entity of vulvovaginitis (2,3). In 1937, Hesseltine used Koch's postulates to demonstrate that he could reproduce the disease by inoculating *Candida* in normal, healthy volunteers (4).

VVC is a common problem in women, especially of reproductive age, and it is often misdiagnosed. Often confused with other causes of vaginitis, it is frequently diagnosed when the woman does not have vaginitis or diagnosed via a telephone conversation between the patient and a nurse, nurse practitioner, or physician. It is included in this book not because the author believes it is a sexually transmitted disease (STD) but because antifungal agents are readily accessible, with or without a prescription, and patients often mistake STD symptoms as symptoms of VVC then seek treatment for the wrong condition.

EPIDEMIOLOGY

Approximately 75% of women experience at least one episode of VVC during their reproductive age. It has been reported that 50% of 25-year-old college women have had one documented yeast infection (5). Several reports also suggest that approximately 72% of women have self-reported at least one episode of VVC (2–6). This frequency of VVC raises interesting questions with regard to transmission and acquisition of yeast, as well as the possibility of the yeast being a member of the endogenous vaginal microflora. Therefore, VVC may be the result of a disturbance in the patient's own vaginal ecosystem.

Vaginal colonization with *Candida* is estimated between 10% and 55% in healthy asymptomatic women (7). However, carefully conducted studies place the colonization rate between 15% and 20% (8–10). Asymptomatic colonization in pregnant women ranges between 30% and 40% (10). Interestingly, higher colonization rates are found among women taking oral contraceptive pills (OCPs), in individuals treated for STDs, and in association with taking antibiotics (11–13). Thus, the theory that symptomatic VVC is caused by a disruption of the vaginal ecosystem, resulting in the patient's own endogenous *Candida* becoming activated to cause symptomatic disease, is interesting. It is also estimated that 45% of patients will experience more than one episode of VVC (14). Approximately 5% will be plagued with recurrent VVC, and probably 1% or more will develop chronic and/or persistent VVC.

There appears to be an association between estrogen and the occurrence of, or risk for developing, VVC. Reproductive-age women, women on OCPs, pregnant women, and postmenopausal women on estrogen replacement therapy are at the highest risk for developing VVC. However, the precipitating factor or factors for developing symptomatic VVC are not known. It is also interesting to note that it is during the previously mentioned periods of a woman's life that she is the most sexually active. The role of sexual activity remains controversial, but there does appear to be a relationship between the frequency of sexual activity and the occurrence of VVC (15,16). Transmission of *Candida* via sexual intercourse, as well as other sexual activity, has been demonstrated (17). However, this in itself does not establish VVC as a STD in the same sense as the venereal diseases like gonorrhea. Another mechanism of VVC transmission is oral-genital contact, which can also serve as a risk factor for the development of VVC (18,19).

The epidemiology of VVC remains somewhat clouded because this is not a reportable disease, it is often self-diagnosed or treated without examination of the patient, and it is frequently overlooked and/or misdiagnosed. The importance of understanding the epidemiology is underscored by both the poor results in treating this disease and our understanding of treatment failures, which often result in chronic recurrence or persistent VVC.

MYCOLOGY

Candida and *Torulopsis* belong to a group of yeasts that do not have a sexual stage and are commonly referred to as asporogenous yeast. Therefore, these yeasts are often classified among the "fungi imperfecti." Yeasts, such as *Saccharomyces,* that produce sexual spores are referred to as ascospores and are classified in the group of fungi known as Ascomycetes. The two genera, *Candida* and *Torulopsis,* are distinguished from one another by their ability to produce pseudohyphae and true hyphae (germ tube formation when grown in the presence of serum). *Candida* species typically produce pseudohyphae, which are elongated chains of yeast cells. The asexual yeasts reproduce by forming buds from ovoid blastospores (yeast cells). *Candida* species have the ability to form pseudohyphae, true hyphae, and chlamydospores (Fig. 8-1). Chlamydospores are attached to a blastospore via a suspension cell and may represent a dormant phase of the yeast. They are spherical and contain a double-layered cell wall. The chlamydospores contain all the structural elements to produce a viable organism. *Torulopsis* does not produce pseudohyphae but does produce blastospores (Fig. 8-2).

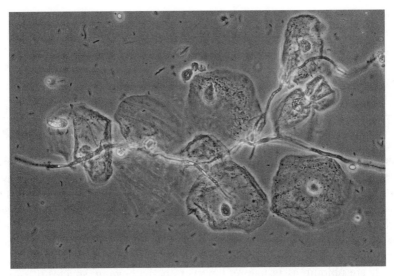

FIG. 8-1. *Candida albicans* hypha associated with squamous cells containing chlamydospores. (See Color Plate 10 following page 148.)

Candida and *Torulopsis* can grow without difficulty at a pH of 3 to 8. Therefore, it is not uncommon to find *Candida* in association with a normal vaginal ecosystem or with bacterial vaginosis (BV), bacterial vaginitis, trichomoniasis, and other STDs.

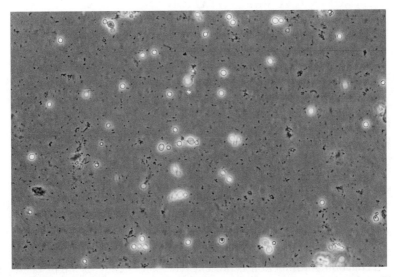

FIG. 8-2. *Candida* (*Torulopsis*) *glabrata*. Note budding cell and no hyphae. (See Color Plate 11 following page 148.)

Candida is a dimorphic yeast. This means that it can either grow as a budding organism or can form pseudohyphae and true hyphae. A blastospore is the unicellular form of the yeast, and it grows by forming buds. The nucleus of the blastospore divides by mitosis and a bud develops in the cell. This is often referred to as the mother cell. The bud is formed by production of both a new cell wall and intracellular constituents. Growth of the budding cell is accompanied by nuclear mitotic division and migration of the nucleus into the bud, creating a daughter cell. The budding process is completed by the development of a septum between the daughter and the mother cell.

The difference between true hyphae and pseudohyphae is that in the former the cell is long and divided by septa containing the fungal elements. The hypha grows at its tip and can give rise to branches. In contrast, a pseudohypha arises from a bud that remains attached to the mother cell. The bud remains elongated and can give rise to another generation of budding cells. The distinguishing characteristic between a true hypha and pseudohypha is that the latter has a constriction at each junction between buds.

Yeasts are ubiquitous in nature; however, the pathogenic species of *Candida* reside within the human host. *Candida* can be recovered from healthy individuals from a variety of sites that include the mouth, feces, vagina, and skin. Because yeasts form part of the normal endogenous microflora of the human, this creates a problem in the management of the patient with VVC, especially the one with recurrent or persistent VVC. When attempting to treat the VVC patient, resolution can be abatement of symptoms, but a mycologic cure may not be achievable.

CLINICAL PRESENTATION AND DIAGNOSIS

The patient with VVC typically presents with vulvovaginal itching. She may also state that she experiences vulvovaginal burning within 24 to 72 hours after sexual intercourse. Her partner may also note transient or persistent burning of the genitalia and pruritus. The patient may complain of a nondescript discomfort in the genitalia with associated swelling of the labia. These symptoms may sound specific, but they are not pathognomonic of VVC.

Clinical examination can reveal a spectrum of presentation from hardly noticeable to severe changes. Typically, the patient may have mild to severe erythema of the external genitalia. Close inspection of the external genitalia may reveal the presence of a white discharge, especially between the labial folds. This discharge is usually thick and easily removed with a cotton-tipped applicator. If yeasts are present, microscopic examination of this discharge will usually reveal fungal elements. In moderate to severe cases, the labia will be swollen and excoriations can be observed.

The vagina can appear erythematous with white discharge, except in cases in which a concomitant infection is present. The consistency of the discharge can range from liquid to thick pastelike discharge, like cottage cheese.

In cases in which no other abnormal condition exists, the pH of the discharge is typically 4.5 or lower. Microscopic analysis can be conducted on either an unaltered specimen of the vaginal discharge diluted with normal saline or by mixing some of the discharge with a drop or two of 10% potassium hydroxide (KOH). The KOH will dissolve almost all other material present in the discharge except the yeasts. This is because of the chitin in the cell walls of the yeast, which is resistant to strong alkali.

Specimens for yeast culture are not usually obtained from patients experiencing their first yeast infection. However, microscopic analysis of the discharge should be conducted because this may be beneficial in determining if the patient's vaginitis is because of a hyphal or budding form. The latter represents *Candida* (*Torulopsis*) *glabrata* and is typically resistant to the standard antifungal medications used to treat vulvovaginal yeast infections.

Specimens for culture are usually obtained from patients with recurrent (more than four) infections during a 12-month period. Identification of the species of yeast causing symptomatic disease may be important because nonalbicans species tend to be resistant to the commonly available antifungal agents used to treat VVC. Determining if the yeast is resistant to those agents may be necessary, but it is rarely done because alternative antifungal agents are used to treat this condition. Culture is important in the patient who presents with symptomatic vaginitis but in whom cause cannot be established. One approach is to obtain a specific culture for yeast in a symptomatic patient whose vaginal pH 4.5 or lower. This pH virtually rules out the presence of BV and other bacterial causes of vaginitis. Patients with a vaginal pH 5 or higher who do not have BV or trichomoniasis should have a culture for both yeast and bacteria. This should be preceded by a microscopic examination of the vaginal discharge. The examination can determine if large bacillary forms are present, indicating the presence or absence of lactobacilli, or if the microflora is dominated by small bacillary forms, like *Escherichia coli,* or cocci, like *Streptococcus agalactiae.* Patients whose pH is 5 or greater and have yeasts identified on microscopic examination of the vaginal discharge should not be considered as solely having yeast vaginitis. This is because the yeasts prefer a pH of 4.5 or less for ideal growth. Therefore, in those instances when the vaginal pH is greater than 4.5 and yeasts are present, the possibility of an associated condition should be sought.

Individuals with recurrent or persistent yeast vaginitis should be screened for diabetes and human immunodeficiency virus (HIV). The patient with diabetes whose blood sugar is not under control will have an elevated glucose concentration in their vagina. Glucose is a carbon source desired by yeasts, and they flourish with an easily accessible source of glucose. Patients who respond to therapy with a typical antifungal but easily relapse should have 3-hour glucose tolerance tests. Patients with a normal 3-hour glucose tolerance test should be tested for HIV. Individuals who have had blood transfusions; who practice high-risk sexual behavior; and who are known to use drugs, including the abuse of alcohol, should be screened for HIV. Individuals taking immunosuppressive drugs are also at risk for recurrent VVC. The yeasts are opportunistic microbes and, therefore, not good competitors. This will become apparent when the host's defenses are significantly weakened.

Once the diagnosis has been established, factors contributing to infection should be considered. Remember the patient may normally be colonized by *Candida;* that is, it may be part of her normal vaginal microflora. There is also a good chance that yeasts make up part of the normal fecal flora, and this may serve as the reservoir for vaginal infection. Another consideration is the male sexual partner. Although the role of sexual transmission has not been clearly established, consideration of its role should be entertained. Spinillo et al. (16) were able to demonstrate a reduction in the recurrence of candidiasis in women whose sexual partners were treated with antifungal agents.

RECURRENT VVC

The patient with recurrent VVC poses a significant problem. If this is her second or third episode of VVC, it should not be thought of as a simple infection. Rather the frequency should signal that this patient might be one of the small number of individuals moving to the group with recurrent, chronic, or persistent disease. The patient with recurrent disease should be thought of as a patient with a complex problem that may involve her vaginal ecology, her local host defense mechanisms, external factors, and her sexual behavior, all of which contribute to recurrent VVC.

When treating a patient with recurrent, chronic, or persistent VVC it is important to consider internal and external factors that may impinge on the patient's risk of experiencing repeated episodes of infection. As stated previously, although sexual transmission remains questionable it must still be considered a possible factor. The reasons that sexual behavior must be considered are (a) an increase in the frequency of VVC coincides with the time women begin having regular sexual intercourse, (b) there may be a relationship between the frequency of coitus and occurrence of VVC, (c) the frequency of oral-genital sex appears to be related to an increase in VVC occurrence, and (d) sexual intercourse is not related to vaginal colonization by *Candida* (20–24). Therefore, the sexual partner should be considered a possible source of reinfection. If the male partner is willing, a culture of the penis surface, especially behind the glans, should be obtained. If the male is not circumcised, strong consideration should be given to his role in reinfecting his partner.

The use of OCPs also appears to increase the woman's risk of acquiring VVC (21,25). Patients taking OCPs containing high doses of estrogen, compared with the lower dose pills, may have a greater risk for developing VVC (25,26). Although sexual intercourse remains a question in regard to transmission of yeasts from one partner to another, when a diaphragm is used with a spermicide there appears to be an increase in the rate of colonization by *Candida* (24). Although an association between spermicide use and VVC has not been found, an association between VVC and the independent use of the vaginal sponge and the intrauterine device has been found (27).

Douching has been hypothesized as a possible factor in the development of pelvic inflammatory disease, but such an association has not been established for VVC (28). However, Spinillo et al. (26) found an association between douching and recurrent episodes of VVC involving *C. glabrata*. However, the use of sanitary napkins and tampons do not appear to be associated with an increased risk of developing VVC (5,28). Much has been said about the wearing of tight-fitting undergarments, especially noncotton ones, and pants as risk factors for developing VVC, but no scientific data is available to substantiate this anecdotal information.

Concerning risk factors, another popular issue is antibiotics and an increased risk of developing VVC. There is no doubt that some women do develop symptomatic VVC during, or following, the use of antibiotics. This is true whether they have received oral, intravenous, or intravaginal antibiotics. It appears that any agent that can affect the balance of the vaginal microflora has the potential to precipitate VVC. This is an interesting observation because it implies that the yeasts are, most likely, already present in the vaginal ecosystem. A situation in which the ecosystem is in balance and then subjected to the pressure of an agent that has antimicrobial activity, but not antifungal activity, can provide a noncompetitive environment for the yeasts and they can then flourish.

An area that has received a great amount of attention, especially in the lay literature, is the link to dietary factors. However, most scientific studies have failed to demonstrate that either dietary excesses or deficiencies have any role in the cause of VVC. The relationship between dietary factors and VVC probably stems from the fact that diabetics, especially those with poor glucose control, commonly develop symptomatic VVC. Although the pathophysiology of VVC in this setting has not been explained, a possible explanation may reside in a deficiency in the vaginal immunologic system.

Thus, the pathophysiology of recurrent VVC remains unclear. Additional research is required to develop an understanding of the role of *Candida* as a member of the normal endogenous vaginal microflora. Currently, factors that can permit *Candida* to overcome the potential antagonistic agents produced by coinhabiting microorganisms are unknown. In addition, the mechanism(s) involved in converting asymptomatic colonization to a symptomatic state are not understood.

TREATMENT

Treatment modalities were initially offered to relieve the symptoms associated with VVC. Hippocrates, Galen, and Pepys were the first to describe what were probably cases of VVC (29–31). In 1792, Frank offered the first written description of VVC (31). These four individuals raised awareness of this malady, and therapeutic attempts were made with aqueous solutions of gentian violet, crystal violet, and brilliant green. This was followed by chemical treatment with agents such as boric acid and dequalinium chloride. In the last 50 years, and more recently, interest in developing antifungal agents has proceeded at a fairly rapid pace. This is especially true since the HIV and AIDS epidemic has come to the forefront throughout the world. This immunosuppressive condition permitted fungi to emerge as common causes of disease.

Nystatin, the first polyene antifungal agent, was approved in the United States in 1955. Nystatin vaginal tablets frequently were used to treat vaginal candidiasis. This agent has a "cure" rate between 70% and 80%. Nystatin and other polyenes interfere with the permeability of the fungal membranes by binding with sterols, especially ergosterol, in the cell membranes. Nystatin does not affect mammalian cellular membranes because they lack ergosterol and contain cholesterol instead.

Azoles were developed and first became available in the 1960s. Since then, a variety of azoles have been developed (Table 8-1). The azoles are divided into two groups of agents, the imidazoles and triazoles. The latter is considered to have a broader spectrum of activity than the imidazoles (Table 8-2). Azoles act by binding with the fungal hemoprotein enzyme cytochrome P-450. The triazoles appear to be more potent than the imidazoles because they bind more efficiently with cytochrome P-450 in the fungal cell wall than the imidazoles (29). Although these agents can affect mammalian cytochrome P-450, the concentration required is much higher than that achieved with the usual dosing of the triazoles. Thus, triazoles and imidazoles act by binding to cytochrome P-450 inhibiting the synthesis of ergosterol, which is an essential constituent in the fungal hyphal wall. This process interferes with chitin synthesis, the carbohydrate polymer that is the main structural component of the hyphal wall, thus resulting in gaps or holes in the fungal cell wall.

Other agents used in the treatment of VVC are flucytosine and boric acid. The fluorinated pyrimidine flucytosine, an anticancer drug not particularly effective as an antineoplastic agent, has been used to treat chronic and/or persistent VVC. It is well absorbed through the gastrointestinal tract and, therefore, can be used to treat systematic candidiasis. This agent has not been widely used because the

TABLE 8-1. *Antifungal agents*

Imidazoles
    Butoconazole vaginal cream—Femstat
    Butoconazole 2% vaginal emulsion—Gynazol-1
    Clotrimazole vaginal cream, vaginal tablets—Gyne-Lotrimin
    Miconazole vaginal cream, vaginal suppository, IV—Monistat
    Tioconazole vaginal ointment—Monistat-1
    Ketoconazole tablets—Nizoral
Triazoles
    Terconazole vaginal cream, vaginal suppositories—Terazol
    Itraconazole capsules—Sporanox
    Fluconazole tablets—Diflucan

TABLE 8-2. *Adverse effects of imidazoles*

Flu-like syndrome
Temperature elevation
Inflammation of the vulva and vagina
Vulvovaginal burning and pruritus
Headache
Myalgias
Dysmenorrhea
Abdominal pain

organism develops resistance to flucytosine rather easily. Flucytosine is typically administered both orally and intravenously, but intravaginal use has been successful (30). Flucytosine activity requires that the drug be actively transported into the fungal cell via cytosine permease. Flucytosine is converted to 5-fluorouracil by cytosine deaminase and is subsequently phosphorylated to 5-FU monophosphate. This phosphorylated compound can then be incorporated into ribonucleic acid (RNA) or converted to 5-fluorodeoxyuridine monophosphate, which can inhibit thymidylate synthetase, in turn preventing deoxyribonucleic acid (DNA) synthesis (31).

Although all these agents have been fairly effective in treating uncomplicated, nonrecurrent VVC, patients suffering with recurrent, chronic, or persistent VVC have not been as fortunate. The latter patients appear to have a complex condition and treatment may well be based on developing an understanding of the organism, the vaginal environment, and the antifungal agent. It is not uncommon to suspect that the patient has resistant yeast, but when antifungal sensitivities are carried out in the laboratory, the yeast is found to be sensitive to the agents. Thus, a factor affecting the efficacy of the drug comes into play. When the antifungal agent is placed in the vaginal environment, a reduction in the bioavailability of the drug may occur; a decrease in permeability may be present because of competing or blocking substances in the vagina; or the drug may be inactivated, to a significant degree, by the vaginal environment.

Studies conducted in patients with complicated VVC found that patients had a better response rate when treatment was extended to 14 days, instead of the conventional dosage regimens (32,33). Once the initial episode is resolved, these patients should be placed on suppressive therapy for a prolonged period. Suppressive therapy is indicated because the patients suffering from recurrent disease are probably not being reinfected but are experiencing relapses of their original condition because of host factors. This hypothesis fits the theory that this condition is more likely the result of an imbalance in the patient's vaginal ecosystem, and suppression of the yeast allows the ecologic system to regain balance.

Several possible regimens can be used to suppress the vaginal yeasts. These regimens include fluconazole 150 mg weekly for 6 weeks or 100 mg weekly for 6 months, ketoconazole 100 mg daily for 6 months, itraconazole 50-100 mg daily for 6 months, and clotrimazole 500 mg vaginal suppositories weekly for 6 months (33–35). Recurrences following suppressive therapy are high, in the range of 30% to 40%. Thus, a patient off suppressive therapy who develops symptoms of vaginitis should be seen and evaluated. Therapy should not be instituted without a thorough evaluation. A culture should be obtained to determine if it is the same species that caused the previous VVC episode. If it is present, isolation of the patient's endogenous *Lactobacillus* should be accomplished to determine if it is a healthy species, that is a species that produces hydrogen peroxide and bacteriocin. Although limited, there is data that suggest women with recurrent VVC may also have a deficiency in healthy lactobacilli that may contribute to their chronic VVC (36).

The nonalbicans species of *Candida* tend to have higher minimum inhibitory concentrations (MICs) to the available imidazoles and triazoles but are still sensitive. However, the concentration of these agents, when applied as intravaginal products, is much higher than the MICs required. Although there appears to be an increase in the number of nonalbicans species causing VVC, this increase still must be established. Thus, treatment should be successful if therapy is prolonged at least 14 days. The approach one can take is to initiate treatment with an available agent such as terconazole, butoconazole (2%), or fluconazole. If this fails, treatment with intravaginal boric acid gelatin capsules or suppositories (600 mg) twice a day for 10 days is recommended (37).

VVC IN THE PREGNANT PATIENT

VVC is common in pregnancy, occurring in 10% to 20% of pregnant women. Although VVC usually remains a localized infection, it can ascend into the intrauterine cavity resulting in chorioamnionitis, intraamniotic infection, placentitis, funisitis, and maternal infection. Postpartum endometritis and sepsis resulting from *Candida,* although uncommon, have also been reported (38–44).

VVC should be treated with intravaginal antifungal agents and the patient should be reevaluated following completion to determine if the treatment was efficacious. Miconazole, terconazole, and probably other azoles are safe to use in the pregnant patient. However, the oral agents should not be administered to pregnant or breast-feeding mothers.

REFERENCES

1. Wilkinson JS. The development of epiphytes. *Lancet* 1849;2:448–451.
2. Plass ED, Hesseltine HC, Borts IH. Monilia vulvovaginitis. *Am J Obstet Gynecol* 1931;21:320–324.
3. Hesseltine HC, Borts IH, Plass ED. Pathogenicity of the *Monilia* (Castellani), vaginitis and oral thrush. *Am J Obstet Gynecol* 1934;27:112–115.
4. Hurely R, Delouvois J. *Candida* vaginitis. *Postgrad Med* J 1979;55:645–647.
5. Geiger AM, Foxman B. Risk factors in vulvovaginal candidiasis: a case-control study among college students. *Epidemiology* 1996;7:182–187.
6. Horowitz B. Edelstein SW, Lippman L. Sexual transmission of *Candida. Obstet Gynecol* 1987;69: 883–886.

7. Drake TE, Maibach HI. *Candida* and candidiasis: cultural conditions, epidemiology, and pathogenesis. *Postgrad Med* 1973;53:83.
8. Fleury FJ. Recurrent *Candida* vulvovaginitis. *Chemotherapy* 1982;28(Suppl):48–52.
9. Odds FC. Genital candidosis. *Clin Exp Dermatol* 1982;7:345–349.
10. Odds FC. *Candida and candidosis*. Baltimore: University Park Press, 1979.
11. Oriel JD, Partridge BM, Denny MJ, et al. Genital yeast infections. *Br Med J* 1972;4:761–764.
12. Caruso LJ. Vaginal moniliasis after tetracycline therapy. *Am J Obstet Gynecol* 1964;90:374–377.
13. Oriel JD, Waterworth PM. Effect of minocycline and tetracycline on the vaginal yeast flora. *J Clin Pathol* 1975;28:403–406.
14. Hurley R. Inveterate vaginal thrush. *Practitioner* 1975;215:753–757.
15. Geiger AM, Foxman B. Risk factors in vulvovaginal candidiasis: a case-control study among college students. *Epidemiology* 1996;55:645–647.
16. Spinillo A, Carrata L, Pizzoli G. Recurrent vulvovaginal candidiasis: results of a cohort study of sexual transmission and internal reservoir. *J Reprod Med* 1992;l37:343–347.
17. Horowitz B, Edelstein SW, Lippman L. Sexual transmission of *Candida. Obstet Gynecol* 1987;60: 883–886.
18. Hellburg D, Zdolsek B, Nilsson S, et al. Sexual behavior in women with repeated bouts of vulvovaginal candidiasis. *Eur J Epidemiol* 1995;11:575–579.
19. Hooten TM, Roberts PL, Stamm WE. Effect of recent sexual activity and use of diaphragm on vaginal flora. *Clin Infect Dis* 1994;19:274–278.
20. Fidel PJ Jr, Sobel JD. Immunopathogenesis of recurrent vulvovaginal candidiasis. *Clin Micro Rev* 1996;9:335–348.
21. Geiger AM, Foxman B. Risk factors in vulvovaginal candidiasis: a case-control study among college students. *Epidemiology* 1996;7:182–187.
22. Hellburg D, Zdolsek B, Nilsson S, et al. Sexual behavior in women with repeated bouts of vulvovaginal candidiasis. *Eur J Epidemiol* 1995;11:575–579.
23. Foxman B. Epidemiology of vulvovaginal candidiasis: risk factors. *Am J Public Health* 1990;80: 329–331.
24. Hooten TM, Roberts PL, Stamm WE. Effect of recent sexual activity and use of diaphragm on vaginal flora. *Clin Infect Dis* 1994;19:274–278.
25. Spinillo A, Capuzzo F, Nicola S, et al. The impact of oral contraception on vulvovaginal candidiasis. *Contraception* 1995;51:293–297.
26. Spinillo A, Capuzzo E, Egbe TO, et al. *Torulopsis glabrata* vaginitis. *Obstet Gynecol* 1995;85: 993–998.
27. Barbone F, Austin H, Louv WC, et al. A follow-up study of methods of contraception, sexual activity and rates of trichomoniasis, candidiasis, and bacterial vaginosis. *Am J Obstet Gynecol* 1990;163: 510–514.
28. Reed BD. Risk factors for *Candida* vulvovaginitis. *Obstet Gynecol Surv* 1992;47:551–560.
29. Cauwenbergh G, Vanden Bossche H. Terconazole, pharmacology of a new agent with antibacterial activity. *Chemotherapy* 1972;17:392–404.
30. Horowitz, BJ, Edelstein SW, Lippman L. *Candida tropicalis* vulvovaginitis. *Obstet Gynecol* 1985;66: 229–232.
31. Kent HL. New therapy for vulvovaginal candidiasis. In: Horowitz BJ, Mardh P-A, ed. *Vaginitis and vaginosis*. New York: Wiley-Liss, 1991:257–268.
32. Sobel JD, Brooker D, Stein GE, et al. Single dose fluconazole compared with conventional topical therapy of *Candida* vaginitis. *Am J Obstet Gynecol* 1995;172:1263–1268.
33. Sobel JD. Recurrent vulvovaginal candidiasis. A prospective study of the efficacy of maintenance ketoconazole therapy. *N Engl J Med* 1986;315:1455–1458.
34. Reef S, Levine WC, McNeil MM, et al. Treatment options for vulvovaginal candidiasis background paper for development of 1993 STD treatment recommendations. *Clin Infect Dis* 1995;20(Suppl): 580–590.
35. Sobel JD. Treatment of recurrent vulvovaginal candidiasis with maintenance fluconazole. *Int J Gynecol Obstet* 1992;37:17–34.
36. Hawes SE, Hillier SL, Beneditti J, et al. Hydrogen peroxide produced lactobacilli and acquisition of vaginal infections. *J Infect Dis* 1996;174:1058–1063.
37. Sobel JD, Chaim W. Treatment of *Candida glabrata* vaginitis: a retrospective review of boric acid therapy. *Clin Infect Dis* 1997;24:649–652.
38. Svensson L, Ingemarsson I, Mardh P. Chorioamnionitis and the isolation of microorganisms from the placenta. *Obstet Gynecol* 1986;67:403–409.

39. Plotkin SA. Routes of fetal infection and mechanisms of fetal damage. *Am J Dis Child* 1975;129: 444–449.
40. Benirschke K, Raphael SI. *Candida albicans* infection of the amniotic sac. *Am J Obstet Gynecol* 1958;75:200–202.
41. Van Winter JT, Ney JA, Ogburn PL Jr, et al. Preterm labor and congenital candidiasis. A case report. *J Reprod Med* 1994;39:987–990.
42. Bruner JP, Elliott JP, Kilbride HW, et al. *Candida* chorioamnionitis diagnosed by amniocentesis with subsequent fetal infection. *Am J Perinatol* 1986;3:213–218.
43. Romero R, Reece EA, Duff GW, et al. Prenatal diagnosis of *Candida albicans* chorioamnionitis. *Am J Perinatol* 1985;2:121–122.
44. Berry DL, Olson GL, Wen TS, et al. *Candida* chorioamnionitis: a report of two cases. *J Mat Fetal Med* 1997;6:151–154.

9

Herpes Simplex

INTRODUCTION

Herpes simplex virus (HSV) is one of the more common sexually transmitted diseases (STDs), only superseded by the human papillomavirus in prevalence. Although HSV was a focus of interest through the 1970s and 1980s, interest has waned in the 1990s because of *Chlamydia trachomatis* and human immunodeficiency virus (HIV), but it is still a common STD causing significant morbidity. The infection also has significant effect on human relationships, pregnancy, and pregnancy outcomes. The fact that HSV infection continues to maintain a position of significance is bolstered by the pharmaceutical industry's continued effort to develop new antiviral agents for the treatment of HSV infection, as well as the development of a vaccine. There continues to be not only difficulty in identifying HSV genital infection but also problems in prescribing appropriate management for both the nonpregnant and pregnant patient.

EPIDEMIOLOGY

HSV was first described in 1736, but the mechanism of transmission was not postulated until the late nineteenth and early twentieth centuries by French and German investigators (1). However, this hypothesis was not widely accepted. In the 1960s, isolation and differentiation of the types of HSV established that HSV-2 was the major cause of genital herpes (1,2). The human is the only natural host of HSV-1 and HSV-2. Therefore, the reservoir is the infected individual, and she is typically asymptomatic. HSV has a unique life cycle; after an incubation period of 3 to 9 days, the initial infection can be followed by the development of numerous lesions at the site of infection. In addition, the organism can assume a latent state. This state of latency following symptomatic or asymptomatic initial infection is a unique and important feature of HSV infection.

HSV-1 and HSV-2 infection can result in a variety of clinical presentations, and each has a distinct epidemiology. Kaposi's varicelliform eruption is seen in individuals with chronic skin disease like atopic eczema or Darier's disease (3–5). Health care professionals frequently develop HSV infection on their fingers (e.g., herpetic whitlow) (6,7), and wrestlers develop a HSV infection referred to as herpes gladiatorum (8,9). Disseminated HSV infection can result in meningitis, which is most frequently seen in young adults (10–13). Most HSV-1 infection results in oral-pharyngeal infections, and HSV-2 infection results in genital disease. However, depending on the sexual practices of the individual, HSV-1 can cause genital infection, and HSV-2 can result in oral infection.

HSV infection is a worldwide problem, and all sexually active individuals are at risk. The risk of acquiring HSV is dependent on the sexual practices of the individual. Individuals at greatest risk are those that have multiple sexual partners. It must be remembered that this infection is for a lifetime, and transmission is a constant concern because the symptomatic patient is capable of transmitting the virus. In a study of more than 5,000 adults, a history of genital herpes was obtained in 25% of Caucasians and in 14% of African Americans (14). Among this group of individuals with a history of genital herpes, 26% of Caucasians and 12% of African Americans did not have antibodies to HSV-2 (14). In a study conducted in the Netherlands, patients were seen by general practitioners, gynecologists, dermatologists, and urologists (15). The most common STD was *C. trachomatis* (46%), followed by condylomata acuminata (28%), genital herpes (17%), and gonorrhea (8%) (15). 2,730 STD cases were reported for a prevalence of 32/10,000 of the population.

Women are more likely to acquire genital herpes than men are. In one study of 95 women who had antibodies to HSV-2, 47 (49%) male partners were also positive; in the males positive for HSV-2 antibodies, 47 (77%) of the female partners were positive (16). In a study of 144 couples, transmission of males to females was 45%, and the rate from females to males was 19% (17). The greater surface area of the endocervical columnar epithelium present on the portio of the cervix in reproductive-aged women, compared with the limited exposure of the urethral epithelium of the male penis, is responsible for this greater propensity for acquisition of STDs in general.

Transmission of HSV-2 among asymptomatic shedders is more likely than among individuals with symptomatic disease. This is because individuals with symptomatic disease are less likely to engage in sexual intercourse. Acquisition is also likely to occur via breaks in the epithelium that are likely during the trauma associated with sexual intercourse. This accounts for the lesion developing in the epithelium of the labia majora, perineum, and perianal area. The presence of lesions on areas of the body, other than the vaginal epithelium and cervix, accounts for the limited effectiveness of condoms in preventing the transmission of herpes.

Genital herpes is a common infection among individuals with acquired immunodeficiency syndrome (AIDS). Recurrence rates in the HIV patient are eight times higher than in the HSV patient who is HIV negative (18). Among the HIV-positive patients, the recurrences appear to be subclinical, and this accounts for a greater risk of HSV-2 transmission between partners. Approximately ⅓ of HIV patients with HSV may have visible lesions when experiencing a recur-

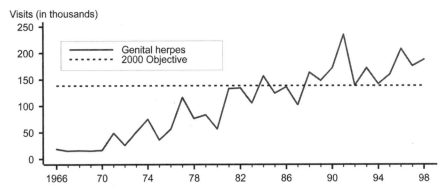

FIG. 9-1. Genital herpes simplex virus infections—initial visits to physicians' offices in the United States from 1966 to 1998 and the Healthy People year 2000 objective. (From *Sexually Transmitted Disease Surveillance, 1998,* U.S. Department of Health and Human Services, Centers for Disease Control, Atlanta, GA, with permission.)

rence. HSV-2 can be isolated from these individuals in the absence of identifiable ulcers (14). There appears to be a synergistic relationship between these two viruses. It is believed that HSV infection upregulates expression of HIV and increases the viral load of HIV associated with HSV recurrences (18,19). The individual who is both HSV-2 and HIV positive with microulcerations or breaks in the skin serves as a transmitter of both infections.

Thus, herpes simplex infection of the genitalia continues to be a significant problem not only in its own right but also as an enhancer of transmitting and acquiring other STDs. The number of genital herpes cases continues to rise (Fig. 9-1). In addition, the number of asymptomatic seropositive cases also appears to be increasing (Fig. 9-2). Awareness on the part of the patients and physicians is extremely important if this disease is to be curtailed.

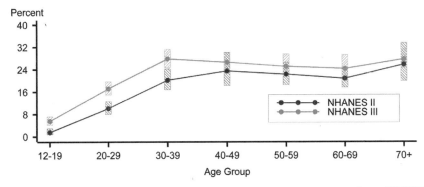

FIG. 9-2. Genital herpes simplex virus type 2—percent seroprevalence according to NHANES* II (1976 to 1980) and NHANES III (1988 to 1994). *NHANES, National Health and Nutrition Examination Survey. (From *Sexually Transmitted Disease Surveillance, 1998,* U.S. Department of Health and Human Services, Centers for Disease Control, Atlanta, GA, with permission.)

VIROLOGY

Herpes simplex types 1 and 2 belong to the genus Simplexvirus in the family Herpesviridae and the subfamily Alphaherpesvirinae. The deoxyribonucleic acid (DNA) of HSV-1 and HSV-2 is similar because they share a significant amount of sequence homology and genome colinearity. Genomic recombination between the two types has been documented (20–23). Although there are genetic similarities between HSV-1 and HSV-2, there are significant differences between the two viruses.

The virus (virion) contains a central DNA core surrounded by an icosahedral protein capsid. The capsid is surrounded by an amorphous protein layer, referred to as the tegument, which is enclosed in a lipid layer. The outer surface of this lipid layer contains glycoproteins (24). At least 11 glycoproteins on the surface of the virus form spikes on the surface. The lipid forming the envelope of the virus is derived from the host cell membrane through budding when the virion is liberated from the infected host cell.

When the virus encounters a susceptible host cell, it attaches to a receptor on the surface of that cell. The viral glycoproteins (gB and gC) bind to heparin sulfate on the host cell receptor. It is believed that this initial binding stimulates further binding to specific proteins activating fusion between the viral envelope and the host cell plasma membrane. This fusion between the viral capsid and host cell membrane results in the formation of a single unit permitting the virus (capsid and tegument) to enter the host cell (Fig. 9-3) (24). The nucleocapsid is carried to the host cell nuclear membrane and the viral DNA enters the host cell nucleus through a pore in the nuclear membrane. The viral DNA is transcribed, in the infected host cell nucleus, by the host ribonucleic acid (RNA) polymerase II permitting expression of the viral genome (24).

The viral genome is divided into three groupings: immediate early, early, and late genes. Early viral genes require prior viral protein synthesis but do not require viral DNA synthesis. Once the virus enters the host cell, there are at least 70 viral proteins expressed, many that are involved in the regulation of gene expression (25). Within 4 hours of infection, the viral immediate early genes responsible for expression of early and late genes are expressed. The immediate early genes ICP4, ICP0, ICP27, ICP22, and ICP47 play a role in expression of all viral genes (26–29). ICP4 is required for expression of all early genes. ICP27 also plays a role in expression of early genes and in several DNA replication proteins (30). An increase in transcription of late genes occurs following completion of viral DNA replication. Once this is complete and the late genes have achieved maximum expression, the viral capsids are formed. The viral DNA is packed into the capsids in the nucleus of the infected cells. Tegument proteins bind to the capsids containing the viral DNA, and this particle binds to the inner membrane of the nuclear envelope (31,32). The actual mechanism by which the virions are released from the infected host cell has not been uncovered. There are two hypotheses. The first hypothesis is that the capsid, enveloped by the host cell inner nuclear membrane, is de-enveloped at the outer nuclear membrane or

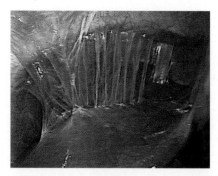

Color Plate 1. Curtis-Fitz-Hugh syndrome. Notice violin-string adhesions from liver capsules to abdominal wall and note liver in the bottom of the image. (See Figure 3-10.)

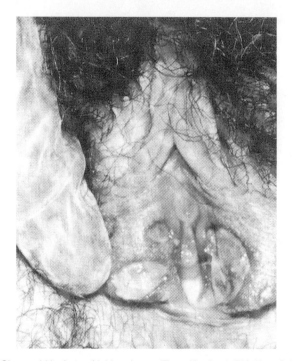

Color Plate 2. Chancroid lesions of labia minora. (From Kaufman RH, Faro S, Friedrich EG Jr, et al. *Benign diseases of the vulva and vagina,* 4th ed. St. Louis: Mosby, 1994, with permission.) (See Figure 4-1.)

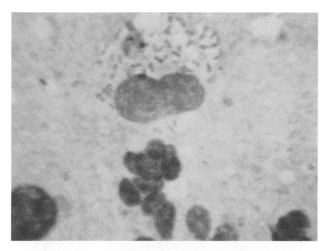

Color Plate 3. Donovan bodies contained within vacuoles of a mononuclear cell. Note the bipolar staining, which is typical of *Calymmatobacterium granuloma.*(See Figure 5-1.)

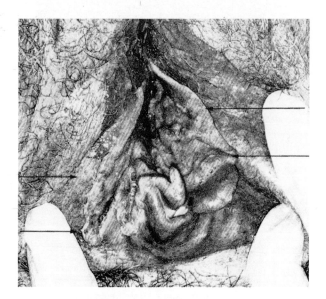

Color Plate 4. Granuloma inguinale large granular, raised ulceration involving extensive areas of the vulva. This lesion has been mistaken for carcinoma of the vulva. (From Kaufman RH, Faro S. *Benign diseases of the vulva and vagina,* 4th ed. St. Louis: Mosby, 1994:62, Figure 5.9 on page 71, with permission.) (See Figure 5-2.)

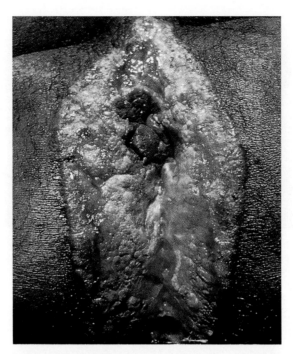

Color Plate 5. Granuloma inguinale large ulceration involving an extensive area in the perianal region. This lesion, most likely, arose by autoinoculation of adjacent areas and coalescence of these lesions. The base is beefy red and friable. (From Lambert HP, Farrar WE. *Infectious disease illustrated. An integrated text and color atlas.* Philadelphia: WB Saunders and London, New York: Gower Medical Publishing, 1982:23, Figure 9.54, with permission.) (See Figure 5-3.)

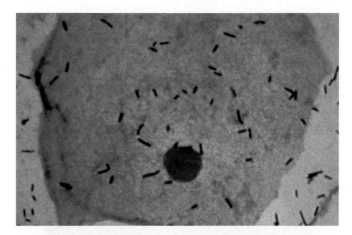

Color Plate 6. Gram stain representation of a healthy vaginal ecosystem. Note: the squamous epithelia cell is well estrogenized, and the dominant bacterium is large gram-positive rods. There is a noticeable absence of other bacteria and white blood cells. (See Figure 6-1.)

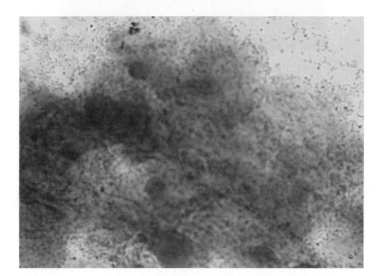

Color Plate 7. Gram stain of vaginal discharge: clue cells. Note: the squamous epithelial cells are obliterated by densely adhering gram-negative rods (*Gardnerella vaginalis*). There are numerous individual free-floating bacteria in the vaginal discharge. There is a noticeable absence of white blood cells. (See Figure 6-3.)

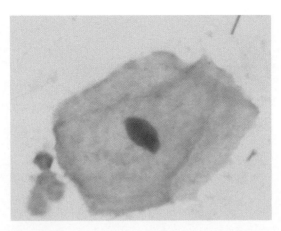

Color Plate 8. Gram stain of vaginal discharge following treatment of a patient with bacterial vaginosis. Note the following: (a) clue cells are absent, (b) a well-estrogenized squamous epithelial cell without adherent bacteria is present, (c) two white blood cells are present, and (d) the dominant bacteria are large gram-positive bacilli consistent with *Lactobacillus*. (See Figure 6-4.)

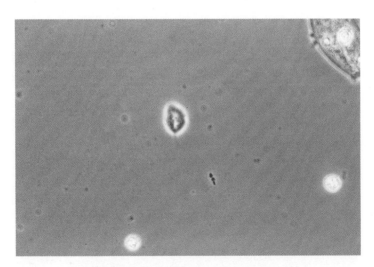

Color Plate 9. Trichomonas. (See Figure 7-1.)

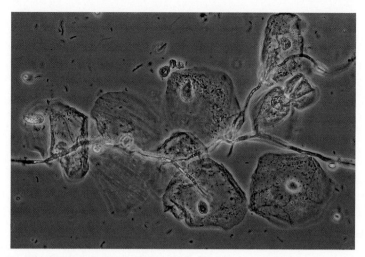

Color Plate 10. *Candida albicans* hypha associated with squamous cells containing chlamydospores. (See Figure 8-1.)

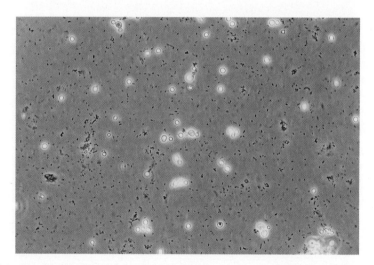

Color Plate 11. *Candida* (*Torulopsis*) *glabrata*. Note budding cell and no hyphae. (See Figure 8-2.)

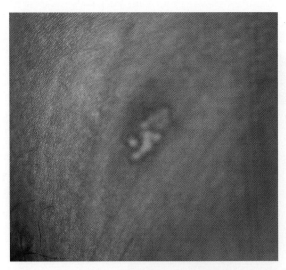

Color Plate 12. Primary herpes with edema of the vulva and a frothy discharge. Patient was found to be positive for *Neisseria gonorrhoeae* and trichomoniasis. (See Figure 9-6.)

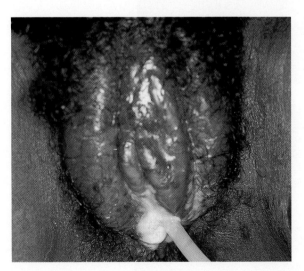

Color Plate 13. Demonstration of purulent herpetic vesicles that are not secondarily infected. (See Figure 9-7.)

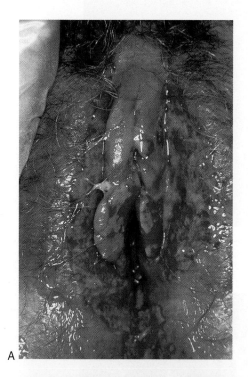

A

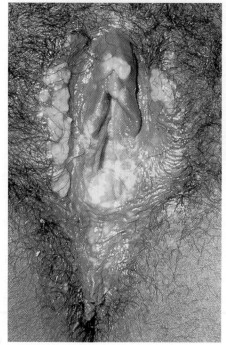

B

Color Plate 14. A: Herpetic ulcers. **B:** Demonstration of herpetic ulcerations that are secondarily infected as noted by purulent exudate covering the ulceration. Obtaining specimen for herpes culture from such a lesion, without removing the purulent exudate, would likely result in a negative culture for herpes. (See Figure 9-8.)

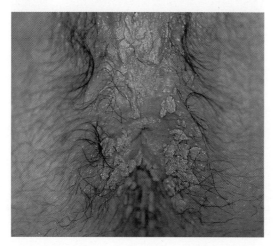

Color Plate 15. Typical lesions of condyloma acuminata. (See Figure 10-2.)

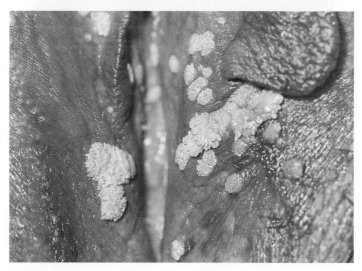

Color Plate 16. Note that the condyloma can form individual lesions or form small and large aggregates. (See Figure 10-3.)

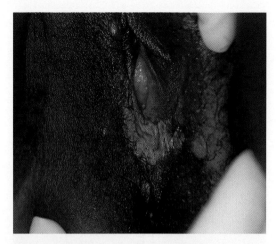

Color Plate 17. Lesions can be distributed over the vulva, the labia majora, and labia minora. These lesions appear gray in color and are dry, in contrast to those in Fig. 10-4, which are white and moist. (See Figure 10-4.)

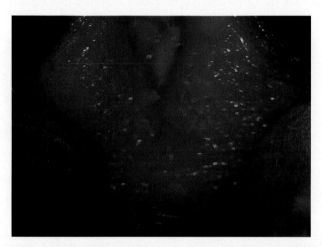

Color Plate 18. Condyloma appear as papillary projections. Although it cannot be seen in this photograph, when the papillary structures are viewed through a colposcope, the vascularity of the lesion can be seen. (See Figure 10-5.)

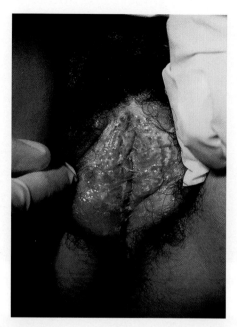

Color Plate 19. The condyloma lesions have to form two large flat moist lesions on the inner aspect of the labia minora. The lesions although flat do not have a waxy appearance and should not be confused with condyloma lata. (See Figure 10-6.)

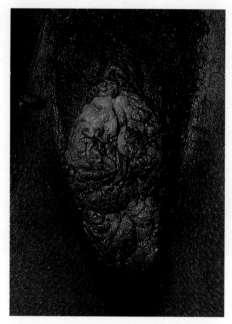

Color Plate 20. The condyloma has replaced almost the entire labia minora and appears brain-like. (See Figure 10-7.)

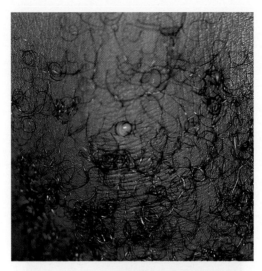

Color Plate 21. Spontaneous rupture of a papule with drainage of thick pus. (See Figure 12-1.)

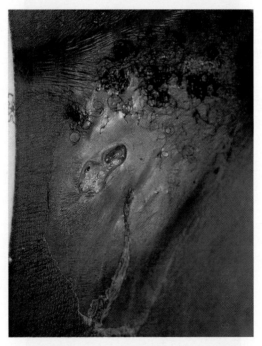

Color Plate 22. Ulceration of bubo. (See Figure 12-2.)

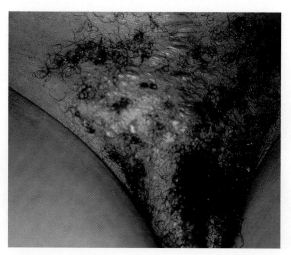

Color Plate 23. Grove sign. Enlargement of inguinal and femoral lymphonodes separated by inguinal ligament. (See Figure 12-3.)

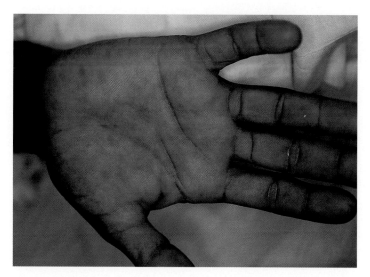

Color Plate 24. Maculopapular rash on the palms of the hand in a patient with secondary syphilis. (See Figure 13-5.)

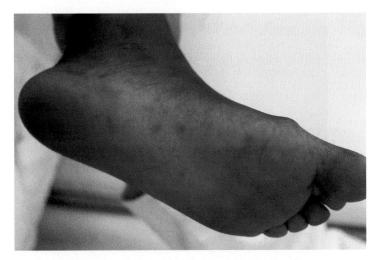

Color Plate 25. Maculopapular rash on the sole of the foot of a patient with secondary syphilis. (See Figure 13-6.)

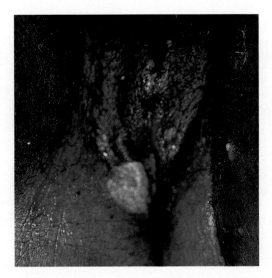

Color Plate 26. Chancre on the inferior aspect of labia in a patient with secondary syphilis. (See Figure 13-7.)

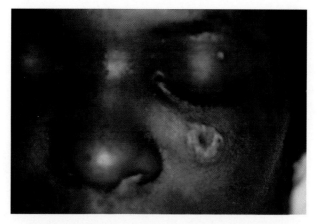

Color Plate 27. Chancre of secondary syphilis occurring on the face of the patient. Lesion is secondarily infected. (See Figure 13-8.)

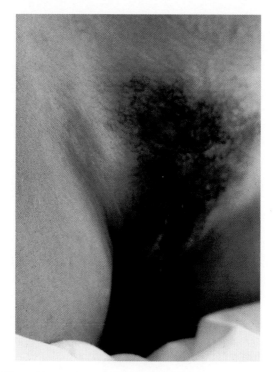

Color Plate 28. Bilateral inguinal adenopathy of patient with secondary syphilis. Patient had temperature of 102°F and a VDRL of 1:128. (See Figure 13-9.)

... .

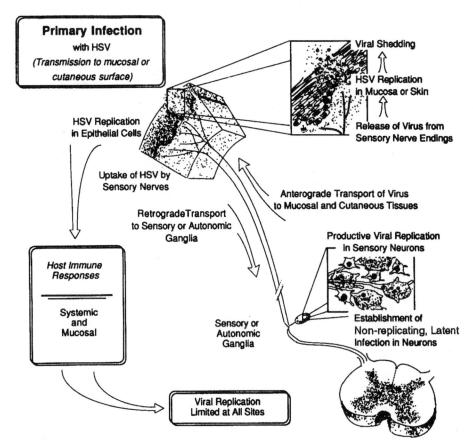

FIG. 9-3. Diagrammatic representation of herpes simplex virus primary infection. (From Stanberry LR. The pathogenesis of herpes simplex virus infections. In: Stanberry LR, ed. *Genital and neonatal herpes.* New York: John Wiley and Sons, 1996:32, with permission.)

endoplasmic reticulum and extruded into the cytoplasm. The Golgi membrane apparatus engulfs the virion and through this membrane channel the virion is brought to the cell surface cytoplasmic membrane (33–35). An alternate hypothesis differs in that once the capsid is enveloped in the host inner nuclear membrane it is not de-enveloped but buds from the outer nuclear membrane and is transported to the Golgi apparatus.

PATHOGENESIS

The herpes virus enters the host through contact with a susceptible site on the host. The most common site for HSV-2 infection is the genitalia. Individuals with oral HSV-1 infection who engage in oral sex can transmit oral HSV-1 infection to the genitalia. Individuals with an active lesion caused by HSV-2 genital disease, who participate in oral sex, can communicate HSV-2 to the oral mucosa. The virus attaches to the host cell via HSV glycoproteins, gB and gC, binding to heparin sulfate proteoglycans on the host cell membrane (34–37). The viral envelope fuses with the host cell membrane permitting the virus entry into the host cell. The virus is transported to the host cell nucleus and simultaneously infects sensory nerve endings present in the genital tract. Once in the sensory nerve endings, the virus travels along the axon to the spinal sensory ganglia (38,39). The difference between replication in epithelial cells and nerve cells is that in the latter the virus requires viral thymidine kinase (40). Replication of the virus in the nerve cells is incomplete. The virus is transported unenveloped along unmyelinated C-type sensory nerve fibers to the distal regions of the axon. Final assembly of the virus occurs just before release from the sensory nerve endings (41). When the virus is released, the neuron dies and the virus enters mucosal and epithelial cells to further replicate (Fig. 9-3). During primary and initial infection, the viral infection results in numerous lesions distributed over the vulva, perineum, perianal area, and buttocks because of the highly branched sensory neurons.

Not all individuals exposed to HSV during sexual activity develop symptomatic disease. Like all infections, there is a required inoculum or viral titer necessary to initiate symptomatic infection. Individuals can be exposed to a titer insufficient to infect the ganglion, but the virus can still infect the mucosal epithelium and stimulate the host to initiate an immune response. Virus in the latent stage is not affected by the immune response, whereas replicating virus is eliminated by the immune system. The latent forms can become active causing recurrent disease. This phenomenon of differentiation between virions, why some virions are actively replicating and others establish latent infection, is not understood. Typically, when the genitalia are infected, the virus takes up residence in the lumbosacral root ganglia (42,43). The virus can also assume a latent stage in vaginal and cervical tissue. Reactivation of virus can occur randomly or coincident with the menses. Ultraviolet radiation, trauma, or stress can reactivate latent virus.

HSV-1 and HSV-2 genital infection produces lesion that are indistinguishable. However, the frequency or recurrences are different. Individuals experiencing a primary genital infection with HSV-1 are unlikely to experience a recurrence, whereas individuals infected with HSV-2 are likely to experience frequent recurrent episodes (44,45). Asymptomatic shedding of HSV-2 is of significant concern because these individuals can pass the virus to their sexual partners. The percentage of women infected with HSV-2 experiencing asymptomatic viral shedding range from 10% to 50% (46–53). Women infected with HSV-2 who shed virus when asymptomatic have been found to shed virus from the cervix, vagina, and vulva. In a study of 27 women with recurrent HSV-2 infection who were cultured 3 times a week, 26% were found to shed virus (54). Women infected with HSV-2 are also more likely to experience a recurrence than women infected with HSV-1 and typically experience their first recurrence within 3

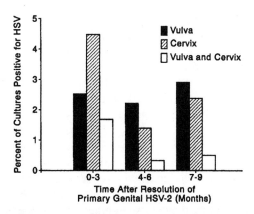

FIG. 9-4. Percent of cultures positive for herpes simplex virus represents the number of days that viral cultures were obtained in the 9 months following resolution of acute primary genital HSV-2. The graph depicts decreasing frequency of shedding from the cervix, and the cervix and vulva, whereas the vulva shedding remains relatively constant. (From Koelle DM, Benedetti J, Langenberg A, et al. Asymptomatic reactivation of herpes simplex virus in women after the first episode of genital herpes. *Ann Intern Med* 1992;116:433–437, with permission.)

months of their primary infection (55,56). Asymptomatic shedding of HSV-2 is important because it is an important factor in the transmission to sexual partners and the newborn (57–59). Although there is asymptomatic shedding from the vulva and cervix, there is a decrease in shedding from the cervix over time (55). Shedding from the vulva appears to remain fairly constant (Fig. 9-4).

The fact that HSV-1 and HSV-2, oral and genital infections, can develop latent and symptomatic infection indicates that the virus has evolved to a highly significant state. The virus has developed the ability to evade the host immune system and reproduce to infect other individuals. Thus, HSV-1 and HSV-2 have the ability to avoid the host immune defenses and, depending on the appropriate triggering mechanism or factor, go from a latent phase to an active phase, which can be asymptomatic or symptomatic (56–59). This is an important aspect of HSV infection because of the ability to transmit the virus and infection to both sexual partners and neonates. It should also be emphasized that both HSV-1 and HSV-2 can occur on other parts of the body; therefore, postpartum women and men handling their newborns must be extremely careful not to transmit the virus through physical contact when holding, changing, or bathing the baby.

DIAGNOSIS AND CLINICAL PRESENTATION

Although HSV-2 occurs primarily on the genitalia, the virus is capable of infecting any site on the human body. This is important to recognize because a mistake in diagnosis can lead to significant consequences and mistreatment.

HSV infection of the hand was first recognized in 1909 and reportedly occurs mainly among health care workers but can occur in any individual (60–63).

Infection of the hand and digits has been referred to as herpetic whitlow, recurrent traumatic herpes, and herpetic paronychia (64–67). Interestingly, in the study by Gill et al. (61) 79 cases were described and 32 of them occurred in individuals 21 to 30 years of age, and 20 cases were attributed to HSV-2. 43 cases of the virus were typed as either HSV-1 or HSV-2. HSV-2 occurred in individuals who were 20 years of age or older and predominantly in those between the ages of 20 and 30. In this age group, infection occurred more frequently in women (the ratio of women to men was 2.3:1) (61). Distribution of cases with regard to health care workers versus non-health care workers revealed that only 7 of the 49 cases occurred among health care workers (61). Among the infected women, it was found that individuals with recurrent infections from HSV-2 had a history of genital herpes. This study confirms that women with genital herpes are at risk for disseminating the disease to other parts of the body and that when lesions occur on other areas, such as the hand, this could potentially serve as a source of transmission to others. HSV has also been reported to cause hemorrhagic cystitis, endometritis, infection of the buttocks, hepatitis, and lymphadenitis (64–72).

Patients contracting genital herpes fall into two infection categories—asymptomatic and symptomatic. Most individuals infected with HSV develop subclinical infection. This can be an asymptomatic infection or the individual can develop a minor or a mild infection that goes unrecognized. The fact that asymptomatic patients can shed virus represents a significant dilemma for the patient and physician. In one study, 70% of patients acquired HSV infection from having sexual contact with individuals shedding the virus, although they did not have any detectable or noticeable lesions (73). These investigators also found that the risk of acquisition was greater for women than for men. In addition, if the woman had a previous HSV-1 infection and manifested antibodies to HSV-1, her risk of developing an HSV-2 infection following exposure was reduced.

Individuals who have never been exposed to the HSV virus, either HSV-1 or HSV-2, and subsequently become infected may develop a true primary infection. This is typically characterized by the development of a flulike syndrome with malaise, myalgias, fever, and frequently pharyngitis. The patient at this time is experiencing a viremia and may report headache and photophobia. The patient should be evaluated for the possibility of meningitis, especially if he or she reports stiffness or pain when turning, flexing, or extending their head. The patient may also develop signs and symptoms of a respiratory infection and should be evaluated for pneumonia. In addition, the patient may also develop hepatitis. The incubation for genital herpes is variable, ranging from 2 to 20 days. Experiments conducted to determine the incubation period in a group of volunteers noted the time from infection to the appearance of lesions was 48 to 72 hours (74). Typically, the prodrome of HSV precedes the appearance of lesions by 1 to 2 days. The life cycle of a lesion is divided into three stages: a vesicular pustule; a wet ulcer; and a dry, crusted over ulcer (Fig. 9-5).

Systemic symptoms and signs of HSV infection may persist for up to a week. Symptoms of meningitis, headache, photophobia, and neck stiffness are likely to

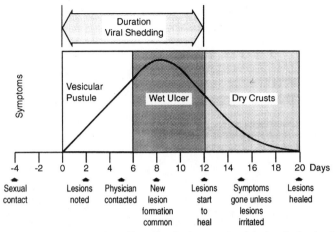

FIG. 9-5. Graphic representation of the life cycle of a herpes simplex virus lesion beginning with sexual contact or inoculation through the prodromal period and the actual changes of a herpetic pustule. (From Wald A, Corey L. The clinical features and diagnostic evaluation of genital herpes. In: Stanberry LR, ed. *Genital and neonatal herpes.* New York: John Wiley and Sons, 1996:115, with permission.)

occur more frequently in women than in men (36% to 11%) (75). Although genital infection by HSV-1 and HSV-2 are clinically indistinguishable, meningeal involvement is more frequently present with HSV-2 (42%) infection than HSV-1 (12%) (76).

The development of symptomatic genital herpes is characterized by the presence of pain, itching, burning, vaginal discharge, and dysuria. The vaginal discharge is typically clear and copious, especially if the cervix is involved. Patients with significant cervical involvement often report that they are incontinent of urine. Examination of the cervix often reveals the presence of diffuse cervical necrosis. The patient also develops bilateral inguinal lymphadenopathy. There are multiple lesions diffusely distributed over the external and internal genitalia, and the labia tends to be swollen and inflamed. The presence of a purulent or dirty gray vaginal discharge should alert the physician that there is likely more than one STD present (Figs. 9-6 and 9-7). Initially the lesions begin as small blisters that can contain either clear or purulent fluid (pustules). The lesions rupture spontaneously leaving behind small painful ulcers. The ulcers are typically clean in appearance but may be secondarily infected (Fig. 9-8). The ulcers have an erythematous base and clean margins. Numerous ulcers may be opposed to fuse and form a large ulcer that can be mistaken for a chancre of syphilis, chancroid, or lymphogranuloma venereum. The lesions continue to form over a 2-day period.

Cervicitis is frequently found in patients experiencing primary infection. Typically, in the patient whose cervix is not necrotic, the cervical discharge reflects acute infection and is purulent. Approximately 80% of women with acute primary genital HSV-2 infection have cervical involvement (76). The patient may note that her pain also involves the lower abdomen. This indicates that the infection has involved the bladder, the uterus, and the fallopian tubes (77).

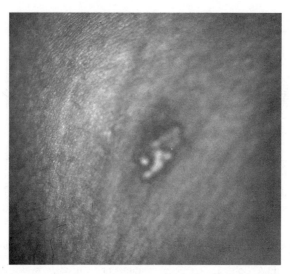

FIG. 9-6. Primary herpes with edema of the vulva and a frothy discharge. Patient was found to be positive for *Neisseria gonorrhoeae* and trichomoniasis. (See Color Plate 12 following page 148.)

Often patients experiencing their primary infection have urinary retention and severe pain. These patients require hospitalization for treatment. Likewise, the patient with headache, photophobia, and neck stiffness should be thoroughly evaluated. If genital lesions are apparent, the patient should be hospitalized and treated with intravenous (IV) antiviral therapy.

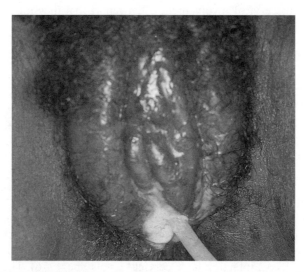

FIG. 9-7. Demonstration of purulent herpetic vesicles that are not secondarily infected. (See Color Plate 13 following page 148.)

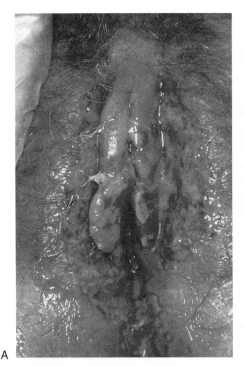
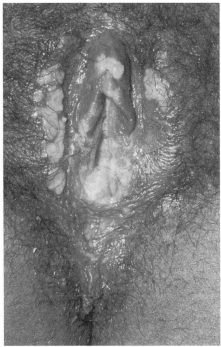

A   B

FIG. 9-8. A: Herpetic ulcers. **B:** Demonstration of herpetic ulcerations that are secondarily infected as noted by purulent exudate covering the ulceration. Obtaining a specimen for herpes culture from such a lesion, without removing the purulent exudate, would likely result in a negative culture for herpes. (See Color Plate 14 following page 148.)

Most patients note that the lesions spontaneously resolve in approximately 17 to 20 days. In a small percentage of patients, the lesions take longer to resolve, more than 35 days, and these patients tend to experience more frequent recurrences. There is also an associated bilateral inguinal lymphadenopathy, and the discomfort may be significant. This tends to last longer in men than in women (76).

Patients with primary herpes, HSV-1 or HSV-2, can also develop nongenital herpes. The lesions can occur on the oral-pharyngeal mucosa, the arm, the leg, and the buttocks (78). When these patients have recurrences, the lesions reappear at these same nongenital sites. The nongenital site infection can result from either autoinoculation or from the distribution of the particular nerve involved; for example, buttock and leg involvement are likely caused by the distribution of sacral innervation.

Recurrent episodes are preceded by a prodrome that is a complex of symptoms that precedes the appearance of the vesicular lesions. The prodrome usually occurs at the site where the vesicular lesion appears. The patient often reports that there is a localized itching, pain, irritation, tingling, or paraesthesias. Patients have also reported that they have a lower backache before the appearance of a lesion. Some patients develop a prodrome but fail to develop lesions. This has been referred as a "false-prodrome" or "nonlesional" episode. Patients who experience prodromal neuralgia but do not develop a lesion often feel more distressed than those who do experience lesional recurrences.

Patients who experience their initial episode are also at risk to develop recurrences. The patient who typically has an initial episode is one who has been exposed to the herpes virus HSV-1, HSV-2, or both and has developed antibodies to the herpes virus. The individual does not experience a viremia and the symptomatic disease is localized. Like the primary episode, the lesions are diffusely located on the external genitalia and can involve the vagina and cervix. However, the lesions are less numerous, and there does tend to be a significant amount of edema. The rate of recurrence between HSV-1 and HSV-2 is not the same. Individuals with HSV-1 genital infection tend not to have a recurrence in the first year of their infection. In contrast, individuals with genital HSV-2 infection do experience recurrences in the first year of infection (79). Patients with HSV-2 genital infection, approximately 89%, experience at least one recurrence, 38% have at least six recurrences, and 20% have more than 10 recurrences in the first year following a primary episode. Patients experiencing recurrent outbreaks usually have one to three lesions that last for 3 to 5 days.

The diagnosis of HSV-1 and HSV-2 infection is typically made on clinical findings. However, because this is an STD, its presence should be confirmed. This can be accomplished either by performing a culture, antigen, or nucleic acid detection. Although the clinical presentation of HSV infection is impressive, a definitive diagnosis cannot be based solely on clinical findings. The differential diagnosis for genital ulcer disease is lengthy (Table 9-1).

There are a variety of diagnostic tests available; however, the most sensitive is polymerase chain reaction (PCR). Viral culture is relatively easy and the cytopathic effect can be detected within 48 to 72 hours. Approximately 85% of cultures will be positive in 3 days and 95% in 5 days. The presence of the virus can be established with monoclonal antibody (80). The percentage of cultures that will be positive is dependent on the stage of the ulcerative disease when the specimen is obtained. Approximately 95% of the specimens will be positive for HSV if obtained during the vesicular stage, whereas when an ulcer is present, only about 70% of the specimens will be positive. If the lesion is crusted, only about 30% of the specimens will yield virus (80).

Patients presenting with their first clinical episode of HSV genital infection may not be having a primary clinical episode and, therefore, should not be thought to have had recent sexual contact with an infected individual. Individuals with primary HSV-2 will not have antibodies to the HSV in acute phase serum samples (81,82). Individuals with their first clinical HSV-2 infection, who do have antibodies to HSV-2, can be considered previously infected with the virus remaining in a latent state. Therefore, these individuals are indeed experiencing their initial clinical infection (81,82). Individuals seen because of suspected genital infection should, in addition to having the infection confirmed as

TABLE 9-1. *Differential diagnosis for genital ulcer disease*

Herpes
Syphilis
Chancroid
LGV
Granuloma inguinale
Fixed drug eruptions
Crohn's disease
Bullous impetigo
Cytomegalovirus
Epstein-Barr virus
Trauma
Scabies
Tuberculosis
Aphthous ulcers

LGV, lymphogranuloma venereum.

HSV-1 or HSV-2, also have serum obtained for the detection of antibodies. This will assist in placing the disease as acquired recently or sometime in the past.

The diagnosis of genital herpes infection is not difficult and can be made on clinical findings, but confirmation should be established. There are basically three modalities available for the detection and confirmation of HSV infection. The first method is culturing of the herpetic vesical and inoculating tissue culture to document the presence of infection. The virus can then be typed as either HSV-1 or HSV-2 by monoclonal antibody. Another method is to use HSV antigen detection tests employing monoclonal and polyclonal antibodies. PCR assays are also available for the detection of HSV DNA.

TREATMENT

Antiviral agents effective against HSV-1 and HSV-2 have been available for a decade; however, there are agents that can effectively rid the patient of latent virus. The best strategy in combating HSV is prevention; however, this is nearly impossible because there is no way of identifying the asymptomatic carrier.

The antiviral agents can be grouped into those administered orally and those applied topically (Table 9-2). Acyclovir is the antiviral agent with the longest history and most use up until the last few years. Valacyclovir and famciclovir, two newer agents, recently became available and are enjoying widespread use.

The following are the treatments for herpes genitalis recommended by the Center for Disease Control and Prevention (83):

First clinical episode (primary or initial):
Acyclovir 400 mg orally three times a day for 7 to 10 days
Acyclovir 200 mg orally five times a day for 7 to 10 days
Famciclovir 250 mg orally three times a day for 7 to 10 days

TABLE 9-2. *Antiviral agents for the treatment of HSV infection*

Acyclovir is available for administration orally, intravenously, and topically for the treatment of genital HSV, chicken pox, herpes zoster, HSV encephalitis, and HSV hepatitis

Valacyclovir is available for oral administration, for the treatment of genital HSV and herpes zoster

Famciclovir is available for oral administration, for the treatment of genital HSV and herpes zoster

Vidarabine is available for topical and IV administration for the treatment of neonatal herpes, herpes encephalitis, herpes zoster, acute keratoconjunctivitis, recurrent epithelial keratitis, and superficial keratitis unresponsive to idoxuridine

Idoxuridine is available as a topical agent for the treatment of HSV keratitis

Trifluridine is available as a topical agent for the treatment of keratoconjunctivitis, recurrent epithelial keratitis, and superficial keratitis unresponsive to idoxuridine

HSV, herpes simplex virus.

Valacyclovir 1 g orally twice a day for 7 to 10 days
Recurrent episodes:
Acyclovir 400 mg orally three times a day for 5 days
Acyclovir 200 mg orally five times a day for 5 days
Acyclovir 800 mg orally twice a day for 5 days
Famciclovir 125 mg orally twice a day for 5 days
Valacyclovir 500 mg orally twice a day for 5 days
Daily suppression:
Acyclovir 400 mg orally twice a day
Famciclovir 250 mg orally twice a day
Valacyclovir 250 mg orally twice a day
Valacyclovir 500 mg orally once a day
Valacyclovir 1g orally once a day
Severe disease:
Acyclovir should be administered intravenously
Dosage 5 to 10 mg/kg of body weight every 8 hours for 5 to 7 days or until clinical signs and symptoms of disease have resolved
Patient should be kept well hydrated

REFERENCES

1. Nahmias AJ, Dowdle WR. Antigenic and biologic differences in *Herpesvirus hominis. Prog Med Virol* 1968;10:110–159.
2. Stanberry LR, Jorgensen DM, Nahmias AJ. Epidemiology of herpes simplex virus 1 and 2. In: Kaslow R, Evans A, eds. *Viral infection of humans,* 4th ed. New York: Plenum Press, 1997.
3. Wheeler CE, Abele DC. Eczema herpeticum, primary and recurrent. *Arch Dermatol* 1966;93: 162–173.
4. Terezhalmy GT, Tyler MT, Ross GR. Eczema herpeticum: atopic dermatitis complicated by primary herpetic gingivostomatitis. *Oral Surg Oral Med Oral Pathol* 1979;48:513–516.
5. Hazen PG, Eppes RB. Eczema herpeticum caused by herpesvirus type 2. A case in a patient with Darier disease. *Arch Dermatol* 1977;113:1085–1086.
6. Stern H, Elek SD, Miller DM, Andersen HF. Herpetic whitlow. A form of cross-infection in hospitals. *Lancet* 1959;2:871–874.
7. Rosato FE, Rosato EF, Plotkin SA. Herpetic paronychia—an occupational hazard of medical personnel. *N Engl J Med* 1970;283:804–805.

8. Selling B, Kibrick S. An outbreak of herpes simplex among wrestlers (herpes gladiatorum). *N Engl J Med* 1964;270:979–982.
9. Wheeler CE, Cabaniss WH. Epidemic cutaneous herpes simplex in wrestlers (herpes gladiatorum). *JAMA* 1965;194:993–937.
10. Craig CP, Nahmias AJ. Different patterns of neurologic involvement with herpes simplex virus types 1 and 2: isolation of herpes simplex virus type 2 from the buffy coat of 2 adults with meningitis. *J Infect Dis* 1973;127:365–372.
11. Hevron JE. Herpes simplex virus type 2 meningitis. *Obstet Gynecol* 1977;49:622–624.
12. Skoldenberg B, Jeansson S, Wolontis S. Herpes simplex virus type 2 and acute aseptic meningitis. Clinical features of cases with isolation of herpes simplex virus from cerebrospinal fluids. *Scand J Infect Dis* 1975;7:227–232.
13. Terni M, Caccialanza P, Cassai E, et al. Aseptic meningitis in association with herpes progenitalis. *N Engl J Med* 1971;285:503–504.
14. Nahmias AJ, Lee FK, Keyserling HL. The epidemiology of genital herpes. In: Stanberry LR, ed. *Genital and neonatal herpes*. New York: John Wiley and Sons, 1996:93–108.
15. Henquet CJ, Jansen MW, Buwalda PJ, et al. Sexually transmitted diseases in Limburg in 1997; prevalence according to a survey of family practitioners and specialists and according to reports from microbiologic laboratories. *Nederlands Tijdschrift voor Geneeskunde* 2000;144:608–612.
16. Keyserling H, Robinowitz M, Ratchford R, et al. Herpes simplex virus type antibodies and history of genital herpes among steady couples. Second World Congress on Sexually Transmitted Diseases, Paris, France, June 1986.
17. Mertz GJ, Benedetti J, Ashley R, et al. Risk factors for the sexual transmission of genital herpes. *Ann Int Med* 1992;116:197–202.
18. Schacker T, Corey L. HSV as a factor in HIV transmission, 2nd National Conference on Human Retroviruses, Washington, DC, 1995.
19. Griffiths PD. Herpesviruses and AIDS. *J Antimicrob Chemother* 1996;37(Suppl B):87–95.
20. Morse LS, Pereira L, Roizman B, et al. Anatomy of herpes simplex virus (HSV) DNA. X. Mapping of viral genes by analysis of polypeptides and functions specified by HSV-I × HSV-2 recombinants. *J Virol* 1978;26:386–410.
21. Morse LS, Buchman TG, Roizman B, et al. Anatomy of herpes simplex virus DNA. IX. Apparent exclusion of some parental DNA arrangements in the generation of intertypic (HSV-1 × HSV-2) recombinants. *J Virol* 1977;24:231–248.
22. Preston VG, Davison AJ, Marsden HS, et al. Recombinants between herpes simplex virus types 1 and 2: analyses of genome structures and expression of immediate early polypeptides. *J Virol* 1978;28:499–517.
23. Marsden HS, Stow ND, Preston VG, et al. Physical mapping of herpes simplex virus-induced polypeptides. *J Virol* 1978;28:624–642.
24. Knipe DM. The replication of herpes simplex virus. In: Stanberry LR, ed. *Genital and neonatal herpes*. New York: John Wiley and Sons 1996:1–29.
25. Shieh MT, WuDunn D, Montgomery RI, et al. Cell surface receptors for herpes simplex virus are heparan sulfate proteoglycans. *J Cell Bio* 1992;116:1273–1281.
26. Knipe DM, Ruyechan WT, Roizman B, et al. Molecular genetics of herpes simplex virus: demonstration of regions of obligatory and nonobligatory identity within diploid regions of the genome by sequence replacement and insertion. *Proc Natl Acad Sci U S A* 1978;75:3896–3900.
27. Preston CM. Control of herpes simplex virus type 1 mRNA synthesis in cells infected with wild-type virus or temperature-sensitive mutant tsK. *J Virol* 1979;29:275–284.
28. Watson RJ, Clements JB. A herpes simplex virus type 1 function continuously required for early and late virus RNA synthesis. *Nature* 1980;285:329–330.
29. Dixon RA, Schaffer PA. Fine-structure mapping and functional analysis of temperature-sensitive mutants in the gene encoding the herpes simplex virus type 1 immediate early protein VP175. *J Virol* 1980;36:189–203.
30. Godowski PJ, Knipe DM. Transcriptional control of herpesvirus gene expression: gene functions required for positive and negative regulation. *Proc Nat Acad Sci U S A* 1986;83:256–260.
31. Stackpole CW. Herpes-type virus of the frog renal adenocarcinoma. I. Virus development in tumor transplants maintained at low temperature. *J Virol* 1969;4:75–93.
32. Whealy ME, Card JP, Meade RP, et al. Effect of brefeldin A on alphaherpesvirus membrane protein glycosylation and virus egress. *J Virol* 1991;65:1066–1081.
33. Jones F, Grose C. Role of cytoplasmic vacuoles in varicella-zoster virus glycoprotein trafficking and virion envelopment. *J Virol* 1988;62:2701–2711.

34. WuDunn D, Spear PG. Initial interaction of herpes simplex virus with cells is binding to heparan sulfate. *J Virol* 1989;63:52–58.
35. Herold BC, WuDunn D, Soltys N, et al. Glycoprotein C of herpes simplex virus type 1 plays a principal role in adsorption of virus to cells and in infectivity. *J Virol* 1991;65:1090–1098.
36. Spear PG. Entry of alphaherpesviruses into cells. *Semin Virol* 1993;4:167–180.
37. Herold BC, Visalli RJ, Susmarski N, et al. Glycoprotein C-independent binding of herpes simplex virus to cells requires cell surface heparan sulfate and glycoprotein B. *J Gen Virol* 1994;75: 1211–1222.
38. Cook ML, Stevens JG. Pathogenesis of herpetic neuritis and ganglionitis in mice: evidence for intra-axonal transport of infection. *Infect Immun* 1973;7:272–288.
39. Stanberry LR, Bourne N, Bravo FJ, et al. Capsaicin-sensitive peptidergic neurons are involved in the zosteriform spread of herpes simplex virus infection. *J Med Virol* 1992;38:142–146.
40. Stanberry LR, Kit S, Myers MG. Thymidine kinase-deficient herpes simplex virus type 2 genital infection in guinea pigs. *J Virol* 1985;55:322–38.
41. Penfold ME, Armati P, Cunningham AL. Axonal transport of herpes simplex virions to epidermal cells: evidence for a specialized mode of virus transport and assembly. *Proc Natl Acad Sci U S A* 1994;91:6529–533.
42. Baringer JR. Recovery of herpes simplex virus from human sacral ganglions. *N Engl J Med* 1974; 291:828–830.
43. Stanberry LR, Kern ER, Richards JT, et al. Genital herpes in guinea pigs: pathogenesis of the primary infection and description of recurrent disease. *J Infect Dis* 1982;146:397–404.
44. Reeves WC, Corey L, Adams HG, et al. Risk of recurrence after first episodes of genital herpes: relation to HSV type and antibody response. *N Engl J Med* 1981; 305:315–319.
45. Lafferty WE, Coombs RW, Benedetti J, et al. Recurrences after oral and genital herpes simplex virus infection: influence of site of infection and viral type. *N Engl J Med* 1987;316:1444–1449.
46. Barton SE, Davis JM, Moss VW, et al. Asymptomatic shedding and subsequent transmission of genital herpes simplex virus. *Genitourin Med* 1987;63:102–105.
47. Rattray MC, Corey L, Reeves WC, et al. Recurrent genital herpes among women: symptomatic vs asymptomatic viral shedding. *Br J Vener Dis* 1978;54:262–265.
48. Adam E, Kaufman RH, Mirkovic RR, et al. Persistence of virus shedding in asymptomatic women after recovery from herpes genitalis. *Obstet Gynecol* 1979;54:171–173.
49. Stenzel-Poore MP, Hallick LM, Fendrick JL, et al. Herpes simplex virus shedding in genital secretions. *Sex Transm Dis* 1987;14:17–22.
50. Barton SE, Wright LK, Link CM, et al. Screening to detect asymptomatic shedding of herpes simplex virus (HSV) in women with recurrent genital HSV infection. *Genitourin Med* 1986;62:181–185.
51. Douglas JM, Critchlow C, Benedetti J, et al. A double-blind study of oral acyclovir for suppression of recurrences of genital herpes simplex virus infection. *N Engl J Med* 1984;310:1551–1556.
52. Willmott FE, Mair HJ. Genital herpesvirus infection in women attending a venereal diseases clinic. *Br J Vener Dis* 1978;54:341–343.
53. Guinan ME, Wolinksy SM, Reichman RC. Genital herpes simplex virus infection. *Epidemiol Rev* 1987;7:127–146.
54. Brock BV, Selke S, Benedetti J, et al. Frequency of asymptomatic shedding of herpes simplex virus in women with genital herpes. *JAMA* 1990;263:418–420.
55. Koelle DM, Benedetti J, Langenberg A, et al. Asymptomatic reactivation of herpes simplex virus in women after the first episode of genital herpes. *Ann Intern Med* 1992;116:433–437.
56. Mertz GJ, Schmidt O, Jourden JL, et al. Frequency of acquisition of first-episode genital infection with herpes simplex virus from symptomatic and asymptomatic source contacts. *Sex Transm Dis* 1985;12:33–39.
57. Stone KM, Brooks CA, Guinan ME, et al. National surveillance for neonatal herpes simplex virus infections. *Sex Transm Dis* 1989;16:152–156.
58. Whitley RJ, Corey L, Arvin A, et al. Changing presentation of herpes simplex virus infection in neonates. *J Infect Dis* 1988;158;109–116.
59. Rooney JF, Felser JM, Ostriove JM, et al. Acquisition of genital herpes from an asymptomatic sexual partner. *N Engl J Med* 1986;314:1561–1564.
60. Adamson HG. Herpes febrilis attacking the fingers. *Br J Dermatol* 1909;21:323–324.
61. Gill JM, Arlette J, Buchan K. Herpes simplex virus infection of the hand. A profile of 79 cases. *Am J Med* 1988;84:98–93.
62. Hamory BH, Osterman CA, Wenzel RP. Herpetic whitlow [Letter]. *N Engl J Med* 1975;292:268.

63. Stern H, Elek SD, Millar DM, et al. Herpetic whitlow: a form of cross-infection in hospitals. *Lancet* 1959;2:871–874.
64. Louis DS, Silva J. Herpetic whitlow: herpetic infections of the digits. *J Hand Surg Am* 1979;4:90–94.
65. Muller SA, Herrmann EC. Association of stomatitis and paronychias due to herpes simplex. *Arch Dermatol* 1970;101:396–402.
66. Findlay GM, MacCullum FO. Recurrent traumatic herpes. *Lancet* 1940;1:259–261.
67. Brightman VJ, Guggenheimer JG. Herpetic paronychia-primary herpes simplex infection of the finger. *J Am Dent Assoc* 1970;80:112–115.
68. DeHertogh DA, Brettman LR. Hemorrhagic cystitis due to herpes simplex virus as a marker of disseminated herpes infection. *Am J Med* 1988;84:632–635.
69. Schneider V, Behm FG, Mumaw VR. Ascending herpetic endometritis. *Obstet Gynecol* 1982;59: 259–262.
70. Suarez M, Briones H, Saaevdra T. Buttock herpes: high risk in pregnancy. *J Reprod Med* 1991;36: 367–368.
71. Baxter RP, Phillips LE, Faro S, et al. Hepatitis due to herpes simplex virus in a non-pregnant patient: treatment with acyclovir. *Sex Transm Dis* 1986;13:174–176.
72. Taxy JB, Tillawi I, Goldman PM. Herpes simplex lymphadenitis. An unusual presentation with necrosis and viral particles. *Arch Pathol Lab Med* 1985;109:1043–1044.
73. Mertz GJ, Benedetti J, Ashley R, et al. Risk factors for the sexual transmission of genital herpes. *Ann Intern Med* 1992;116:197–202.
74. Blank H, Haines HG. Experimental human reinfection with herpes simplex virus. *J Invest Dermatol* 1973;61:223–225.
75. Wald A, Corey L. The clinical features and diagnostic evaluation of genital herpes. In: Stanberry LR, ed. *Genital and neonatal herpes.* New York: John Wiley and Sons, 1996:108–137.
76. Corey L, Adams HG, Brown ZA, et al. Genital herpes simplex virus infections: clinical manifestations, course, and complications. *Ann Intern Med* 1983;98:958–972.
77. Lehtinen M, Rantala I, Teisala K, et al. Detection of herpes simplex virus in women with acute pelvic inflammatory disease. *J Infect Dis* 1985;152:78–82.
78. Benedetti JK, Zeh J, Selke S, et al. Frequency and reactivation of nongenital lesions among patients with genital herpes simplex virus. *Am J Med* 1995;98:237–242.
79. Reeves WC, Corey L, Adams HG, et al. Risk of recurrence after first episodes of genital herpes. Relation to HSV type and antibody response. *N Engl J Med* 1981;305:315–319.
80. Ashely RL. Laboratory techniques in the diagnosis of herpes simplex infection. *Genitourin Med* 1993;69:174–183.
81. Bryson YJ, Dillon M, Lovett M, et al. Treatment of first episodes of genital herpes simplex virus infection with oral acyclovir. A randomized double-blind controlled trial in normal subjects. *N Engl J Med* 1983;308:916–921.
82. Nahmias AJ, Danneenbarger J, Wickliffe C, et al. Clinical aspects of infection with herpes simplex virus 1 and 2. In: Nahmias AJ, ed. *The human herpesviruses, an interdisciplinary perspective.* New York: Elsevier Science, 1981:3–9.
83. Anonymous. 1998 guidelines for the treatment of sexually transmitted diseases. Centers for Disease Control and Prevention. *MMWR* 1998;47:20–23.

10

Human Papillomavirus

INTRODUCTION

The papillomaviruses are deoxyribonucleic acid (DNA) viruses responsible for the development of cutaneous and mucosal warts. In 1907, Ciuffo (1) demonstrated that common warts can be transmitted by using cell-free extracts of warts. In 1933, Schope and Hurst (2) were the first to report that cutaneous warts observed in the cottontail rabbit were caused by papillomavirus infection. The human papillomavirus (HPV) is probably the most common sexually transmitted viral organism in the United States. HPV is found in 20% to 60% of sexually active women in America (3–8). It is estimated that there are more than 1 million cases in the United States each year. This virus is of particular concern because of its association with significant benign and malignant disease. It commonly infects the vulva, vagina, and cervix and can be transmitted to the newborn. Newborn infection can result in infection of the genitalia and the bronchial tree. Although the development of bronchial tree condyloma in children can cause significant morbidity and mortality, it has not received a great deal of attention from the obstetric community.

The association between HPV, vulvar and cervical dysplasia, and cancer is alarming because the infection is extremely common in young sexually active women and can persist for a lifetime. Individuals between 15 and 30 years of age are the most vulnerable because these women are likely to either have multiple sexual partners or be exposed to multiple contacts indirectly. However, older women with multiple sexual partners are at similar risk. Women diagnosed with HPV infection often become distraught, especially after learning more about the infection from the Internet and by reading lay literature. HPV is similar to herpes simplex infection in that once either infection is acquired it can remain with the individual for life.

Like all sexually transmitted diseases (STDs) diagnosis should be confirmed and not based solely on clinical appearance. However, condyloma acuminata is not likely to be confused with other STDs or infections with the possible exception of condyloma lata, an expression of secondary syphilis. Therefore, screening for other STDs, including human immunodeficiency virus (HIV), is recommended when making an initial diagnosis of HPV. The first diagnosis may not always be made based on the presence of a verrucous lesion but might be reported on a Papanicolaou smear or after finding an acetowhite area on examination of the vulva (flat condylomatous lesion). This finding is extremely unsettling to the patient because it may appear later in life, at a time when she is not participating in risky behavior. This creates a particularly stressful situation because, if she believes she is in a monogamous relationship, she immediately suspects that her partner or husband has breached their relationship. However, the physician must go over the patient's history, beginning with her first sexual contact, to determine the potential risk and expose her to the possibility that she may have acquired the infection before entering into her current relationship. The physician should explain that this virus has the unique ability to assume a latent phase for a long period and becomes activated for unknown reasons.

When inquiring into the patient's sexual history it is important to determine the age of her first sexual experience, the degree of contact, and whether she has had multiple partners over the years. The total number of sexual partners is important because it determines her real relative risk of acquiring a STD. A review of STDs should also be conducted to explain the characteristics of each to help the patient understand the questions. It is not uncommon for the patient to recall that she had genital warts or a "sore" in her teens or twenties that was treated with some liquid. Often this treatment was considered insignificant at the time.

When a diagnosis of HPV is made, another difficulty confronting the patient and the physician is that there are currently no satisfactory treatments to eradicate the virus from the patient. Although the disease may spontaneously resolve, this is not reassuring to the patient. Because the patient is told or learns of the relationship between HPV and cancer of the genital tract, she often feels that she has a "time bomb" waiting to explode and that she will inevitably develop cancer.

The psychologic trauma is usually significant when the patient receives a diagnosis of HPV because she is often caught by surprise. Such a diagnosis was not suspected and the patient often feels taken advantage of, betrayed, or violated. The patient's reaction is similar to the reaction seen when a patient finds out that she has herpes. It is not uncommon for these patients to become angry and depressed. Thus, it is difficult for physicians to inform patients that they have HPV because of the following:

1. HPV may be a lifetime disease
2. It can remain dormant for years
3. HPV often makes its appearance at a time when it is difficult to satisfactorily explain it to a partner or husband
4. It can cause congenital infection in the newborn
5. HPV can cause cancer of the genital tract

The immunosuppressed patient with HPV presents an extremely difficult management problem, more so than the nonimmunosuppressed patient. This large group of patients includes transplant patients, patients with collagen vascular disease being treated with steroids, patients with chronic skin conditions who require long-term use of oral steroids, and patients with HIV. HPV exacerbations appear to be common in the immunosuppressed. It is a long-held belief that pregnancy is an immunosuppressed state, although mild. HPV often worsens during pregnancy, causing pregnant patients to experience a HPV bloom. It is not uncommon for patients to experience multiple lesions and rapid growth of their lesions during pregnancy.

All patients diagnosed with HPV, regardless of age and especially if it is their initial diagnosis, should be screened for other STDs. This includes testing for *Neisseria gonorrhoeae, Chlamydia trachomatis, Treponema pallidum,* herpes simplex, HIV, hepatitis B and C, and *Trichomonas vaginalis.*

EPIDEMIOLOGY

Reporting of HPV infection is not a requirement; therefore, the Centers for Disease Control and Prevention (CDC) can only estimate the prevalence of this disease. Approximately 1 to 2 million sexually active individuals have genital warts; it is also estimated that 26 to 29 million people have molecular evidence of HPV (HPV DNA) infection. The CDC estimates that there are approximately 750,000 new cases of condyloma acuminata each year (9). There has been a steady rise in the number of physician visits for HPV from 1966 to 1988 (Fig. 10-1). There does appear to be a decline in the number of visits throughout the 1990s; however, this could be because of inaccuracy in computing the number of cases because this is a nonreportable disease.

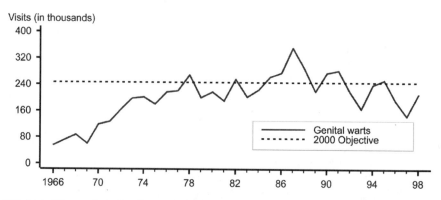

FIG. 10-1. The graph depicts the number of initial visits to physicians' offices for HPV from 1966 to 1998. It should be noted that there is a steady increase in the number of visits to physician offices from 1966 to 1986. Then there appears to be a decrease in office visits because of condyloma acuminata. (National Disease and Therapeutic Index [IMS America, Ltd])

HPV infections can be grouped into three categories:

1. Cutaneous infections not involving the genital areas, typically benign warts, which usually involve types 1, 2, 3, 4, and 10.
2. Cutaneous infection in patients with epidermodysplasia verruciformis (EV). These patients tend to have widespread chronic disease (10). HPV types 3 or 10 are commonly involved, and patients can be infected with more than one type. Patients with EV who are infected with type 5 and/or type 8 have significant potential for malignant disease.
3. Genitomucosal infection is caused by a variety of types. HPV 6 and 11 are referred to as low-risk types because they are associated with benign lesions or low-grade malignancies. Types 16, 18, 31, and 33 are referred to as high-risk types because of the strong association with genital cancer.

Infection with HPV is categorized as follows: clinical infection defined as the presence of genital warts; subclinical infection lesions not easily visible to the naked eye but detected by specific tests; and latent infection, which is defined as the detection of HPV DNA in cells with no detectable abnormal appearance.

The clinical course following exposure can be variable. The patient may develop lesions or clinical infection after an incubation period of 4 to 8 weeks. These patients typically develop the characteristic warts (Fig 10-2). Some individuals may develop a subclinical infection that is usually detected on a Papanicolaou (Pap) smear by the presence of atypia or low-grade squamous intraepithelial lesion (LGSIL) and can be confirmed by DNA tests. Others may not manifest any clinical or subclinical lesions so the infection is unknown for years until the virus is activated and moves from a latent infection to a detectable state. The mechanism that results in activation of latent virus is unknown. The course

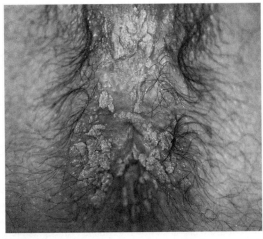

FIG. 10-2. Typical lesions of condyloma acuminata. (See Color Plate 15 following page 148.)

of a HPV infection over time is variable. Some individuals experience constant infection with rather limited involvement of the genital area, others experience spontaneous regression of their disease, and some experience progression with extensive involvement of the genitalia.

The variability or presentation of HPV infection and the inability to measure exposure and determine actual infection makes estimating the prevalence of this disease difficult. There is no serologic test or culture available to determine HPV infection. Attempts to determine the prevalence are further hampered because many patients are treated in private offices and, therefore, not tracked or reported to a central registry. However the National Disease and Therapeutic Index, an organization that surveys private practices, did report a 4.5 fold increase in initial physician visits for HPV between 1966 and 1984 (11). The prevalence of HPV in the population can be detected by: genital warts, cytologic abnormalities found on Pap smear or colposcopy, or the presence of HPV DNA by specific test. (Table 10-1).

HPV is widespread throughout the world and common in the United States. It appears to be increasing as young women and men practice promiscuous sexual behavior. An increase in HPV acquisition is associated with younger age, Hispanic and African-American ethnicity, an increase in the number of sexual partners, anal sex, alcohol use, and partners with multiple sexual partners (12) (Table 10-2).

Sometimes it is difficult to determine if a patient who has been treated and goes for a period without disease, but later returns with clinical disease, has recurrent or new disease. Ho et al. (12) found that an individual was likely to experience spontaneous resolution of HPV infection, if it was a new infection. They also found that persistence of infection was related to its duration. These investigators found that the probability that the infection would resolve spontaneously within the first 6 months was 31% and 39% in the second 6 months. If the infection persisted for the first 12 months, the probability of resolution in the third 6 months was 11%. This pattern of spontaneous resolution or persistence of infection resembles that of squamous intraepithelial lesions (13,14). Franco et al. (15) studying spontaneous resolution of HPV analyzed 1,425 low-income women in São Paulo, Brazil, and found 357 to be positive for HPV. They enrolled 177 of the women with HPV in the study and found that after 12 months only 62 (35%) remained positive. Interestingly, these investigators also found that the monthly clearance rate was higher for nononcogenic types (12.2%) than for oncogenic types (9.5%).

TABLE 10-1. *Estimated prevalence of HPV in women and men in 1994[a]*

Clinically apparent disease—genital warts—1% (1.4 million cases)
Infection detected by cytology or colposcopy—4% (5 million cases)
Infection detected by DNA or RNA amplification tests—10% (14 million cases)
Prior infection—60% (81 million cases)
No prior or current infection but at risk—25% (34 million cases)

[a]Adapted from Koutsky LA, Galloway DA, Holmes KK. Epidemiology of genital papillomavirus infection. *Epidemiol Rev* 1988;10:122–163, with permission.

TABLE 10-2. *Risk factors associated with the acquisition of HPV in college women[a]*

Risk factor	Relative risk	P value	(95% CI)
Time-independent variables			
Age (per additional year)	0.9 (0.8–0.9)	0.001	
Racial or ethnic group			
White, Asian, & others	1.0		
Hispanic	2.1 (1.2–3.7)	0.009	
Black	4.4 (2.2–7.2)	<0.001	
Time-dependent variables			
Frequency of alcohol			
Consumption			
<1 time/month	1.0	0.005	
1–3 times/month	1.3 (0.9–2.1)		
≥4 times/month			
# of male vaginal sex partners in previous 7–12 months			
0–3	1.0	<0.001	1.7 (0.9–3.2)
2–3	3.0 (1.6–5.8)		
>4	4.2 (1.5–2.4)		
Had anal sex with any regular partners. Total frequency of vaginal sex with all regular partners			
<2–6 times/wk	1.0		
≥2–6 times/wk	1.5 (1.1–2.3)	0.02	
# of lifetime sexual partners of main regular partner			
1	1.0	<0.001	
2–5	5.8 (2.1–16.0)		
≥6	10.1 (3.6–28.4)		
Main regular partner was currently in school		0.6 (0.4–0.9)	0.01

CI, confidence interval.

[a]Adapted from Ho GY, Bierman R, Beardsley L, et al. Natural history of cervicovaginal papillomavirus infection in young women. *N Engl J Med* 1998;338:423–428, with permission.

Another important area with regard to HPV infection is pregnancy and vertical transmission to the newborn. Schneider et al. (16) reported that the prevalence of infection was higher in pregnant women compared with nonpregnant women (28.3% vs. 12.5%). However, in a similar study, Kemp et al. (17) did not find a significant relationship between pregnancy and HPV infection. These authors studied 115 pregnant patients, 100 postpartum patients, and 160 patients that were neither pregnant nor postpartum. They did not find any association between the prevalence of HPV and pregnancy, race, smoking, or number of sexual partners (17). This divergent opinion with regard to HPV and pregnancy has been debated for several years. However, the data seems to support the conclusion that pregnancy does not impose an independent risk factor for the acquisition of HPV infection. In 1985, Garry and Jones (18) reported that HPV occurs more frequently and may worsen in pregnancy. Several investigators have come to similar conclusions, suggesting that pregnancy may enhance acquisition and progression of infection (19–21). However, other investigators reported a lower prevalence or no differences in pregnant women (22–25). Tenti et al. (26) studied large populations of pregnant (752) and nonpregnant (504) women in a family planning clinic, and 560 women who visited a vaginitis clinic, using polymerase chain reaction (PCR) to detect HPV. These authors found no difference in the prevalence of HPV in pregnant and nonpregnant women. However, the risk for HPV was 50% less in women without vaginitis than in women with symptomatic vaginitis (26). Interestingly, the prevalence of oncogenic types 16 and 18 was lower in pregnant women ($p = 0.015$ and $p = 0.0018$, respectively) (26).

A significant complication of HPV in pregnancy is the potential for vertical transmission of the virus to the newborn, resulting in laryngeal papillomatosis. Papillomas of the larynx were first reported in 1871 and are considered the most common benign tumor of the larynx and respiratory tract in children (27–29). In 1956, Hajek (30) reported that of the cases of laryngeal papillomas occurring in small children and adolescents, HPV could be found in 20% of these cases at birth.

Children with laryngeal papillomatosis appear to contract the virus as they pass through the birth canal during delivery and come in contact with HPV. Typically, the disease regresses spontaneously when the child reaches puberty; however, spread of the disease into the trachea and bronchi does occur, although rarely. It has been reported that progression into the trachea and proximal bronchi occurs in 2% to 5% of infected individuals, and in less than 1% of patients the lung parenchyma is involved (31–33). Pulmonary involvement can result in chronic obstructive pneumonia, bronchiectasis, hemoptysis, lower airway obstruction, and malignant transformation (34).

Acquisition of HPV by the newborn with subsequent development of laryngeal papillomatosis appears to occur during the birthing process; however, transplacental infection cannot be ruled out. Children, born to HPV infected women, who develop juvenile respiratory papillomatosis have been found to have the same HPV type in their buccal mucosa as that recovered from the mother's cervix (35–37). Interestingly, HPV DNA has been recovered from the vaginas of virginal women (36). HPV DNA has also been detected in amniotic fluid, neonatal cord blood, and the peripheral mononuclear cells of pregnant women (38–41). Puranen et al. (42) studied the possible vertical transmission of HPV from maternal cervical infection to the neonate. These investigators studied 105 mothers and 106 infants. Women with no history or clinical findings of HPV infection delivered 60 infants vaginally and 26 by cesarean section; mothers with clinical findings of cervical HPV infection gave birth to 18 infants vaginally and one set of twins by cesarean section. Twenty-nine mother-infant pairs were found to be positive for the HPV types, and five infants delivered by cesarean section had the same HPV type found in their mother's cervix. The overall concordance between HPV type in mother and child was 69% (29/42). Overall, HPV DNA was found in 37% (39/106) of the infants.

The data regarding vertical transmission from mothers with HPV infection of the cervix to their newborn infants is not conclusive but does raise significant concern about the route of delivery for infants born to HPV-infected mothers. Prospective studies are needed to bring some degree of resolution to this problem. Studies involving infants delivered both vaginally and by cesarean section are needed. Amniocentesis data are also needed to determine if transplacental migration of the virus occurs. Until this data is available, it might be in the pregnant patient's best interest to discuss the available information, the possibility of cesarean delivery, the morbidity associated with cesarean delivery, and the possibility of *in utero* infection with her physician.

Sexual transmission of HPV is not restricted to women who have sex with men but can also occur between lesbians. There are approximately 2.3 million lesbian women in the United States (43). It is estimated that 4.3% of all women have had same gender sex since puberty (44–46). Marrazzo et al. (47) studied 149 lesbians, 21 of whom reported no prior sexual contact with men. Among those 21 women, 19% had HPV DNA and 14% had squamous intraepithelial lesions. Overall, HPV DNA was detected in 30% of the individuals. Of the 30% found to have HPV DNA, 20% had types 31, 33, 35, and 39; 18% had type 16; and 2% had types 6 and 11. The sexual transmission of HPV between women raises concern for the development of squamous intraepithelial lesions and cervical cancer. Therefore, these women should have routine Pap smears and examinations just as frequently as heterosexual women. The sexual practices of lesbian women include contact of external genitalia, the use of sexual toys, and digital-to-genital contact. This contact is not without potential consequence; for example, the sharing of sexual toys can lead to transmission of HPV to an uninfected individual (48). Because genital types of HPV have been detected on human fingers, it is plausible that the virus can be transmitted to the genitalia by either autoinoculation or genital contact between partners (49). An important aspect in the epidemiology of HPV for lesbian women is that many of their partners have had sex, and continue to have sex, with men. It is estimated that 53% to 99% of lesbians have had sex with men, and 21% to 30% continue to participate in bisexual behavior (50,51). This bisexuality raises concern for transmission of a variety of STDs like genital and oral herpes, genital and oral HPV, and HIV. Bisexual women can transmit some of these STDs to their female partners.

Thus, for all women, pattern of sexual behavior is the major risk factor for acquiring HPV. This includes the number of sexual partners and the frequency of sexual intercourse (Table 10-3). If the individual's sexual partner or contact has genital warts, then the woman's risk is significantly increased. Another signifi-

TABLE 10-3. *Risk factors for the acquisition of HPV*

Sexual intercourse
Frequency of sexual intercourse
Having 4 or more partners
A sexual partner who has genital warts
Immunosuppression
Failure to use condoms
Significant alcohol consumption
Race: African American > Hispanic > Caucasian

cant risk factor for the acquisition and progression of HPV is immunosuppression in the patient. The immunosuppressed patient has a more than 17-fold incidence of genital HPV infection.

VIROLOGY

HPV is a DNA virus that belongs to the family Papovaviridae. The genome consists of circular, double-stranded DNA encased in a protein icosahedral capsid. Electron microscope studies revealed that the capsid consists of 12 five-coordinated and six-coordinated capsomers on the surface of the virion arranged in a lattice (52,53). The capsid consists of two proteins termed a major and minor component, with the former accounting for 80% of the total viral protein (54). There are approximately 80 HPV types, and new types continuously are discovered. Some types are significant because of their association with genital tract cancers (Table 10-4). In a study of 2,624 women, 6% of cytologically and colposcopically normal cervices were found to contain latent HPV 16 (55).

Viral types 1, 2, 3, 4, and 10 are associated with nongenital, cutaneotropic disease such as benign skin warts. HPV types 3, 5, 8, 10, and 18 are associated with EV, an autosomal recessive disease (10,56,57). A total of approximately 50 HPV types have been isolated in patients with EV.

EV is a rare disease characterized by disseminated flat warts and pityriasis versicolor-like skin lesions. Skin lesions occur in approximately 75% of the cases, and approximately 30% of the patients develop skin cancers (58,59). The development of skin cancer related to sun exposure is associated with HPV types 5, 6, and 14. The affected individual can develop either EV or squamous cell cancer. EV typically begins at an early age, infancy or childhood, and occurs almost exclusively in Caucasians (60,61). The disease that occurs in African Americans is usually benign, and cancer has not been found in association with EV. HPV and cancer can, and does, occur in non-African-American women with genital HPV. A variety of HPV types have been found to be associated with epidermodysplasia and HPV genital disease, but only a few are associated with cancer (Table 10-5).

Benign HPV disease is associated with HPV types 6 and 11 and is typically seen in association with raised genital warts. HPV types 16 and 18 are more frequently associated with flat condyloma, and approximately 90% of cervical cancer is associated with HPV 16 (62). It does not appear that the virus is independently oncogenic but actually requires a cofactor to initiate abnormal cellular

TABLE 10-4. *HPV types and their association with genital tract cancer*

Low-risk types—6, 11, 42, 43, 44
Intermediate-risk types—31, 33, 35, 51, 58
High-risk types—16, 18, 45, 56

TABLE 10-5. *Classification of HPV types*

Nongenital disease
Typical skin warts—1, 2, 3, and 4
Epidermodysplasia verruciformis associated with malignancy—5, 8, and 14
Genital mucocutaneous disease
Low malignant potential—6, 11, 42, 43, and 44
Intermediate malignant potential—31, 33, 35, 51, 52, and 58
High malignant potential—16, 18, 45, and 56

growth and division. These malignancies develop in areas of the skin exposed to sunlight, suggesting that ultraviolet light may serve as the cofactor or cocarcinogen that upregulates an area of the genome in HPV 5.

The viral genome is divided into three regions: (a) regulatory region that controls the expression of the viral genes, (b) an early region containing the genes that encode for proteins that are not part of the viral particle (these early proteins are involved in viral DNA replication and the malignant process), and (c) the late region that encodes for the major and minor proteins of the virus.

Incorporation of the viral DNA into the host DNA is associated with late viral protein synthesis (major and minor proteins). Deletion of the late viral proteins, the major and part of the minor proteins, results in the inability to encode for the viral structural proteins. Thus, infected host cells that become dysplastic and malignant do not produce viral particles. Incomplete differentiation found in dysplastic and malignant cells is associated with the inhibition of viral replication.

When the viral DNA becomes integrated into the host cell DNA it is transferred to progeny cells. Another change that occurs after integration is that cells infected with HPV oncogenic types appear to have a significantly increased lifespan. Cells infected with nononcogenic HPV types do not have an increased life span (63–67).

Increased cellular life or immortalization by high-risk viral types found in cervical cancer requires the presence and function of two early genes, E6 and E7 (68,69). E6 and E7 genes encode for proteins that inactivate two tumor suppressor genes thus enhancing cell growth. These genes are more active in HPV strains associated with cancer. The E6 gene product inactivates the host p53 protein and E7 inactivates the retinoblastoma susceptibility protein, Rb (70,71).

Thus, all HPV viruses replicate in the host cell nucleus as extrachromosomal plasmids, as in benign lesions, or they become integrated into the host chromosome. In malignant transformed cells, such as those associated with HPV 16 and 18, the viral DNA becomes integrated onto the host chromosome (72,73). When the virus is in the host cell, it may assume a latent or active phase. Once the virus is activated and causes host cell transformation a wart appears. All cells that make up the wart are derived from a single infected basal cell (74). The lesions produced by HPV can assume a raised pyriform or cauliflower form commonly referred to as condylomata acuminata, popular warts, or flat warts. A subclinical presentation has also been noted and is detected by the presence of koilocytosis on biopsy specimens containing HPV DNA. The characteristic lesions can resolve spontaneously and can, subsequently, be followed by a period of latency. The patient can experience exacerbations of her disease in which crops of warts appear repeatedly with intermittent periods of absence of warts. The lesions can persist and require a combination of therapeutic agents to achieve resolution, and they may reappear following therapy.

CLINICAL PRESENTATION

Clinical presentations of HPV vary from grossly apparent disease to histologic and molecular evidence of infection. Low-risk types, such as HPV 6 and 11, are commonly associated with benign disease and appear as condylomata acuminata (Figs. 10-3 to 10-6). These lesions are typically pyriform but may coalesce to form large raised flattened lesions. The condyloma may become extremely large in size, resembling a pedunculated tumor, or it may replace the entire labia appearing brainlike (Fig. 10-7). Low-risk HPV types (6, 11, 42, 43, and 44) can be found in association with LGSIL cervical lesions but are rarely found in high-grade squamous intraepithelial lesion (HGSIL) (75). The intermediate-risk HPV types (31, 33, 35, 51, and 52) are commonly associated with HGSIL and less frequently found with LGSIL and cancer (75). High-risk HPV types (16, 18, 45, and 56) are commonly found in association with HGSIL and cervical cancer (75). All HPV types can be found in association with atypia and LGSIL. Wallin et al. (76) demonstrated that the presence of HPV types 16, 18,

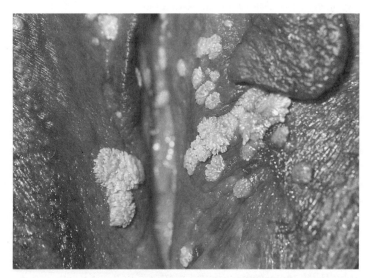

FIG. 10-3. Note that the condyloma can form individual lesions or form small and large aggregates. (See Color Plate 16 following page 148.)

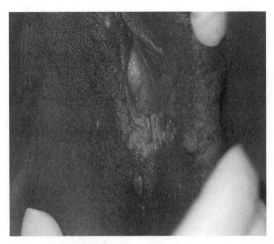

FIG. 10-4. Lesions can be distributed over the vulva, the labia majora, and labia minora. These lesions appear gray in color and are dry, in contrast to those in Fig. 10-4, which are white and moist. (See Color Plate 17 following page 148.)

31, and 33 strongly correlated with the development of cervical cancer. These authors studied 118 women ages 25 to 29 with invasive cervical disease who had a normal Pap smear between 1969 and 1995. For individuals who had multiple normal Pap smears, the smear taken closest to the diagnosis of cervical cancer was used. The control group was matched for age, the time a normal Pap smear was obtained, and the time a normal smear was obtained after cancer had been

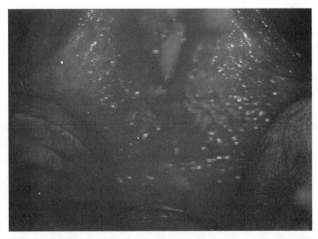

FIG. 10-5. Condyloma appear as papillary projections. Although it can not be seen in this photograph, when the papillary structures are viewed through a colposcope, the vascularity of the lesion can be seen. (See Color Plate 18 following page 148.)

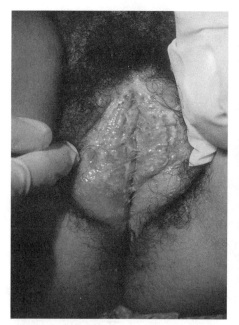
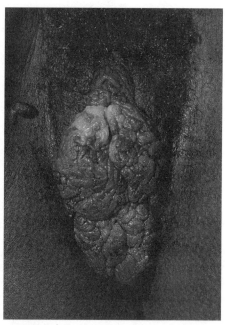

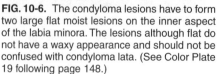

FIG. 10-6. The condyloma lesions have to form two large flat moist lesions on the inner aspect of the labia minora. The lesions although flat do not have a waxy appearance and should not be confused with condyloma lata. (See Color Plate 19 following page 148.)

FIG. 10-7. The condyloma has replaced almost the entire labia minora and appears brainlike. (See Color Plate 20 following page 148.)

diagnosed in the study patient. HPV DNA was detected in the Pap smears of 35 women with cancer (30%) and 3 controls (3%). In the cervical cancer group, HPV DNA was detected in 77% of the patients and in 4% of the controls. The average time from normal Pap smear (subsequently found to have HPV DNA) to cancer was 5.6 years. These authors concluded that a finding of HPV DNA in a Pap smear increases risk for the development of invasive cervical cancer (76).

One concern in the management and treatment of genital HPV is the suspected presence of HPV in normal tissue adjacent to infected and transformed tissue. Thus, latent or occult infection in cells without an abnormal morphologic appearance is of concern because of its potential to transform healthy cells into dysplastic or cancerous cells. One study found that 28% of women with HPV-positive Pap smears developed cervical intraepithelial neoplasia (CIN) (77). The hypothesis that the virus assumes latency in normal squamous epithelial cells is the cornerstone for the assumption that the virus is not eliminated from the normal epithelium and is responsible for subsequent recurrences following therapy (78,79). The hypothesis that the virus can assume a posture of latency in healthy host cells is an issue that has complicated therapeutic regimens; if HPV can indeed assume a state of latency in cells that have no morphologic appearance, treatments will undoubtedly fail and recurrence will likely occur. Using PCR techniques, studies have documented that HPV DNA can be detected in 2% to 60% of exfoliated cervical cells (6,80,81). Thus, the hypothesis that latent virus can persist in morphologically normal cells following treatment of a diseased area is responsible for recurrence of clinical disease. However, following treatment of cervical HPV, there have been reports that HPV types, other than those causing the original lesion, caused recurrent disease. These reports also state that HPV DNA is not commonly found in normal appearing squamous epithelium adjacent to morphologically abnormal cells infected with HPV (82,83). Tate et al. (83) concluded that occult infection could go undetected when treating patients with CIN resulting from HPV; however, when treating CIN, occult infection is not normally maintained in morphologically normal appearing cells. This conclusion is supported by the absence of HPV DNA in normal cells adjacent to CIN and the low recurrence rate following treatment (84). This question of latent virus infection in morphologically normal cells remains unsettled because the possibility still exists. In a study by Czeglédy et al. (85), 108 women wearing an intrauterine device (IUD) had a Pap smear, colposcopic examination, and their cervical cells harvested and subjected to *in situ* hybridization for the detection of HPV DNA. No evidence of HPV was found in 86 of the patients. However, 22 patients were found to have evidence of HPV types 6, 11, 16, and 18. When treating patients for HPV-related cervical disease, the patient should not be reassured that "all virus" has been eliminated and that there is no need for close follow-up examinations. The patient can be reassured that it is unlikely that she will experience recurrent disease because of latent infection, but she is still at risk for acquiring new infection if she participates in high-risk behavior.

The diagnosis of HPV infection can be obvious or not so obvious depending on the clinical manifestation of disease. As stated earlier, it is often diagnosed by the presence of pyriform moist lesions, papillary lesions containing a central vessel, flat raised white coarse lesions, or subtle lesions revealed by applying 5% acetic acid to the tissue to be examined. Cells containing HPV can be detected by microscopic examination of stained cells looking for characteristic nuclear and cytoplasmic changes referred to as koilocytosis, detection of HPV DNA by *in situ* hybridization, or PCR. HPV DNA has also been detected in urine obtained from men with urethral condyloma and in men without clinical signs or symptoms of HPV infection (86–88).

DIAGNOSIS

There is no doubt that clinically apparent condyloma can easily be recognized and not mistaken for another disease, except perhaps condyloma lata. However, less obvious lesions often go undiagnosed; therefore, more sensitive and specific tests are indicated. The detection of HPV and its association with genital cancer necessitated the development of such tests to detect DNA or ribonucleic acid

(RNA), like filter hybridization (Southern blot and slot blot hybridization), *in situ* hybridization, and PCR (Table 10-6).

The typical condyloma acuminata lesion is piriform, growing outward from the skin. These lesions are referred to as exophytic and tend to be white, granular, and moist. The lesions may coalesce to form large lesions and may appear flat and raised above the level of normal tissue. The lesion may not be clinically apparent or detectable with either the unaided eye or the colposcope. Painting the tissue with 5% acetic acid enhances the lesion, causing it to become white and distinguishing it from uninfected tissue (89).

The Pap smear is the most common cytologic method of identifying HPV-infected cells. Typically the nucleus of the infected cell is enlarged and dark, has an irregular border, and is surrounded by a clear cytoplasmic ring referred to as koilocytosis. Koilocytosis is not equivalent to cells containing latent virus because those cells do not show signs of koilocytosis (90). The Pap smear only detects from 15% to 50% of patients with HPV infection (91,92). The most commonly used test for detecting HPV DNA in clinical specimens is *in situ* hybridization (commercially available, Digene Diagnostics, Inc.). There has also been considerable discussion regarding whether or not the patient with HPV should have the virus type determined. The question the physician must ask is whether or not this information will change the management of the patient. Most likely patients diagnosed with HPV infection and cellular abnormalities will be managed in the same fashion as patients with dysplasia who do not have HPV. All dysplasia patients will also require management and follow-up to prevent severe disease, including cancer.

TABLE 10-6. *Comparison of different methods of diagnosing HPV[a]*

Test	Sensitivity	Specificity	Comments
Visual inspection	Low	High	Can identify only gross disease
Colposcopy	Moderate	Low	Can detect clinical lesions not observed by visual inspection
Pap smear	Low	High	
Southern blot	High	High	Not good for clinical use
Dot blot	Moderate	High	Rapid, inexpensive
In situ hybridization	Moderate	High	Can detect HPV DNA in tissue
Filter *in situ* hybridization	Poor	Poor	
PCR	High	High	Extremely sensitive, but high risk of false positives

HPV, human papillomavirus; PCR, polymerase chain reaction.

[a]Adapted from Johnson K. Canadian Task Force on the Periodic Health Examination. Periodic health examination, 1995 update: 1. Screening for human papillomavirus infection in asymptomatic women. *Can Med Assoc J* 1995;152:483–493.

Reid R, Lorincz AT. Human papillomavirus tests. *Bailliére's Clin Obstet Gynaecol* 1995;9: 65–103.

Trofatter KF. Diagnosis of human papillomavirus genital tract infection. *Am J Med* 1997;102: 21–27.

THERAPY

There are a variety of therapeutic agents available for the treatment of HPV infection. Treatments for condylomata acuminata and HPV disease are listed in Table 10-7. Basically all therapeutic regimens for the treatment of genital warts are not extremely efficacious, have a significant recurrence rate, and transmission is likely. Because of the lack of understanding of the role of latency in this infection, speculation with regard to recurrences continues to occur. Is it a recurrence of a new infection? If virus is present in an epithelium that appears normal, should the tissue adjacent to the infected area also be treated?

A standard treatment since the 1940s has been to paint the condylomata with podophyllin (93). Podophyllin is a resin derived from *Podophyllin* or *Podophyllin peltatum* that contains biologically active lignans such as podofilox or podophyllotoxin, α-peltatin, β-peltatin, and 43-demethyl-podophyllotoxin (94,95). Podofilox is the most active compound found in podophyllin and is marketed under the trade name Condylox. Podofilox has a variety of biologic activities resulting in tissue necrosis (Table 10-8).

Podofilox is prepared in a 0.5% formulation that is applied by the patient twice daily for 3 days, followed by 4 days of no treatment. This regimen is repeated for a total of four cycles. Several studies have demonstrated that podofilox is efficacious and systematically safe; however, the local side effects may be rather high (Table 10-9).

Other adverse reactions reported were erythema, dryness, irritation, and nausea. Because the treatment regimens for condylomata acuminata have not met

TABLE 10-7. *Treatment modalities for HPV[a]*

Therapy	Average # Rx	Success rates	Recurrence rates	References
Chemotherapeutic agents				
TCA	4	64–81%	36%	93, 94
Podophyllin	3.4–6.7	38–79%	21–65%	95
Podofilox	3.2 Rx cycles	68–88%	16–34.5%	96–102
5-Fluorouracil	2–2.5 Rx cycles	68–97%	0–8%	103, 104
Interferon-α				
Topical		33%	21–25.5%	105, 106
Intralesional		36–53%	210–25%	107
Systemic		7–82%	23.5%	108–110
Imiquimod		50%		111
Destructive methods				
Cryotherapy	2.6–3.2	70–96%	25–39%	112
CO_2 laser	1–2	72–96%	25–39%	113–116
Electrodesiccation	1.3	94%	25.5%	98
LEEP		72%	51%	97
Surgical				
Excision	1.1	89–93%	19–22%	99

LEEP, loop electrosurgical excision procedure; TCA, trichloroacetic acid.
[a]Adapted from references 101, 102, 106, 112–133.

TABLE 10-8. *Biologic activity of podofilox*

Inhibits mitosis[a]
Damages dermal circulation[b]
Causes cell necrosis[c]
Inhibits nucleoside transport[a]
Inhibits the mitogen response of human lymphocytes[a]
Induces production of interleukin-1 by human monocytes[a]
Induces production of interleukin-2 by human lymphocytes[a]
Enhance macrophage proliferation[a]

[a]Loike JD, Horowitz SB. Effects of podophyllotoxin and VP-16-23 on microtubule assembly in vitro and nucleoside transport in He La cells. *Biochemistry* 1976;15:5435–5443.
[b]von Krogh G, Maibach HI. Cutaneous cyto destructive potency of lignars I. A comparative evaluation of epidermal and dermal DNA synthesis on dermal microcirculation in the hairless mouse. *Arch Dermatol Res* 1982;274:9–20.
Zheng QY, Wiranowska M, Sadlik JR, et al. Purified podophyllotoxin (CPH-86) inhibits lymphocyte proliferation but augments macrophage proliferation. *Int J Immunopharmacol* 1987;9: 539–549.
[c]Wade TR, Ackerman AB. The effects of resin of podophyllin on condyloma acuminatum. *Am J Dermatol* 1984;6:109–122.

with great success, therapeutic agents continue to be sought. One group of agents that appeared promising was the interferons. Discovered over 40 years ago, interferons are part of the body's natural defensive mechanisms to combat viral infection, tumors, and antigens (96,97). Interferons are proteins that react with host cells making them resistant to viruses. In addition, these proteins can affect the body's metabolism, cell proliferation, hormone stimulation, immunity, and tumor development (98-100). Interferons (INF-alph-2a and INF-γ) have

TABLE 10-9. *Adverse effects associated with topically applied podofilox*

Inflammation	40% to 64%[a]
Erosion	48% to 63%[a]
Pain	38% to 67%[a]
Burning	52% to 93%[a]
Itching	31% to 65%[a]

[a]Baker DA, Douglas JM, Buntin DM, et al. Topical podofilox for the treatment of condylomata acuminata in women. *Obstet Gynecol* 1990;76:656–659.
Baron S. Mechanism of recovery from viral infection. In: Smith DM, Lauffer MA, eds. *Advances in virus research*. New York: Academic Press, 1963;39–60.
Baron S, Diazani F, Stanton GJ, et al., eds. *The interferon system: a current review to 1987*. Austin: University Texas Press, 1987.
Ferenczy A. Comparison of 5-fluorouracil and CO_2 laser for treatment of vaginal condylomata. *Obstet Gynecol* 1984;64:773–778.
Isaacs A, Lindermann J. Virus interferons. I: the interferon. *Proc R Soc Ser B* 1957;147:258–267.
Kirby P, Dunne A, King DH, et al. Double-blind randomized clinical trial of self administered podofilox solution versus vehicle in the treatment of genital warts. *Am J Med* 1990;88:465–469.
Pride GL. Treatment of large lower genital tract condylomata acuminata with topical 5-fluorouracil. *J Reprod Med* 1990;35:384–387.
Taylor JL, Grossberg SE. Recent progress in interferon research: molecular mechanisms of regulation, action, and virus circumvention. *Virus Res* 1990;15:1–25.

been effective when injected intralesionally or systemically causing regression or partial resolution of condyloma acuminata (101-105).

Treatment of condylomata acuminata with interferon has demonstrated a reasonable rate of success. Friedman-Kien et al. (106) treated 86 patients with interferon alfa, a natural leukocyte (alfa) interferon, injected into the base of each lesion, 2.5 to 5×10^5 IU/25 mm^2 of wart-area index. These authors achieved a 62% success rate for complete elimination of the warts. Leventhal et al. (107) also reported success in the treatment of respiratory papillomatosis with systemic administration of lymphoblastoid interferon alfa-n1 in a dose of 2,000,000 U per square meter every day or 4,000,000 U per square meter every other day. The condyloma international collaborative group conducted a double-blind placebo-controlled clinical trial with recombinant interferon alfa-2a administered systemically in doses of 3,000,000 or 9, 000,000 U three times a week for 4 weeks (108). This study, however, did not find a satisfactory response to either dosing regimen. The recurrence rates at the end of 9 months in the group receiving 3,000,000 U was 9%, and in the group receiving 9,000,000 U was 36%. Thus, when examining all studies, it appears that treatment with interferon may be useful in some instances but should not be a first-line therapy or be used on a wide scale. Perhaps interferon treatment should be reserved for individuals who are not immunosuppressed but who have a significant amount of disease. It probably should be used in conjunction with ablative therapy. Trizna et al. (109) examined IFN-α and IFN-γ alone and in combination for the treatment of anogenital condylomata acuminata. These authors injected interferon into the subcutaneous tissue in the groin as follows: IFN-α 3×10^6 U, IFN-γ 3×10^6 U, IFN-α 1.5×10^6 U plus IFN-γ 1.5×10^6 U, and IFN-α 3×10^6 U plus IFN-γ 1.5×10^6 U, three times a week for 6 weeks. All patients were considered to have recalcitrant anogenital condylomata acuminata. The response rates were 13.6%, 18.5%, 16%, and 3.8% respectively. However, the authors felt that when partial and complete responses were taken together, the group receiving IFN-α (3×10^6 U) plus IFN-γ (1.5×10^6 U) had a success rate of 73%. These authors concluded that regional administration of interferon was moderately effective for the treatment of recalcitrant condylomata acuminata. Interferon is relatively safe and well tolerated; however, there are adverse effects, the most common is a flu-like syndrome (Table 10-10). Other less frequent side effects are arthralgias, muscle stiffness, blurred vision, and cold sweats (109).

A new agent that has been approved for the treatment of vulvar condylomata and HPV is imiquimod (imidazoquinolin heterocyclic amine), an immune-modulating agent. Imiquimod stimulates the production of cytokines and appears effective against viruses and tumors (110,111). Systemic toxicity is unusual because this agent is a 5% cream topically applied to the affected area. Local adverse reactions include erythema, ulceration, edema, pain, and bleeding. Treatment with imiquimod cream appears to be as effective as any other treatment. For vulvar condylomata treatment, imiquimod is applied 3 times a week for 4 to 16 weeks. Clearance rates in women were 72% with a recurrence rate of 13% (112).

TABLE 10-10. *Adverse effects associated with interferon therapy*

Flu-like syndrome—40%
Fever/chills—30%
Myalgias—30%
Headaches—40%
Malaise—20%
GI—10%
Fatigue—5%
Nausea/vomiting—12%
Diarrhea—18%
Dizziness—8%
Pain at the injection site—5%

GI, gastrointestinal.

TABLE 10-11. *Treatment regimens for anogenital condylomata acuminata and vulvovaginal and cervical HPV-associated dysplasia*

1. Caustic treatment
   a. Podophyllin—success rates 22% to 77%, recurrence rates as high as 74%. Adverse reactions—pain, erythema, itching, burning, swelling, ulcerations. Can be absorbed systemically, contraindicated in pregnancy. Should be washed off in 4 to 6 hours, is not likely to cause ulceration. Not suitable for extensive treatment, old lesions, or hyperkeratotic lesions. Requires multiple treatments.
   b. Podofilox—similar to podophyllin
   c. Trichloroacetic & bichloracetic acid—success rate approaches 80%, recurrence rate up to 35%. Not suitable for large lesions, numerous lesions, or hypkeratinized lesions. May cause significant pain, burning, erythema, and ulcerations. Requires multiple treatments.
   d. 5-Fluorouracil—for treatment of small, nonkeratinized vaginal warts. Adverse reactions are irritation, intense inflammation, burns, and ulcerations.
2. Ablative treatment
   a. Surgical incision—recurrence rate of 30%
   b. Cryotherapy—recurrence rate of approximately 40%
   c. Laser vaporization—recurrence rate of up to 95%
   d. Electric cauterization
   e. Loop diathermy
3. Chemotherapeutic agents
   a. Interferons—recurrence rate of 60%
   b. Imiquimod—recurrence rate of 13%

The treatment and management of anogenital condylomata acuminata is based on the distribution, number, and size of the lesions. The treatment and management of HPV is dependent on the location and stage of dysplasia. Table 10-11 summarizes the available treatment regimens.

REFERENCES

1. Ciuffo G. Imnfesto positivo con filtrato di verruca volgare. *Italn Mal Venerol* 1907;48:12–17.
2. Schope RE, Hurst EW. Infectious papillomavirus of rabbits; with a note on histopathology. *J Exp Med* 1933;58:607–624.
3. Anonymous. 1989 Sexually transmitted diseases treatment guidelines. *MMWR* 1989;38(Suppl 8): 1–43.

4. American College of Obstetrics and Gynecology. Sexually transmitted diseases. In: Precis V, ed. *An update in obstetrics and gynecology.* Washington DC: American College of Obstetrics and Gynecology, 1994:87–91.
5. Bauer HM, Ting Y, Greier CE, et al. Genital human papillomavirus infection in female university students as determined by PCR-based method. *JAMA* 1991;265:472–477.
6. Ley C, Bauer HM, Reingold A, et al. Determinants of genital human papillomavirus infection in young women. *J Natl Cancer Inst* 1991;83:997–1003.
7. Franco EL, Villa LL, Richardson H, et al. Epidemiology of cervical human papillomavirus infection. In: Franco EL, Monsonego J, eds. *New developments in cancer cervical screening and prevention.* Oxford, United Kingdom: Blackwell Science, 1997:14–22.
8. Schiffman MH, Brinton LA. The epidemiology of cervical carcinogenesis. *Cancer* 1995;76: 1888–1901.
9. Centers for Disease Control and Prevention. Annual report. Atlanta, GA: Department of Health and Human Services, 1994.
10. Orth G. Epidermodysplasia verruciformis. In: Salzman NP, Howely PM, eds. *The Papovaviridae: the papillomaviruses.* New York: Plenum Press, 1987:199–243.
11. Becker TM, Stone KM, Alexander ER. Genital human papillomavirus infection. A growing concern. *Obstet Gynecol Clin North Am* 1987;14:389–396.
12. Ho GY, Bierman R, Beardsley L, et al. Natural history of cervicovaginal papillomavirus infection in young women. *N Engl J Med* 1998;338:423–428.
13. Richart RM, Barron BA. A follow-up study of patients with cervical dysplasia. *Am J Obstet Gynecol* 1969;105:386–393.
14. Nasiell K, Roger V, Nasiell M. Behavior of mild cervical dysplasia during long-term follow-up. *Obstet Gynecol* 1986;67:665–669.
15. Franco EL, Villa LL, Sobrinho JP, et al. Epidemiology of acquisition and clearance of cervical human papillomavirus infection in women from a high-risk area for cervical cancer. *J Infect Dis* 1999;180:1415–1423.
16. Schneider A, Hotz M, Gissmann L. Increased prevalence of human papillomavirus in the lower genital tract of pregnant women. *Int J Cancer* 1987;40:198–203.
17. Kemp EA, Hakenewerth AM, Laurent SL, et al. Human papillomavirus prevalence in pregnancy. *Obstet Gynecol* 1992;79:649–656.
18. Garry R, Jones R. Relationship between cervical condyloma, pregnancy and subclinical papillomavirus infection. *J Reprod Med* 1985;30:393–399.
19. Fife KH, Rogers RE, Zwickl BW. Symptomatic and asymptomatic cervical infections with human papillomavirus during pregnancy. *J Infect Dis* 1987;156:904–911.
20. Rando RF, Lindheim S, Hasty L, et al. Increased frequency of detection of human papillomavirus deoxyribonucleic acid in exfoliated cervical cells during pregnancy. *Am J Obstet Gynecol* 1989;161: 50–55.
21. Fife KH, Katz BP, Roush J, et al. Cancer-associated human papillomavirus types are selectively increased in the cervix of women in the first trimester of pregnancy. *Am J Obstet Gynecol* 1996;174: 1487–1493.
22. Peng TC, Searle CP, Shah KV, et al. Prevalence of human papillomavirus infections in term pregnancy. *Am J Perinatol* 1990;7:189–192.
23. Smith EM, Johnson SR, Jiang D, et al. The association between pregnancy and human papillomavirus prevalence. *Cancer Detect Prev* 1991;15:397–402.
24. de Roda Husman AM, Walboomers JM, Hopman E, et al. HPV prevalence in cytomorphologically normal cervical scrapes of pregnant women as determined by PCR: the age-related pattern. *J Med Virol* 1995;46:97–102.
25. Chang-Claude J, Schneider A, Smith E, et al. Longitudinal study of the effects of pregnancy and other factors on detection of HPV. *Gynecol Oncol* 1996;60:355–362.
26. Tenti P, Zappatore R, Migliora P, et al. Latent human papillomavirus infection in pregnant women at term: a case-control study. *J Infect Dis* 1997;176:277–280.
27. Mackenzie M. *Essays in growth in the larynx with reports of analysis of 100 consecutive cases treated by the author.* London: J & A Churchill, 1871.
28. Glazer G, Webb WR. Laryngeal papillomatosis with pulmonary spread in a 69-year-old man. *AJR* 1979;132:820–822.
29. Fearon B, MacRae D. Laryngeal papillomatosis in children. *J Otolaryngol* 1976;5:493–496.
30. Hajek EF. Clinical records: contribution to the etiology of laryngeal papilloma in children. *J Laryngol Otol* 1956;70:166–168.

31. Anderson KC, Roy TM, Fields CL, et al. Juvenile laryngeal papillomatosis: a new complication. *South Med J* 1993;86:447–449.
32. Mounier-Kuhn P, Gaillard J, Dumolard P, et al. Papilloma of the larynx and trachea in children. *Int Surg* 1974;59:483–486.
33. Smith L, Gooding CA. Pulmonary involvement in laryngeal papillomatosis. *Pediatr Radiol* 1974;2: 161–166.
34. Weiss MD, Kashima HK. Tracheal involvement in laryngeal papillomatosis. *Laryngoscope* 1983;93: 45–48.
35. Fredericks BD, Balkin A, Daniel HW, et al. Transmission of human papillomaviruses from mother to child. *Aust N Z J Obstet Gynaecol* 1993;33:30–32.
36. Parkarian F, Kaye J, Cason J, et al. Cancer associated with human papillomaviruses: perinatal transmission and persistence. *Br J Obstet Gyneacol* 1994;101:514–517.
37. Puranen M, Yliskoski M, Saarikoski S, et al. Vertical transmission of human papillomavirus from infected mothers to their newborn babies and persistence of the virus in childhood. *Am J Obstet Gynecol* 1996;174:694–699.
38. Tang CK, Shermeta DW, Wood C. Congenital condylomata acuminata. *Am J Obstet Gynecol* 1978; 131:912–913.
39. Rogo KO, Nyansera PN. Congenital condylomata acuminata with meconium staining of amniotic fluid and fetal hydrocephalus: case report. *East Afr Med J* 1989;66:411–413.
40. Tseng C-J, Lin CY, Wang RL, et al. Possible transplacental transmission of human papillomaviruses. *Am J Obstet Gynecol* 1992;166:35–40.
41. Armbruster-Moraes E, Ioshimoto LM, Leao E, et al. Presence of human papillomavirus DNA in amniotic fluids of pregnant women with cervical lesions. *Gynecol Oncol* 1994;54:152–158.
42. Puranen MH, Yliskoski MH, Saarikoski SV, et al. Exposure of an infant to cervical human papilloma infection of the mother is common. *Am J Obstet Gynecol* 1997;176:1039–1045.
43. O'Hanlan KA. Lesbian health and homophobia. *Curr Prob Obstet Gynecol Fertil* 1995;18:92–136.
44. Laumann EO, Gagnon JH, Micheal RT, et al. *The social organization of sexuality: sexual practices in the United States.* Chicago: University of Chicago Press, 1994:295.
45. Diamond M. Homosexuality and bisexuality in different populations. *Arch Sex Behav* 1993;22: 291–310.
46. Anonymous. Health care needs of gay men and lesbians in the United States. Council on Scientific Affairs, American Medical Association. *JAMA* 1996;275:1354–1359.
47. Marrazzo JM, Koutsky LA, Stine KL, et al. Genital human papillomavirus infection in women who have sex with women. *J Inf Dis* 1998;178:1604–1609.
48. Ferenczy A, Bergeron C, Richart RM. Human papillomavirus DNA in fomites on objects used for the management of patients with genital human papillomavirus infections. *Obstet Gynecol* 1989;74: 950–954.
49. Sonnex C, Strauss S, Gray JJ. Detection of human papillomavirus DNA on the fingers of patients with genital warts. *Sex Transm Infect* 1999;75:317–319.
50. Einhorn L, Polgar M. HIV-risk behavior among lesbians and bisexual women. *AIDS Educ Prev* 1994;6:514–523.
51. Marrazzo JM, Stine K, Koutsky LA. Genital human papillomavirus infection in women who have sex with women: a review. *Am J Obstet Gynecol* 2000;183:770–774.
52. Klug A, Finch JT. The structure of viruses of the papilloma-polyoma type III. Structure of rabbit papillomavirus with an appendix on the topography of contrast in negative-staining for electron-microscopy. *J Mol Biol* 1965;13:1–12.
53. Klug A, Finch JT. Structure of viruses of the papilloma type I. Human wart virus. *J Mol Biol* 1963; 11:403–423.
54. Favre M. Structural polypeptides of rabbit, bovine, and human papillomaviruses. *J Virol* 1975;15: 1239–1247.
55. Lorincz AT, Reid R, Jenson AB, et al. Human papillomavirus infection of the cervix: relative risk associations of 15 common anogenital types. *Obstet Gynecol* 1992;79:328–337.
56. Pfister H, Nurnberger F, Gissmann L, et al. Characterization of human papillomavirus from epidermodysplasia verruciformis lesions of a patient from Upper-Volta. *Int J Cancer* 1981;27:645–650.
57. Claudy AL, Touraine JL, Mitanne D. Epidermodysplasia verruciformis induced by a new human papillomavirus (HPV-8). Report of a case without immune dysfunction. *Arch Dermatol Res* 1982; 274:213–219.
58. Durst M. Physical state of papillomavirus DNA in tumors. In: Syrjanen K, Gissman L, Koss LG, eds. *Papillomaviruses and human disease.* New York: Springer Verlag, 1987:403.

59. Lutzner MA. Epidermodysplasia verruciformis. An autosomal recessive disease characterized by viral warts and skin cancer. A model for viral oncogenesis. *Bull Cancer* 1978;65:169–182.
60. Haustein UF. Epidermodysplasia verruciformis Lewandowsky-Lutz with multiple squamous epithelium and Bowen's carcinomas. *Dermatol Montatssch* 1992;168:821–828.
61. Ruiter M. On the histomorphology and origin of malignant cutaneous changes in epidermodysplasia verruciformis. *Acta Derm Vener* 1973;53:290–298.
62. zur Hausen H. Human papillomaviruses in the pathogenesis of anogenital cancer. *Virology* 1991; 184:9–13.
63. Werner BA. Role of human papillomavirus oncoproteins in transformation and carcinogenic progression. In: DeVito JT, ed. *Important advances in oncology.* Philadelphia: JB Lippincott, 1991:3.
64. Weinberg RA. *Oncogenes and their molecular origins of cancer.* Cold Spring Harbor, NY: Cold Spring Harbor Laboratory, 1989.
65. Feldman SR, Yaar M. Oncogenes. The growth control genes. *Arch Dermatol* 1991;127:707–711.
66. Marshall CJ. Tumor suppressor genes. *Cell* 1991;64:313–326.
67. Weinberg RA. Tumor suppressor genes. *Science* 1991;254:1138–1146.
68. Schiffman MH. Recent progress in defining the epidemiology of human papillomavirus infection and cervical neoplasia. *J Natl Cancer Inst* 1992;84:394–398.
69. Barbosa MS, Vass WC, Lowy DR, et al. In vitro biological activities of the E6 and E7 genes vary among human papillomaviruses of different oncogenic potential. *J Virol* 1991;65:292–298.
70. Huibregtse JM, Scheffner M, Howley PM. A cellular protein mediates association of p53 with E6 oncoprotein of human papillomavirus types 16 or 18. *EMBO J* 1991;10:4129–135.
71. Hubbert NL, Sedman SA, Schiller JT. Human papillomavirus type 16 E6 increases the degradation rate of p53 in human keratinocytes. *J Virol* 1992;66:6237–6241.
72. Durst M, Schwarz E, Gissman L. Integration and persistence of human papillomavirus DNA in genital tumors. *Banbury Rep* 1986;21:273–280.
73. Durst M, Kleinheinz A, Hotz M, et al. The physical state of human papillomavirus type 16 DNA in benign and malignant genital tumours. *J Gen Virol* 1985;66:1515–1522.
74. Murray RF, Hobbs J, Payne B. Possible clonal origin of common warts (verruca vulgaris). *Nature* 1971;232:51–52.
75. Manos MM, Ting Y, Wright DK, et al. The use of polymerase chain reaction amplification for the detection of genital human papillomavirus. *Molecular Diagnosis of Human Cancer, Cancer Cells* 1989;7:209–214.
76. Wallin KL, Wiklund F, Ångström T, et al. Type-specific persistence of human papillomavirus DNA before the development of invasive cervical cancer. *N Engl J Med* 1999;341:1633–1638.
77. Koutsky LA, Holmes KK, Critchlow CW, et al. A cohort study of the risk of cervical intraepithelial neoplasia grade 2 or 3 in relation to papillomavirus infection. *N Engl J Med* 1992;327:1272–1278.
78. Steinberg BM, Topp WC, Schneider PS, et al. Laryngeal papillomavirus infection during clinical remission. *N Engl J Med* 1983;308:1261–1264.
79. Ferenczy A, Mitao M, Nagai N, et al. Latent papillomavirus and recurring genital warts. *N Engl J Med* 1985; 313:784–748.
80. Melkert PW, Hopman E, van den Brule AJ, et al. Prevalence of HPV in cytomorphologically normal cervical smears, as determined by polymerase chain reaction, is age-dependent. *Int J Cancer* 1993; 53:919–923.
81. Rosenfeld WD, Rose E, Vermund SH, et al. Follow-up evaluation of cervicovaginal human papillomavirus infection in adolescents. *J Pediatr* 1992;121:307–311.
82. Nuovo GJ, Pedemonte BM. Human papillomavirus types and recurrent cervical warts. *JAMA* 1990; 263:1223–1226.
83. Tate JE, Resnick M, Sheets EE, et al. Absence of papillomavirus DNA in normal tissue adjacent to most cervical intraepithelial neoplasms. *Obstet Gynecol* 1996;88:257–260.
84. Richart RM, Townsend DE, Crisp W, et al. An analysis of "long term" follow-up results in patients with cervical intraepithelial neoplasia treated by cryotherapy. *Am J Obstet Gynecol* 1980;137: 823–826.
85. Czeglédy J, Gergely L, Batár I. Human papillomavirus in cervical smears taken from women wearing an intrauterine contraceptive device. *Arch Gynecol Obstet* 1989;244:87–89.
86. Melchers WJ, Schift R, Stolz E, et al. Human papillomavirus detection in urine samples from male patients by the polymerase chain reaction. *J Clin Microbiol* 1989;27:1711–1714.
87. Forslund O, Hansson BG, Rymark P, et al. Human papillomavirus DNA in urine samples compared with that simultaneously collected urethra and cervix samples. *J Clin Microbiol* 1993;31: 1975–1979.

88. Iwasawa A, Hiltunen-Back E, Reunala T, et al. Human papillomavirus DNA in urine specimens of men with condyloma acuminatum. *Sex Transm Dis* 1997;24:165–168.
89. Reid R, Laverty CR, Coppleson M, et al. Noncondylomatous cervical wart virus infection. *Obstet Gynecol* 1980;55:476–483.
90. Brown DR, Fife KH. Human papillomavirus infections of the genital tract. *Med Clin North Am* 1990; 74:1455–1485.
91. Schneider A, Meinhardt G, De-Villiers EM, et al. Sensitivity of the cytologic diagnosis of cervical condyloma in comparison with HPV-DNA hybridization studies. *Diagn Cytopathol* 1987;3: 250–255.
92. Reid R, Greenberg MD, Lorincz A, et al. Should cervical cytologic testing be augmented by cervicography or human papillomavirus deoxyribonucleic acid detection? *Am J Obstet Gynecol* 1991; 164:1461–1471.
93. Kaplan JW. Condylomata acuminata. *New Orleans Med Surg J* 1942;94:388–390.
94. von Krogh G, Maibach HI. Cutaneous cyto destructive potency of lignans. II. A comparative evaluation of macroscopic-toxic influence on rabbit skin subsequent to repeated 10-day applications. *Dermatologica* 1983;167:70–77.
95. von Krogh G. Topical treatment of penile condylomata acuminata with podophyllin, podophyllotoxin and colchicine. A comparative study. *Acta Derm Venereol (Stockh)* 1978;58:163–168.
96. Isaacs A, Lindermann J. Virus interferons, I: the interferon. *Proc R Soc Ser B* 1957;147:258–267.
97. Baron S. Mechanism of recovery from viral infection. In: Smith DM, Lauffer MA, eds. *Advances in virus research.* New York: Academic Press, 1963:39–60.
98. Baron S, Diazani F, Stanton GJ, et al., eds. *The interferon system: a current review to 1987.* Austin: University Texas Press, 1987.
99. Taylor JL, Grossberg SE. Recent progress in interferon research: molecular mechanisms of regulation, action, and virus circumvention. *Virus Res* 1990;15:1–25.
100. Baron S, Tyring SK, Fleischmann WR, et al. The interferons. Mechanisms of action and clinical applications. *JAMA* 1991;266:1375–1383.
101. Schonfeld A, Nitke S, Schattner A, et al. Intramuscular human interferon-beta injections in treatment of condylomata acuminata. *Lancet* 1984;1(8385):1038–1042.
102. Damstra RJ, van Vloten WA. Cryotherapy in the treatment of condylomata acuminata: a controlled study of 64 patients. *J Dermatol Surg Oncol* 1991;17:273–276.
103. Gall SA, Hughes CE, Trofatter K. Interferon for the therapy of condyloma acuminatum. *Am J Obstet Gynecol* 1985;153:157–163.
104. Gall SA, Hughes CE, Mounts P, et al. Efficacy of human lymphoblastoid interferon in the therapy of resistant condyloma acuminata. *Obstet Gynecol* 1986;67:643–651.
105. Gross G, Ikenberg H, Roussaki A, et al. Systemic treatment of condylomata acuminata with recombinant interferon-alpha-2a: low-dose superior to high-dose regimen. *Chemotherapy* 1986;32: 537–541.
106. Friedman-Kien AE, Eron LJ, Conant M, et al. Natural interferon alfa for treatment of condylomata acuminata. *JAMA* 1988;259:533–538.
107. Leventhal BG, Kashima HK, Mounts P et al. Long-term response of recurrent respiratory papillomatosis to treatment with lymphoblastoid interferon alfa-N1. *N Engl J Med* 1991;325:613–617.
108. Anonymous. Recurrent condylomata acuminata treated with recombinant interferon alfa-2a. A multi-center double-blind placebo-controlled clinical trial. Condylomata International Collaborative Study Group. *JAMA* 1991;265:2684–2687.
109. Trizna Z, Evans T, Bruce S, et al. A randomized phase II study comparing four different interferon therapies in patients with recalcitrant condylomata acuminata. *Sex Transm Dis* 1998:25:361–365.
110. Testerman TL, Gerster JF, Imbertson IM, et al. Cytokine induction by the immunomodulators imiquimod and S-27609. *J Leukoc Biol* 1995;58:365–372.
111. Reiter MJ, Testerman TL, Miller RL, et al. Cytokine induction in mice by the immunomodulator imiquimod. *J Leukoc Biol* 1994;55:234–240.
112. Baggish MS. Carbon dioxide laser treatment for condylomata acuminata venereal infections. *Obstet Gynecol* 1980;55:711–715.
113. Abdullah AN, Walzman M, Wade A. treatment of external genital warts comparing cryotherapy (liquid nitrogen) and trichloroacetic acid. *Sex Transm Dis* 1993;20:344–345.
114. Bashi SA. Cryotherapy versus podophyllin in the treatment of genital warts. *Int J Dermatol* 1985; 24:535–536.
115. Beutner KR. Therapeutic approaches to genital warts. *Am J Med* 1997;102:28–37, with permission.

116. Beutner KR, Conant MA, Friedman-Kien AE, et al. Patient-applied podofilox for treatment of genital warts. *Lancet* 1989;1:831–834.

117. Calkins JW, Masterson BJ, Magrina JF, et al. Management of condylomata acuminata with the carbon dioxide laser. *Obstet Gynecol* 1982;59:105–108.

118. Douglas JM, Eron LJ, Judson FN, et al. A randomized trial of combination therapy with intralesional interferon alpha 2b and podophyllin versus podophyllin alone for the therapy of anogenital warts. *J Infect Dis* 1990;162:52–59.

119. Eron LJ, Judson F, Tucker S, et al. Interferon therapy for condylomata acuminata. *N Engl J Med* 1986;315:1059–1064.

120. Edwards A, Atma-Ram A, Thin RN. Podophyllotoxin 0.5% v podophyllin 20% to treat penile warts. *Genitourin Med* 1988;64:263–265.

121. Edwards L, Ferenczy A, Eron L, et al. Self-administered topical 5% Imiquimod cream for external anogenital warts. The HPV Study Group. *Arch Dermatol* 1998;134:25–30.

122. Ferenczy A. Comparison of 5-fluorouracil and CO_2 laser for treatment of vaginal condylomata. *Obstet Gynecol* 1984;64:773–778.

123. Ferenczy A. Laser therapy of genital condylomata acuminata. *Obstet Gynecol* 1984;63:703–707.

124. Ferenczy A, Behelak Y, Haber G, et al. Treating vaginal and external anogenital condylomas with electrosurgery vs CO_2 laser ablation. *J Gynecol Surg* 1995;11:41–50.

125. Godley MJ, Bradbeer CS, Gellan M, et al. Cryotherapy compared with trichloroacetic acid in treating genital warts. *Genitourn Med* 1987;63:390–392.

126. Greenberg MD, Rutledge LH, Reid R, et al. A double-blind, randomized trial of 0.5% podofilox and placebo for the treatment of genital warts in women. *Obstet Gynecol* 1991;77:735–739.

127. Jensen SL. Comparison of podophyllin application with simple surgical excision in clearance and recurrence of perianal condylomata acuminata. *Lancet* 1985;2(8465):1146–48.

128. Keay S, Teng N, Eisenberg M, et al. Topical interferon for treating condyloma acuminata in women. *J Infect Dis* 1988;158:934–939.

129. Khawaja HT. Podophyllin versus scissor excision in the treatment of perianal condylomata acuminata: a prospective study. *Br J Surg* 1989;76:1067–1068.

130. Kirby PK, Kiviat N, Beckman A, et al. Tolerance and efficacy of recombinant human interferon gamma in the treatment of refractory genital warts. *Am J Med* 1988;85:183–188.

131. Pride GL. Treatment of large lower genital tract condylomata acuminata with topical 5-fluorouracil. *J Reprod Med* 1990;35:384–387.

132. Stone KM, Becker TM, Hadgu A, et al. Treatment of external genital warts: a randomized clinical trial comparing podophyllin, cryotherapy, and electrodesiccation. *Genitourin Med* 1990;66:16–19.

133. Vance JC, Bart BJ, Hansen RC, et al. Intralesional recombinant alpha-2 interferon for the treatment of patients with condyloma acuminatum or verruca plantaris. *Arch Dermatol* 1986;122:272–277.

11

Human Immunodeficiency Virus

EPIDEMIOLOGY

Human immunodeficiency virus (HIV), a lymphotropic virus, was first isolated from patients with acquired immunodeficiency syndrome (AIDS) and AIDS-related complex in 1983 (1,2). HIV is closely related to human T-cell lymphotropic virus, type-1, and type-2. Since the first case among adults was diagnosed 15 years ago, the number of cases reported in the United States exceeds 501,310, and the mortality rate is 62% (311,381 deaths) (3). The Centers for Disease Control and Prevention (CDC) reported in 1995 that 67,211 persons were infected with HIV, and 178,550 individuals were living with AIDS (4). AIDS is the leading cause of death among adults between the ages of 25 and 44 (5).

The AIDS epidemic may appear to plateau during the next 5 years; however, there is evidence that a second-wave epidemic may occur among young male homosexuals (3). There is also an increase in the number of cases among women, minorities, adolescents, and young adults ages 13 to 29 caused by heterosexual intercourse and injectable illicit drug use (4,6). The epidemic has spread from the Northeast and West to smaller communities in the South and Midwest, as well as to rural areas.

Unfortunately, the number of cases continues to increase among injectable drug users and heterosexuals. The CDC reported an increase of 17% among injectable drug users from 1981 to 1987 and a 27% increase from 1993 to 1995 (3). Between 1993 and 1995 there was a 7% increase among heterosexuals (3). The number of cases in women is increasing faster than in men and has tripled since 1985 (6). The concern over this increase is that women do not consider themselves to be at risk. This results in women failing to submit to HIV testing, which, in turn, causes a delay in establishing the diagnosis (7). Many of these women do not know or are unaware of their partners' high-risk behavior. Approximately 84% of the cases among women occur in the 15- to 44-year-old age group, with the median age of 35 (6). Most cases, 77%, occurred among African-American and Hispanic women (6).

VIROLOGY AND PATHOPHYSIOLOGY

HIV is a cytopathic virus with a central diploid ribonucleic acid (RNA) core surrounded by a lipid envelope. The serologic marker p24 is an antigen located in the central core of the virus. The HIV binds to T-lymphocytes via the viral glycoprotein, gp120, to the CD+ receptor on the host cell (8). The CD4 receptor-binding site interacts with the viral envelope protein associated with gp120, thus allowing the virus to fuse with the T-lymphocyte cell membrane. The virus then enters the host cell and the viral RNA becomes exposed. Deoxyribonucleic acid (DNA) is made from the viral RNA via reverse transcription. The infected cells remain in a dormant state for an unknown period. Activation stimulates proviral DNA to transcribe genomic and messenger RNA. Once new viral proteins are synthesized, new virions are assembled. The new virions bud from the infected cell, and, once released, the viruses circulate in the blood stream until they come into contact with other target cells (Table 11-1).

The decrease in CD4 lymphocytes is a prognostic marker for the progression of the disease. Acquisition of the virus may result in dissemination of the virus, which is associated with a viremia and a drop in CD4 lymphocytes (9–11). The decrease in CD4 lymphocytes may result in the viral killing of these cells or a redistribution of circulating CD4 lymphocytes to lymphoid tissue (11,12). The decrease in viral burden observed in the plasma and peripheral blood mononuclear cells may be caused by the development of humoral and cellular immune response to the infection (13–15). Reestablishment of the immune response is associated with a rebound in CD4 lymphocyte count but not to preinfection levels.

Following the decrease in the viral burden found after primary infection, there is a resolution in the clinical symptoms initially observed. The HIV-infected individual then enters the latent stage of the disease. Although the viral load in the peripheral mononuclear lymphocytes is decreased, the lymphoid tissue contains a high number of virions (16,17). The lymph nodes of asymptomatic HIV-

TABLE 11-1. *Target cells susceptible to HIV[a]*

Hematopoietic cells	Neurologic cells
CD4 T-lymphocytes	Astrocytes
Monocytes	Oligodendrocytes
Macrophages	
B lymphocytes	Skin
Promyelocytes	Langerhans' cells
	Fibroblasts
Other cells	
Gastrointestinal epithelium	
Cervical epithelium	
Tumor cells	
Renal epithelium	

[a]Adapted from Boswell SL. Pathophysiology and natural history. In: Libman H, Witzburg PA, eds. *HIV infection.* New York: Little, Brown and Company, 1996:3–17, with permission.

infected patients sequester virus on the surface of follicular cells, thus allowing the antigen to be presented to immune-competent cells. This may be the route by which new cells become infected.

Decreasing CD4 lymphocytes is associated with a declining immune system, which becomes clinically apparent by noting the emergence of opportunistic infections that are rarely observed in the immune-competent individual. Infections such as cytomegalovirus, toxoplasmosis, fungal infections, and disseminated *Mycobacterium avium* complex are rarely seen in patients with CD4 counts above 100 cells/mm^3 (18).

NATURAL HISTORY

HIV infection is a progressive disease that can be divided into four stages: primary, early HIV infection (CD4 count greater than 500 cells/mm^3), intermediate HIV infection (CD4 count 200 to 500 cells/mm^3), and late HIV infection or AIDS (CD4 count less than 200 cells/mm^3). Primary infection begins 2 to 4 weeks after acquisition of the virus and lasts for 1 to 2 weeks. Primary infection is characterized by an acute mononucleosis-like syndrome and is often mistaken for mononucleosis (Table 11-2).

Patients with primary HIV infection develop a lymphopenia that is not long lasting and is followed by a lymphocytosis. The lymphocytosis largely consists of CD8 lymphocytes; however, CD4 lymphocytes decrease to levels resembling advanced HIV infection. CD4 lymphocyte counts increase within 2 to 3 weeks but not to preinfection levels (19,20). The clinical presentation of primary infection is multisystem; therefore, it is important that the physician consider HIV infection when patients present with any of the clinical signs or symptoms listed in Table 11-3.

In addition, laboratory tests typically reflect a thrombocytopenia, leukopenia, and an increase in liver function. The thrombocytopenia is transient and spontaneously resolves. Although the patient may develop an increase in hepatic transaminase levels, the patient does not usually manifest hepatitis (21,22).

Early HIV infection is typically asymptomatic, and the CD4 counts are usually greater than 500 cells/mm^3. A small percentage of infected individuals may develop a persistent generalized lymphadenopathy, seborrheic dermatitis, shingles, and folliculitis. Laboratory tests reveal a leukopenia and/or a thrombocy-

TABLE 11-2. *Clinical characteristics of primary infection*

Fever	Maculopapular rash
Lethargy	Myalgia
Lymphadenopathy	Arthralgia
Pharyngitis	Headaches
Photophobia	Diarrhea
Meningoencephalitis	Myelopathy
Peripheral neuropathy	Guillain-Barré syndrome

TABLE 11-3. *Signs and symptoms of primary HIV infection*

Elevated body temperature	Hepatosplenomegaly
Lymphadenopathy	Oropharyngeal candidiasis
Fatigue	Meningoencephalitis
Malaise	Peripheral neuropathy
Myalgia	Truncal maculopapular rash
Arthralgia	Mucocutaneous ulcers
Headache	
Pharyngitis	
Diarrhea	
Nausea	
Vomiting	

topenia. Individuals with intermediate disease usually are asymptomatic or have minimal symptoms but have CD4 counts between 200 and 500 cells/mm^3. Individuals with symptoms that developed during the early phase of infection may experience an increase in severity of symptoms. Symptomatic individuals may experience new problems such as diarrhea, recurrent herpetic infection, oropharyngeal-esophageal and vaginal candidiasis, bacterial sinusitis, and respiratory and skin infections.

AIDS is defined by a CD4 lymphocyte count less than 200 cells/mm^3 or the presence of opportunistic infection such as *Pneumocystis carinii* and *Toxoplasmosis gondii*. Conditions, which constitute AIDS, are listed in Table 11-4.

TABLE 11-4. *Case definition for AIDS[a]*

Candidiasis of bronchi, trachea, lungs, or esophagus
Cervical cancer, invasive
Coccidioidomycosis, disseminated or extrapulmonary
Cryptococcosis, extrapulmonary
Cryptosporidiosis, chronic intestinal (>1-month duration)
Cytomegalovirus disease (other than liver, spleen, or nodes)
Encephalopathy, HIV related
Herpes simplex: chronic ulcer(s) (>1-month duration), bronchitis, pneumonitis, or esophagitis
Histoplasmosis, disseminated or extrapulmonary
Isosporiasis, chronic intestinal (>1-month duration)
Kaposi's sarcoma
Lymphoma, Burkitt's (or equivalent term)
Lymphoma, immunoblastic (or equivalent term)
Lymphoma, primary in the brain
Mycobacterium avium complex or *Mycobacterium kansasii,* disseminated or extrapulmonary
Mycobacterium tuberculosis, any site (pulmonary or extrapulmonary)
Pneumocystis carinii pneumonia
Pneumonia, recurrent
Salmonella septicemia, recurrent
Toxoplasmosis of the brain
Wasting syndrome, HIV-related

[a]Adapted from Centers for Disease Control and Prevention. Revised classification system for HIV infection and expanded surveillance case definition for AIDS among adolescents and adults, 1993. *MMWR* 1992;41(RR-17):15, with permission.

Increase in diseases related to HIV infection is dependent on the CD4 count. Decreases in the CD4 counts below 100 cells/mm^3 place the patient at risk for CMV retinitis, disseminated *M. avium* complex infection, cryptococcal meningitis, progressive multifocal leukoencephalopathy, invasive aspergillosis, disseminated coccidioidomycosis, and disseminated histoplasmosis.

HIV AND AIDS IN WOMEN

The first case of AIDS described in a woman in the United States was reported in 1981 (23). The first 43 cases of AIDS among women were reported in 1983 and approximately 30% acquired the disease through heterosexual intercourse, whereas 70% contracted the infection through illicit injectable drug use (24). A major route of transmission of HIV in women continues to be illicit intravenous drug use either by needle sharing or through sexual intercourse with drug-using males. An important epidemiologic marker for the number of cases in women is the number of pediatric cases because the latter serves as a source of unrecognized cases in women.

In 1993, the CDC published a revision of the surveillance definition of AIDS in the United States based on a laboratory definition (Table 11-4). However, the laboratory definition excludes conditions, especially gynecologic diseases, that occur at CD4 levels greater than 200 cells/mm^3 that would not be considered AIDS-related or AIDS-defining conditions (25). The new surveillance definition does, however, allow physicians greater freedom in diagnosing AIDS; for example, in Table 11-5, all individuals in column C and all those in row 3 are now classified as having AIDS. Category B includes conditions that can be attributed to HIV infection such as those associated with a defect in cell-mediated immunity or those that require management complicated by HIV infection (e.g., persistent, frequently recurrent, or poorly responsive to therapy vulvovaginal candidiasis; cervical dysplasia—moderate or severe; and carcinoma in situ). Category C conditions are those that have been defined as clinical AIDS with the addition of pulmonary tuberculosis, recurrent pneumonia, and invasive cervical carcinoma.

TABLE 11-5. *1993 Revised classification for HIV infection and AIDS expanded surveillance case definition*

CD4 T-cell categories	(A) Asymptomatic HIV or PGL	(B) Symptomatic, acute (primary) not (A) or (C) conditions	(C) AIDS-indicator conditions
(1) >500	A1	B1	C1
(2) 200–499	A2	B2	C2
(3) <200	A3	B3	C3

PGL, persistent generalized lymphadenopathy.
From Centers for Disease Control and Prevention. Revised classification system for HIV infection and expanded surveillance case definition for AIDS among adolescents and adults, 1993. *MMWR* 1992;41(RR-17), with permission.

Although the overall mortality rate because of AIDS is decreasing, it continues to be a major killer among young women in the United States (26,27). Deaths in males decreased in 1996 and were 13% lower than in 1995; however, mortality increased by 3% in women. In 1985, the number of women diagnosed with AIDS accounted for 7% of the cases, whereas in 1996 women accounted for 20% of the cases (28). According to the latest data, 85,000 women in the United States have AIDS. Heterosexual transmission accounts for the largest increase in cases among women. From 1995 to 1996, there has been a 17% increase in women, a 2% increase in cases among homosexual males, and a 2% increase among illicit intravenous drug users.

Sexual contact accounts for 75% to 85% of 28 million cases of HIV; however, the probability of acquiring the virus via sexual contact is lower than through other routes of transmission (29). Infectivity depends on the ability of the virus to enter host cells via attachment to CD4 and chemokine surface receptors (CC-CKR-5) (30,31). Receptive host cells include CD4 T lymphocytes, Langerhans, cells, and other macrophages. HIV receptive cells have been found in the lamina propria of oral, cervicovaginal, foreskin, urethral, and rectal epithelia in other primate models (32). In women, the endocervical columnar epithelium within the transformation zone is the susceptible area for HIV acquisition (33). The presence of an infection within the reproductive tract is strongly associated with susceptibility to HIV (e.g., chancroid, syphilis, or herpes) (34). The presence of a genital tract ulcer and acquisition of HIV has a relative risk of 1.5 to 7.0 for both men and women (35–38). Other sexually transmitted diseases such as gonorrhea and chlamydia, as well as bacterial vaginosis, have been associated with an increased risk for HIV acquisition (39,40). Investigations in women have revealed a two-fold increase in HIV infection associated with sexually transmitted diseases or purulent cervical secretions (41,42). Cervical ectopy has been found to place the individual at risk (relative risk 1.7 to 5.0) for acquisition of HIV in some but not all studies (43–45). Detection of HIV is five times more likely in women with eversion of the endocervical columnar epithelium than in women without ectopy (41). Women whose sexual partners are not circumcised are at higher risk to acquire HIV infection than women whose partners are circumcised (46,47). Women can protect themselves from infection by requiring that their male partners wear a condom or by using the female condom during sexual intercourse (48,49). Other methods of contraception—nonoxynol-9, intrauterine devices, and oral contraceptives—do not afford the individual any degree of protection against acquiring HIV infection. The data regarding these methods of contraception and HIV infection is somewhat confusing. Some studies suggest a protective effect, whereas other studies do not (50).

Transmission of HIV from infected women to uninfected men seems to be increased during menstruation. Men who have sexual intercourse with HIV-positive women who are menstruating are almost four times more likely to acquire infection than men having sex with infected women who are not. This increase in risk during menstruation occurs although infected women will intermittently secrete virus throughout the menstrual cycle (51,52). Uninfected women who are menstruating and have sex with HIV-positive males also increase their risk of acquiring HIV (odds ratio 1.5) (53). Women who are not infected, experience bleeding during sexual intercourse, and have sex with a HIV-positive male are at an increased risk for acquiring infection (odds ratio 4.9) (36).

CLINICAL PROGRESSION OF INFECTION IN WOMEN

The research emphasis has been on vertical transmission from an HIV-infected mother to the fetus or neonate. It is more common to detect the presence of HIV in a woman who is pregnant than in a woman who is not (54). In the gynecologic patient who is HIV positive, infection is usually not diagnosed until the patient develops signs and symptoms of AIDS, because the gynecologist is unlikely to suspect HIV infection when a patient is seen for a gynecologic problem.

HIV infection is likely to lead to a decrease in the patient's cellular immune response to additional infections. The level of the CD4 cell count (Table 11-6) determines the likelihood of an HIV-infected woman developing AIDS.

The average number of CD4 lymphocytes in a healthy immunocompetent woman is approximately 1,000 cells/mm^3. An HIV-infected individual will have a reduction of the CD4 lymphocytes of about 200 to 300 cells in the first year of infection, with a decrease of 50 to 100 CD4 lymphocytes each year. Thus, by the tenth year the patient's CD4 count will be greater than 200 cells/mm^3 (55,56).

Progression of disease in HIV-infected women has not been studied as well as it has been studied in men, but such studies are currently underway. Thus far it does not appear that there are any significant differences with regard to acquisition of opportunistic infection when stratified by CD4 count (57,58). However, when a woman's CD4 count is less than 100 cells/mm^3, disease progression is more rapid and survival is shorter than in a male. In two other studies, no gender differences were found with regard to frequency of opportunistic infections,

TABLE 11-6. *Relationship of developing AIDS with respect to the patient's CD4 cellular count[a]*

CD4 cell count	18-month probability of developing AIDS
100	60%
200	30%
300	15%
400	8%
500	3%

[a]Adapted from Stein DS, Korvick JA, Vermund SH. CD4+ lymphocyte cell enumeration for the prediction of clinical course of human immunodeficiency virus disease: a review. *J Infect Dis* 1992; 165:352, with permission.

survival, or disease progression (58,59). Chaosson et al. (61) studied progression of HIV infection and survival in 1,372 patients of which 538 were women. These investigators did not find any gender differences in disease progression or survival.

DIAGNOSIS

In the acute primary stage, patients typically have very high levels of virus and viral replication but usually no significant immune response (61). During this phase of the disease, the plasma HIV RNA levels are between 105 to 108 copies of virus/mL, the p24 antigen levels are greater than 100 pg/mL, and peripheral blood cultures of mononuclear cells demonstrate an increase of viral titers of 100 to 10,000 tissue culture-infecting doses per 1 million cells (62–64). It is interesting to note that this period of high viral titers occurs in the absence of detectable antibody. This period is referred to as the "window of infectivity."

Detection of HIV RNA in the plasma is more sensitive than the detection of p24 antigen (62). Primary infection can be established by the detection of HIV RNA, which can be determined 3 to 5 days earlier than p24 antigen (65,66). In contrast, p24 antigen detection can be accomplished in only 75% of primary HIV infections, whereas HIV RNA can be detected in all seroindeterminate specimens collected before seroconversion (61). Diagnosing acute HIV is important to explain a patient's undiagnosed acute illness, to counsel patients appropriately, to prevent transmission, to learn more about the natural history of HIV infection, and to institute treatment early in the course of the infection.

During the early course of infection, the viral load is highest (more than 106 RNA copies/mL of blood), and, therefore, transmission is likely. Genital secretions contain a high viral load at this time (66). A mathematical model suggested that between 56% and 92% of all HIV infections might be transmitted during this period of acute infection (67).

A variety of tests are available for determining the presence of HIV. The tests have been divided into screening tests [enzyme-linked immunosorbent assay (ELISA) for HIV-1, HIV-2 or both, latex agglutination for HIV-1, ELISA for HIV-1 detection in urine or saliva], confirmatory tests (Western blot assay for HIV-1and HIV-2, indirect immunofluorescence antibody assay for HIV-1), and supplemental tests (ELISA for HIV p24 antigen, culture, and polymerase chain reaction for HIV-1). The ELISA is the most commonly used screening test to detect the presence of HIV-1 antibodies. This test is inexpensive and has a sensitivity and specificity of 99% (68). If the test is negative, no further testing is performed; however, if the test is positive, the specimen is retested to establish that the initial test was not a false positive. The specimen is then subjected to Western blot analysis to confirm that the initial test was not a false positive (Table 11-7).

The Western blot assay is the most used confirmatory test for the detection of HIV-specific antibodies. Although the Western blot is a more specific test than

TABLE 11-7. *Conditions that will yield a false-positive ELISA for HIV-1*

Human leukocyte antigen (HLA) DR antibodies (multiparous women,
    multiple transfusions)
Autoimmune diseases
HIV-2 infection
Multiple myomas
Alcoholic hepatitis
Recent immunization with the influenza vaccine
Hemodialysis
Positive rapid plasma reagin (RPR)
Mislabeled specimen

ELISA, enzyme-linked immunosorbent assay.

the ELISA, it is more costly, more time consuming, and requires more expertise to perform.

The p24 antigen detection test is used for individuals suspected of having acute or recent onset HIV infection. The test is dependent on the presence of a high level of viremia, which is measured as p24 antigenemia even in the absence of HIV antibody (62,63). The disadvantage of the p24 antigen test is that once antibodies form, p24 antibody-antigen complexes make detection of the antigen (p24) more difficult.

The key to prevention is dependent on two factors: (a) educating the public on transmission and acquisition and (b) diagnosis of primary infection. Although the disease may have plateaued in the homosexual population, it is on the rise among women. Because of the nonspecific nature of the disease, clinicians often overlook this infection in its initial phase. In a retrospective study of 2,120 individuals found to be antibody-negative or Western blot-indeterminate, six (0.28%) had detectable levels of p24 antigen (69). HIV was later confirmed either when patients were hospitalized or at the time of follow-up. In a second study of 46 recently seroconverted individuals, 41 had an acute retroviral syndrome, but only 25% had been diagnosed at the time of their initial examination (70). Although the HIV RNA test is more sensitive, it is also more expensive, and, therefore, the p24 antigen is an affordable assay for the detection of primary infection.

One key to the management and prevention of HIV infection is to provide testing to all patients who are risk to implement treatment. In response to this need an oral test has been developed that is highly accurate. An oral test has appeal because the patient obtains the specimen and the health care provider is not at risk. In addition, viral transmission through contact with saliva from an HIV-infected individual is unlikely because infectious virus is rarely isolated in saliva (71–73). Oral diagnostic testing has advantages over blood testing: it does not require a phlebotomist, and it facilitates specimen collection from children, obese individuals, hemophiliacs, and individuals with compromised venous access (74,75). An oral test is available that has a sensitivity of 99.9% and specificity of 100%—OraSure HIV-1 Oral Specimen Collection Device (Epitope; SmithKline Beecham) (75,76).

TABLE 11-8. *Laboratory tests for HIV-infected patients*

Complete blood count	Prothrombin time
WBC differential	Fibrinogen
Platelet count	Hepatitis serology B, C
CD4 and CD8 counts	Serum lactate dehydrogenase
Serum electrolytes, BUN, creatine	RPR, FTA-ABS
Total bilirubin	Toxoplasmosis IgM_1, IgG
Alkaline phosphatase	PPD
AST, ALT	Chest x-ray film
Albumin	

ALT, alanine transaminase; AST, aspartate transaminase; BUN, blood urea nitrogen; FTA-ABS, fluorescent treponemal antibody–absorption test; PPD, purified protein derivative; RPR, rapid plasma reagin; WBC, white blood cell.

The oral test is based on the presence of IgG antibodies to the virus, and this immunoglobulin is present in relatively high concentrations in the gingival crevicular fluid or transudate (77). The gingival crevice can be identified as a specific anatomic site and provides an assayable source of IgG. Comparative studies have demonstrated that the concentration of IgG in gingival cervical fluid is comparable to serum in HIV patients (75,76). The test is based on obtaining the specimen from the gingival crevice and not saliva because the latter does not contain a high concentration of IgG.

The presence of chronic or acute diseases did not produce false-positive results (Table 11-8). In addition, there are no false-positive results when HIV-positive individuals are tested shortly after eating, smoking, or taking anti-cholinergic medications or after recent use of oral hygiene agents (75,76,78).

TREATMENT OF HIV AND AIDS

HIV is initially a silent or asymptomatic infection that can progress over time to a state in which the immunologic system is severely damaged—AIDS. The development of AIDS occurs over a period of years and is associated with a variety of clinical syndromes. Thus, the goal of therapy is to show this progression from asymptomatic HIV to AIDS.

Following acquisition of the HIV virus, the organism replicates in CD4 lymphocytes, which leads to the appearance of HIV antigens in the peripheral blood. Typically, antibody detection is possible at the time the host's immune system is responsive. Before this time, anti-HIV-antibodies are not detected, and this period is referred to as the "window" when standard screening tests do not detect anti-HIV-antibodies and infection. Most infected patients will be anti-HIV-antibody positive within 6 months of acquiring infection. There have been cases of HIV-infected individuals testing negative for anti-HIV-antibodies for up to 35 months. (79,80).

The appearance of HIV antigens occurs within several weeks following inoculation. The infected individual, at this point, mounts an immune response and produces antibodies resulting in clearance of HIV from the bloodstream. This is misleading because it is at this point that the infection becomes well-established in lymphoid tissue and the virus replicates at a high level.

During the period from acquisition of infection through the establishment of lymphoid infection, the individual manifests a clinical picture of a limited viral syndrome. (81) The spectrum of clinical manifestations range from fever, fatigue, malaise, myalgias, arthralgias, lymphadenopathy, splenomegaly, anorexia, nausea, and vomiting. Some individuals can develop diarrhea, pharyngitis, headache, retroorbital pain, meningitis, encephalitis, neuropathy, myelopathy, maculopapular rash, and mucocutaneous ulceration. During the second week of the syndrome, many infected patients develop a generalized lymphadenopathy or lymphadenopathy may be limited to the occipital, axillary, and cervical regions. HIV infection and disease leading to AIDS can be divided up into the following stages: infection; incubation; and early, middle, and late disease. The duration of incubation to early disease is 6 weeks. The time span from acute infection (early disease) to the establishment of lymphoid infection (middle disease) is within 6 months of the initial infection. The onset of late disease is denoted by a decrease in CD4 counts, and typically the amount of time from the middle to late stage is approximately 10 years (82–84).

During the period of lymphoid involvement, the lymphadenopathy may regress because of the destruction of this tissue by viral replication and immune response. The patient's CD4 count drops below 200 cells/mm^3 and the patient often develops clinical disease of severe immunocompromise often defined as CDC-defined AIDS. CD4 counts below 50 cells/mm^3 are associated with late-stage HIV disease and death is imminent.

Patients first diagnosed with HIV infection should have screening laboratory tests (Table 11-8). Patients should have the tests in Table 11-8 performed every 6 to 12 months. If the CD4 counts are more than 600 cells/mm^3, the tests should be repeated every 6 months. If the CD4 count is less than 600 cells/mm^3, the tests should be repeated every 3 months. Anytime that antiretroviral therapy is administered, the CD4 count should be monitored at least every 3 months.

Management of patients whose CD4 counts are more than 500 cells/mm^3 should be based on specific needs. These individuals rarely require medical therapy and it should only be administered for specific conditions such as vulvovaginal candidiasis, oral and/or esophageal candidiasis, recurrent herpes, vulvovaginal-cervical condyloma acuminata, bacterial vaginosis, and so forth. These individuals typically require counseling, psychologic support, and assistance in understanding HIV disease. The latter may require a significant investment in time spent educating the patient with regard to treatment, options, transmission, prevention, and long-term prognosis.

Patients requiring antiretroviral therapy should be managed by physicians who specialize in AIDS management. Because antiviral treatment changes rapidly with the development of new agents, the patient's best chance is to be under the care of physicians who keep current and are familiar with the various nuances

TABLE 11-9. *Antiretroviral therapy for nonpregnant and pregnant patient*

Nucleoside analogues	Pregnancy categories
Reverse transcriptase inhibitors	
Zidovudine (AZT)	C
Zalcitabine (ddC)	C
Didanosine (ddl)	B
Stavudine (d4T)	C
Lamivudine (3TC)	C
Nonnucleoside reverse transcriptase inhibitors	
Nevirapine	C
Delavirdine	C
Protease inhibitors	
Indinavir	C
Ritonavir	B
Saquinavir	B
Nelfinavir	B

and manifestations of HIV and AIDS. There are a variety of agents available for the treatment of patients with HIV and AIDS (Table 11-9).

PREGNANCY

More than 80% of HIV infections in women occur during the childbearing years (85). An increase in the incidence of HIV in women is associated with an increase in HIV in pregnant women, which results in an increase in the incidence of infected infants. Approximately 1 in 57 pregnant women from inner city environments in the United States deliver babies infected with HIV (86).

Pregnancy is associated with an alteration in the individual's immune status. In the HIV-infected patient, there may be a change in lymphatic response and a decrease in CD4 cell counts (87). However, this does not result in a rapid progression of HIV (88,89).

Transmission of HIV can occur throughout the pregnancy, during the birthing process, and via breast milk (90–92). Transmission is greatest during the intrapartum period (93,94). Transmission to the fetus can be differentiated into early or *in utero* acquisition (the presence of HIV in the infant's blood within the first 2 days of life) and late or intrapartum infection (i.e., the absence of HIV in the infant's blood at 2 days of life) (95–97). Current data indicates that transmission occurs at higher rates in symptomatic HIV-infected pregnant women and those with advanced disease (96,97). Another factor in the transmission rate is prematurity (97).

Pregnant patients with HIV should be screened for tuberculosis, syphilis, chlamydia, gonorrhea, and hepatitis B. In addition, antibody titers to cytomegalovirus and toxoplasmosis should also be performed. CD4 lymphocyte counts should be determined during each trimester and more frequently in patients whose counts decrease below 500 cells/mm^3.

TABLE 11-10. *Risk factors for contracting HIV infection*

Sexually promiscuous
Illicit drug use
History of a sexually transmitted disease
Exposure to an individual known to have a sexually transmitted disease
Recipient of a blood transfusion before 1990
Sexual contact with an individual who received a blood transfusion before 1990
Health care worker

Treatment in the Pregnant Patient

Pregnant women found to be HIV positive should be afforded the same optimal management and therapeutic options as nonpregnant women. The use of antiretroviral therapy should be based on need; however, if possible, the risk to the fetus must be born in mind without compromising the life of the mother. Therefore, for treatment of pregnant women with HIV infection, monoantiretroviral therapy is now considered suboptimal and combination drug therapy is the current standard of care (98).

The pregnant patient with HIV should be administered zidovudine to prevent transmission to the fetus. In a study comparing zidovudine with placebo, there was a significant reduction in transmission of HIV in the treatment group compared with placebo, 8.3% versus 25.5% (99). Therefore, all pregnant women should be assessed for risky behavior, and all pregnant women who are at risk or suspected to be at risk should be screened for HIV (Table 11-10). Zidovudine should be administered to all pregnant women found to be HIV positive regardless of their CD4 count.

Intrapartum and Postpartum Management

Management of the HIV-infected pregnant patient during the intrapartum period is based on the principal that the greatest opportunity for transmission is during the birthing process. Therefore, amniotomy, use of scalp electrodes, and scalp sampling should be avoided. These procedures should be employed only when they are essential to the management of the patient and the fetus.

Women receiving zidovudine before pregnancy should be continued on the drug when becoming pregnant and during the intrapartum period. During the intrapartum period, the patient should be given a loading dose of zidovudine 2 mg/kg/hr followed by an infusion of 1 mg/kg/hr until the fetus is delivered.

The pregnant and nonpregnant patient infected with HIV is at risk for contracting a variety of infectious diseases (Table 11-11). The difficulty with the pregnant patient is the reluctance to administer therapeutic agents prophylactically because of the potential for adverse effects on the fetus.

Chemoprophylaxis for *P. carinii* should be administered to all HIV-infected women. If trimethoprim-sulfamethoxazole is to be withheld in the first trimester, aerosolized pentamidine can be administered because it is not absorbed system-

TABLE 11-11. *Infectious diseases associated with HIV*

Disease	Prophylactic agent
Pneumocystis carinii pneumonia	Trimethoprim-sulfamethoxazole or intravenous pentamidine
Candidiasis of the pharynx or vagina	Topical imidazoles or azoles. Resistant cases—fluconazole or ketoconazole (should also be used for treatment of esophagitis)
Cryptococcus or other life-threatening fungal infections	Amphotericin B
Toxoplasmosis	Pyrimethamine + sulfadiazine + folinic acid Clindamycin can be substituted for patients who cannot tolerate sulfadiazine
Herpes simplex	Acyclovir or valacyclovir or famciclovir
Cytomegalovirus	Ganciclovir or foscarnet (safety in pregnancy not known)
Syphilis	Penicillin (patients allergic to penicillin should be desensitized)
Tuberculosis	Initial management—isoniazid, ethambutol, and rifampin
Mycobacterium avium complex	Clarithromycin, azithromycin, rifabutin

ically. HIV-infected women, pregnant and nonpregnant, should be tested for IgG antibody to *T. gondii* to determine if latent infection is present. The patient should be counseled as to how toxoplasmosis is contracted and be advised not to eat raw or undercooked meat, to wash her hands after handling raw meat, to wear gloves when gardening or handling garden soil, and not to change cat litter. If the patient owns a cat, the animal should be tested for the presence of toxoplasmosis.

HIV AND THE GYNECOLOGIC PATIENT

The gynecologic patient is at risk for all the same opportunistic infections as any HIV-infected patient. However, several investigators have found that transmission of HIV is more likely to occur from men to women than from women to men (53,100,101).

The nonpregnant woman with HIV is at risk for the same genital tract infections as the non-HIV-infected individual. Up to 30% of healthy women have *Candida albicans* as a normal inhabitant in the genital tract. However, vulvovaginal candidiasis may be the presenting symptom in the HIV-infected woman. Typically, therapy with intravaginal imidazoles or azoles is effective. Oral agents such as fluconazole or ketoconazole may also be used. The HIV-infected individual is subject to frequent relapses. The frequent use of antifungal therapy raises the concern of the possible emergence of resistance. The HIV-infected woman with vulvovaginal candidiasis is at risk for relapse, chronic infection, and development of resistant strains, especially if she is receiving long-term fluconazole therapy.

The HIV-infected woman who contracts pelvic inflammatory disease often has a clinical presentation that differs from the non-HIV-infected patient. The HIV-infected woman with pelvic inflammatory disease tends to have less abdominal tenderness, lower white blood cell counts, lower rates of isolation of *Neisseria gonorrhoeae,* and higher rates of operative intervention (102,103).

Herpes simplex is an independent risk factor for the acquisition of HIV, and HIV-positive patients with herpes simplex may have frequent severe recurrences of herpes (104,105). Treatment usually requires higher doses of acyclovir or the newer agents, famciclovir and valacyclovir. Individuals with frequent recurrences may respond to suppressive therapy. Strains resistant to acyclovir have been isolated from HIV-infected women who received long-term treatment (106).

Syphilis is an independent risk factor for the acquisition of HIV infection, secondary to the development of genital ulcers (104,107). Syphilis has also increased among women, especially pregnant women, and this accounted for the increase in congenital syphilis. The incidence of nonulcerative sexually transmitted diseases, gonorrhea, chlamydia, and trichomoniasis, has also increased the transmission of HIV (108,109). Of all the sexually transmitted diseases, the one that has had the most impact in conjunction with HIV infection is the human papillomavirus (HPV). This common sexually transmitted virus has been demonstrated to be a precursor to cervical squamous intraepithelial lesions (SIL) also referred to as cervical intraepithelial neoplasia (CIN). This is also a precursor to cervical cancer. Although HPV in the absence of HIV is associated with an increased risk for the development of cervical dysplasia and cancer, women infected with HIV and HPV are at a 12-fold increased risk for developing CIN and cancer than women not infected with HIV (110–113).

HIV-infected women coinfected with HPV who develop cervical cancer appear to experience a more rapid course to invasive disease than the non-HIV-infected women. In one study of women younger than 50 years, women with invasive cervical squamous cell cancer presented with a more advanced stage of disease, responded poorly to treatment, and had higher rates of recurrences and higher death rates (114–116). Patients coinfected with HIV and HPV whose CD4 counts were less than 500 cells/mm^3 were found to be at higher risk (115).

REFERENCES

1. Barre-Sinoussi F, Chermann JC, Rey F, et al. Isolation of T-lymphotropic retrovirus from a patient at risk for acquired immune deficiency syndrome (AIDS). *Science* 1983;220:868–871.
2. Gallo S, Salahuddin SZ, Popovic M, et al. Frequent detection and isolation of cytopathic retroviruses (HTLV-III) from patients with AIDS and at risk for AIDS. *Science* 1984;224:500–503.
3. Anonymous. First 500,000 AIDS cases—United States, 1995. *MMWR* 1995;44:849–853.
4. Centers for Disease Control. *HIV/AIDS surveillance report mid-year edition* 1995;7:1.
5. National Center for Health Statistics. Annual summary of births, marriages, divorces, and deaths: United States, 1993, *Monthly vital health statistics.* Hyattsville, MD: Public Health Service, 1994; 42 (No.13):18.
6. Anonymous. Update: AIDS epidemic in the United States, 1994. *MMWR* 1995;44:81.

7. Wortley PM, Chu SY, Diaz T, et al. HIV testing patterns: where, why and when were persons with AIDS tested for HIV? *AIDS* 1995;9:487–492.

8. Zhu T, Mo H, Wang N, et al. Genotypic and phenotypic characterization of HIV-1 patients with primary infection. *Science* 1993;261:1179–1181.

9. Clark SJ, Saag MS, Decker WD, et al. High titers of cytopathic virus in plasma of patients with symptomatic primary HIV-1 infection. *N Engl J Med* 1991;324:954–960.

10. Daar ES, Moudgil T, Meyer RD, et al. Transient high levels of viremia in patients with primary human immunodeficiency virus type I infection. *N Engl J Med* 1991;324:961–964.

11. Tindall B, Cooper DA. Primary HIV infection: host response and intervention strategies. *AIDS* 1991; 5:1.

12. Mackay CR, Marston W, Dudler L. Altered patterns of T cell migration through lymph nodes and skin following antigen challenge. *Eur J Immunol* 1992;22:2205–2210.

13. Boucher CA, de Wolf F, Houweling JT, et al. Antibody response to a synthetic peptide covering a LAV-1/HTLV-IIIB neutralization epitope and disease progression. *AIDS* 1989;3:71–76.

14. Albert J, Abrahamsson B, Nagy K, et al. Rapid development of isolate-specific neutralizing antibodies after primary HIV-1 infection and consequent emergence of virus variants which resist neutralization by autologous sera. *AIDS* 1990;4:107–112.

15. Ariyoshi K, Harwood E, Cheingsong-Popov R, et al. Is clearance of HIV-1 viremia at seroconversion mediated by neutralizing antibodies? *Lancet* 1992;340:1257–1258.

16. Pantaleo G, Graziosi C, Butini L, et al. Lymphoid organs function as major reservoirs for human immunodeficiency virus. *Proc Natl Acad Sci U S A* 1991;88:9838–9842.

17. Pantaleo G, Graziosi C, Demarest JF, et al. HIV infection is active and progressive in lymphoid tissue during the clinically latent stage of disease. *Nature* 1993;362:355–358.

18. Jacobson MA, Mills J. Serious cytomegalovirus disease in the acquired immunodeficiency syndrome (AIDS). Clinical findings, diagnosis, and treatment. *Ann Intern Med* 1998;108:585–594.

19. Horsburgh CR Jr. *Mycobacterium avium* complex infection in the acquired immunodeficiency syndrome. *N Engl J Med* 1991;324:1332–1338.

20. Stein DS, Korvick JA, Vermund SH. CD4+ lymphocyte cell enumeration for prediction of clinical course of human immunodeficiency virus disease: a review. *J Infect Dis* 1992;165:352–363.

21. Gaines H, von Sydow M, Pehrson PO, et al. Clinical picture of primary HIV infection presenting as a glandular-fever-like illness. *Br Med J* 1988;297:1363–1368.

22. Sinicco A, Fora R, Sciandra M, et al. Risk of developing AIDS after primary acute HIV-1 infection. *J Acquir Immune Defic Syndr* 1993;6:575–581.

23. Anonymous. Follow-up on Kaposi's sarcoma and *Pneumocystis* pneumonia. *MMWR* 1981;30: 409–410.

24. Anonymous. Immunodeficiency among female sexual partners of males with acquired immune deficiency syndrome (AIDS)—New York. *MMWR* 1983;31:697–698.

25. Centers for Disease Control. 1993 revised classification system for HIV infection and expanded surveillance case definition for AIDS among adolescents and adults. *MMWR* 1992;41(RR-17):1–19.

26. Centers for Disease Control. Update: mortality attributable to HIV infection/AIDS among persons Aged 25–44—United States, 1990–1991. *MMWR* 1983;42:481.

27. Centers for Disease Control. Update: mortality attributable to HIV infection among persons 25–44 years—United States, 1991–1992. *MMWR* 1993;42:869.

28. Phillips P. No plateau for HIV/AIDS epidemic in U.S. women. *JAMA* 1997;277:1747–1748.

29. Joint United Nations Programme on HIV/AIDS. The HIV/AIDS situation in mid 1996: global and regional highlights. *UNAIDS Fact Sheet* July 1, 1996. New York: United Nations, 1996.

30. Weiss RA. HIV receptors and the pathogenesis of AIDS. *Science* 1996;272:1885–1886.

31. Dragic T, Litwin V, Allaway GP, et al. HIV-1 entry into CD4+ cells is mediated by the chemokine receptor CC-CKR-5. *Nature* 1996;381:667–673.

32. Hussain LA, Lehner T. Comparative investigation of Langerhans' cells and potential receptors for HIV in oral, genitourinary and rectal epithelia. *Immunology* 1995;85:475–484.

33. Nuovo GJ, Forde A, MacConnell P, et al. In situ detection of PCR-amplified HIV-1 nucleic acids and tumor necrosis factor cDNA in cervical tissues. *Am J Pathol* 1993;143:40–48.

34. Wasserheit JN. Epidemiological synergy. Interrelationships between human immunodeficiency virus infection and other sexually transmitted diseases. *Sex Transm Dis* 1992;19:61–77.

35. de Vincenzi I. A longitudinal study of human immunodeficiency virus transmission by heterosexual partners. European Study Group on Heterosexual Transmission of HIV. *N Engl J Med* 1994;331: 341–346.

36. Ghys PD, Diallo MO, Ettiegne-Traore V, et al. Genital ulcers associated with human immunodeficiency virus-related immunosuppression in female sex workers in Abidjan, Ivory Coast. *J Infect Dis* 1995;172:1371-1374.

37. Lazzarin A, Saracco A, Musicco M, et al. Man-to-woman sexual transmission of the human immunodeficiency virus. Risk factors related to sexual behavior, man's infectiousness, and woman's susceptibility. Italian Study Group on HIV Heterosexual Transmission. *Arch Intern Med* 1991;151: 2411–2416.

38. Plummer FA, Simonsen JN, Cameron DW, et al. Cofactors in male-female sexual transmission of human immunodeficiency virus type 1. *J Infect Dis* 191;163:233–239.

39. Laga M, Manoka A, Kivuvu M, et al. Non-ulcerative sexually transmitted diseases as risk factors for HIV-1 transmission in women: results from a cohort study. *AIDS* 1993;7:95–102.

40. Cohen CR, Duerr A, Pruithithada N, et al. Bacterial vaginosis and HIV seroprevalence among female commercial sex workers in Chiang Mai, Thailand. *AIDS* 1995;9:1093–1097.

41. Kapiga SH, Shao JF, Lwihula GK, et al. Risk factors for HIV infection among women in Dar-es-Salaam, Tanzania. *J Acquir Immune Defic Syndr* 1994;7:301–309.

42. Clemetson DB, Moss GB, Willerford DM, et al. Detection of HIV DNA in cervical and vaginal secretions. Prevalence and correlates among women in Nairobi, Kenya. *JAMA* 1993;269:2860–2864.

43. Henin Y, Mandelbrot L, Henrion R, et al. Virus excretion in the cervicovaginal secretions of pregnant and non-pregnant HIV-infected women. *J Acquir Immune Defic Syndr* 1993;6:72–75.

44. Plourde PJ, Pepin J, Agoki E, et al. Human immunodeficiency virus type I seroconversion in women with genital ulcers. *J Infect Dis* 1994;170:313–317.

45. Nicolosi A, Correa Leite ML, et al. The efficiency of male-to-female and female-to-male sexual transmission of the human immunodeficiency virus: a study of 730 stable couples. *Epidemiology* 1994;5:570–575.

46. Mati JK, Hunter DJ, Maggwa BN, et al. Contraceptive use and the risk of HIV infection in Nairobi, Kenya. *Int J Gynaecol Obstet* 1995;48:61–67.

47. Seidlin M, Vogler M, Lee E, et al. Heterosexual transmission of HIV in a cohort of couples in New York City. *AIDS* 1993;7:1247–1254.

48. Hunter DJ. AIDS in sub-Saharan Africa: the epidemiology of heterosexual transmission and the prospects for prevention. *Epidemiology* 1993;4:63–72.

49. Daly CC, Helling-Giese GE, Mati JK, et al. Contraceptive methods and the transmission of HIV: implications for family planning. *Genitourin Med* 1994;70:110–117.

50. Feldblum PJ, Morrison CS, Roddy RE, et al. The effectiveness of barrier methods of contraception in preventing the spread of HIV. *AIDS* 1995;9A:s85–93.

51. Royce RA, Sena A, Cates W Jr, et al. Sexual transmission of HIV. *N Engl J Med* 1997;336: 1072–1078.

52. Kreiss J, Willerford DM, Hensel M, et al. Association between cervical inflammation and cervical shedding of human immunodeficiency virus DNA. *J Infect Dis* 1994;170:1597–1601.

53. Vogt MW, Witt DJ, Craven DE, et al. Isolation patterns of the human immunodeficiency virus from cervical secretions during the menstrual cycle of women at risk for the acquired immunodeficiency syndrome. *Ann Intern Med* 1987;106:380–382.

54. Anonymous. Comparison of female to male and male to female transmission of HIV in 563 stable couples. *BMJ* 1992;304:809–813.

55. Barbacci MB, Dalabetta GA, Repke JT, et al. Human immunodeficiency virus infection in women attending an inner-city prenatal clinic: ineffectiveness of targeted screening. *Sex Transm Dis* 1990; 17:122–126.

56. Stein DS, Korvick JA, Vermund SH. CD4+ lymphocyte cell enumeration for the prediction of clinical course of human immunodeficiency virus disease: a review. *J Infect Dis* 1992;165:352–363.

57. Nieman RB, Fleming J, Coker RJ, et al. The effect of cigarette smoking on the development of AIDS in HIV-1-seropositive individuals. *AIDS* 1993;7:705–710.

58. Cozzi Lepri A, Pezzotti P, Dorrucci M, et al. HIV disease progression in 854 women and men infected through injecting drug use and heterosexual sex and followed for up to nine years from seroconversion. Italian Seroconversion Study. *BMJ* 1994;309:1537–1542.

59. Carpenter CC, Mayer KH, Stein MD, et al. Human immunodeficiency virus infection in North American women: experience with 200 cases and a review of the literature. *Medicine* 1991;70: 307–325.

60. Szabo S, Miller LH, Sacks S, et al. Gender differences in the natural history of HIV infection (Abstract MoC0030), 8th International Conference on AIDS, Amsterdam, The Netherlands, 1992: M010.

61. Chaisson RE, Keruly JC, Moore RD. Race, sex, drug use and progression of HIV disease. *N Engl J Med* 1995;333:751–756.
62. Quinn TC. Acute primary HIV infection. *JAMA* 1997;278:58–62.
63. Clark SJ, Saag MS, Decker WD, et al. High titers of cytopathic virus in plasma of patients with symptomatic primary HIV-1 infection. *N Engl J Med* 1991;324:954–960.
64. Daar ES, Moudgil T, Meyer RD, et al. Transient high levels of viremia in patients with primary human immunodeficiency virus type 1 infection. *N Engl J Med* 1991;324:961–964.
65. Piatak M Jr, Saag MS, Yang LC, et al. High levels of HIV-1 in plasma during all stages of infection determined by competitive PCR. *Science* 1993;259:1749–1754.
66. Henrard DR, Phillips J, Windsor I, et al. Detection of human immunodeficiency virus type 1 p24 antigen and plasma RNA: relevance to indeterminate serologic tests. *Transfusion* 1994;34:376–380.
67. Henrard DR, Phillips JF, Muenz LR, et al. Natural history of HIV-1 cell-free viremia. *JAMA* 1995; 274:554–558.
68. Cates W Jr, Cohen MS. Early treatment of HIV infection. *N Engl J Med* 1995;333:1783.
69. Celum CL, Coombs RR, Jones M, et al. Risk factors for repeatedly reactive HIV-1 EIA and indeterminate Western blots. *Arch Intern Med* 1994;154:1129–1137.
70. Clark SJ, Kelen GD, Henrard DR, et al. Unsuspected primary human immunodeficiency virus type 1 infection in seronegative emergency department patients. *J Infect Dis* 1994;170:194–197.
71. Schacker T, Collier AC, Hughes J, et al. Clinical and epidemiologic features of primary HIV infection. *Ann Intern Med* 1996;125:257–264.
72. Barr CE, Miller LK, Lopez MR, et al. Recovery of infectious HIV-1 from whole saliva. *J Am Diet Assoc* 1992;123:36–37, 39–48.
73. Ho DD, Byington RE, Schooley RT, et al. Infrequency of isolation of HTLV-III virus from saliva in AIDS. *N Engl J Med* 1985;313:1606.
74. O'Shea S, Cordery M, Barrett WY, et al. HIV excretion patterns and specific antibody responses in body fluids. *J Med Virol* 1990;31:291–296.
75. Archibald DW, Farely JJ Jr, Hebert CA, et al. Practical applications for saliva in perinatal HIV diagnosis. *Ann N Y Acad Sci* 1993;694:195–201.
76. Emmons WW, Paparello SF, Decker CF, et al. A modified ELISA and western blot accurately determine anti-human immunodeficiency virus type 1 antibodies in oral fluids obtained with a special collecting device. *J Infect Dis* 1995;171:406–410.
77. Gallo D, George JR, Fitchen JH, et al. Evaluation of a system using oral mucosal transudate for HIV-1 antibody screening and confirmatory testing. *JAMA* 1997;277:254–258.
78. Roitt I, Lehner T. Oral immunity. In: Black JF, ed. *Immunology of oral diseases,* 2nd ed. Oxford, United Kingdom: Blackwell Scientific, 1983;279.
79. Granade TC, Parekh B, Phillips SK, et al. Prospective evaluation of optimized methods for the detection of HIV-1 antibodies in oral fluids (abst). Presented at the 2nd national conference on human retroviruses and related infections, January 29–February 2, 1995.
80. Inagawa DT, Lee MH, Wolinsky SM, et al. Human immunodeficiency virus type 1 infection in homosexual men who remain seronegative for prolonged periods. *N Engl J Med* 1989;320: 1458–1462.
81. Ranki A, Valle S, Krohn M, et al. Long latency precedes overt seroconversion in sexually transmitted human-immunodeficiency-virus infection. *Lancet* 1987;2:589–593.
82. Tindall B, Cooper DA. Primary HIV infection: host responses and intervention strategies. AIDS 1991;5:1–14.
83. Bacchetti P, Moss AR. Incubation period of AIDS in San Francisco. *Nature* 1989;338:251-53.
84. Munoz A, Wary AC, Bass S, et al. Acquired immunodeficiency syndrome (AIDS)-free time after human immunodeficiency virus type 1 HIV-1- seroconversion in homosexual men. *Am J Epidemiol* 1998;130:530–539.
85. Longini IM Jr, Clark WS, Byers RH, et al. Statistical analysis of the stages of HIV infection using a Markov model. *Stat Med* 1989;8:831–843.
86. Anonymous. AIDS in women—United States. *MMWR* 1990;39:845–846.
87. Hoff R, Berardi VP, Weiblin B, et al. Seroprevalence of human immunodeficiency virus among childbearing women. Estimation by testing samples of blood from newborns. *N Engl J Med* 1988; 318:525–530.
88. Strelkauskas AJ, Davies IJ, Dray S. Longitudinal studies showing alterations in the levels and functional response of T and B lymphocytes in human pregnancy. *Clin Exp Immunol* 1978;32:531–539.
89. Berrebi A, Chraibi J, Kobuch WE, et al. Influence of pregnancy on HIV disease (abst). Seventh international conference on AIDS, Florence, Italy, June 1991.

90. Hocke C, Morlat P, Chene G, et al. Influence of pregnancy on the progression of HIV infection: a retrospective cohort study (abst). Ninth international conference on AIDS, Berlin, Germany, June 1993.
91. Hill WC, Bolton V, Carlson JR. Isolation of acquired immunodeficiency syndrome virus from the placenta. *Am J Obstet Gynecol* 1987;157:10–11.
92. Lapointe N, Michaud J, Pevovic D, et al. Transplacental transmission of HTVL-III virus. *N Engl J Med* 1985;312:1325–1326.
93. Van de Perre P, Simonon A, Misellati P, et al. Postnatal transmission of human immunodeficiency virus type 1 from mother to infant. *N Engl J Med* 1991;325:593–598.
94. Dunn DT, Newell ML, Ades AE, et al. Risk of human immunodeficiency virus type 1 transmission through breastfeeding. *Lancet* 1992;340:585–588.
95. Ehrnst A, Lindgren S, Dictor M, et al. HIV in pregnant women and their offspring: evidence for late transmission. *Lancet* 1991;338:203–207.
96. Bryson YJ, Luzuriaga K, Sullivan JL, et al. Proposed definitions for in utero versus intrapartum transmission of HIV-1. *N Engl J Med* 1992;327:1246–1247.
97. Anonymous. Risk factors for mother-to-child transmission of HIV-1. *Lancet* 1992;339:1007–1012.
98. Blanche S, Rouzioux C, Moscato ML, et al. A prospective study of infants born to women seropositive for human immunodeficiency virus type 1. *N Engl J Med* 1989;320:1643–1648.
99. Office of Public Health and Sciences, Department of Health and Human Services. Guidelines for use of anti-retroviral agents in HIV-infected adults. *Federal Register* 1997;62:33417–33418.
100. Connor EM, Sperling RS, Gelber R. Reduction of maternal-infant transmission of human immunodeficiency virus type 1 with zidovudine treatment: Pediatric AIDS Clinical Trails Protocol 076 Study Group. *N Engl J Med* 1994;331:1173–1180.
101. Padian NS, Shiboski SC, Jewell NP. Female-to-male transmission of human immunodeficiency virus. *JAMA* 1991;266:1664–1667.
102. Wenstrom KD, Gall SA. HIV infection in women. *Obstet Gynecol Clin North Am* 1989;16:627–643.
103. Korn AP, Landers DV, Green JR, et al. Pelvic inflammatory disease in human immunodeficiency virus-infected women. *Obstet Gynecol* 1993;82:765–768.
104. Hoegsberg B, Abulafia O, Sedlis A, et al. Sexually transmitted disease and human immunodeficiency virus infection among women with pelvic inflammatory disease. *Am J Obstet Gynecol* 1990; 163:1135–1139.
105. Quinn TC, Glasser D, Cannon RO, et al. Human immunodeficiency virus infection among patients attending clinics for sexually transmitted diseases. *N Engl J Med* 1988;318:197–203.
106. Hook EW III, Cannon RO, Nahmias AJ, et al. Herpes simplex virus infection as a risk factor for human immunodeficiency virus infection in heterosexuals. *J Infect Dis* 1992;165:251–255.
107. Erlich KS, Mills J, Chatis P, et al. Acyclovir-resistant herpes simplex virus infections in patients with the acquired immunodeficiency syndrome. *N Engl J Med* 1989;320:293–296.
108. Kreiss JK, Coombs R, Plummer F, et al. Isolation of human immunodeficiency virus from genital ulcers in Nairobi prostitutes. *J Infect Dis* 1989;160:380–384.
109. Laga M, Nzila N, Manoka AT, et al. Non ulcerative sexually transmitted diseases (STD) as risk factors for HIV infection (abst). Seventh international conference on AIDS, Florence, Italy, June 1991.
110. Dolei A, Sertra C, Mattana A, et al. In vitro interactions between HIV and *Trichomonas vaginalis* (abst). Seventh international conference on AIDS, Florence, Italy, June 1991.
111. Sillman FH, Sedlis A. Anogenital papillomavirus infection and neoplasia in immunodeficient women. *Obstet Gynecol Clin North Am* 1987;14:537–558.
112. Vermund SH, Kelley KF, Klein RS, et al. High risk of human papillomavirus infection and cervical squamous intraepithelial lesions among women with symptomatic human immunodeficiency virus infection. *Am J Obstet Gynecol* 1991;165:392–400.
113. Mandelblatt JS, Fahs M, Garibaldi K, et al. Association between HIV infection and cervical neoplasia: implications for clinical care of women at risk for both conditions. *AIDS* 1992;6:173–178.
114. Marte C, Kelly P, Cohen M, et al. Papanicolaou smear abnormalities in ambulatory care sites for women infected with the human immunodeficiency virus. *Am J Obstet Gynecol* 1992;166: 1232–1237.
115. Maiman M, Fruchter RG, Guy L, et al. Human immunodeficiency virus infection and invasive cervical carcinoma. *Cancer* 1993;71:402–406.
116. Maiman M, Fruchter R, Serur E, et al. Recurrent cervical intraepithelial neoplasia in human immunodeficiency virus-seropositive women. *Obstet Gynecol* 1993;82:170–174.

12

Lymphogranuloma Venereum

First described in 1883 by Wallace, lymphogranuloma venereum (LGV) is one of the classical sexually transmitted diseases. Durand, Nicholas, and Favre initially described the clinical manifestations of LGV in 1913 (1). Halberstaedter and Prowazek identified *Chlamydia trachomatis* in cells obtained from conjunctival scrapings of patients suffering from trachoma in 1907 (2). Frei (3), in 1925, developed a skin test for the detection of LGV, which gave the clinician an opportunity to diagnose LGV serologically, and established that the etiologic agent was C. trachomatis.

EPIDEMIOLOGY

LGV is not common in the United States but does occur and should be considered in any patient who presents with inguinal lymphadenopathy and fever. In 1991, the Centers for Disease Control and Prevention (CDC) reported 471 cases of LGV in the United States (4). The disease is endemic to Africa, India, several areas of South America, the Caribbean, and Indochina (5–8). The ease of travel, especially the need for business travel to developing countries, is a significant factor in contracting rare sexually transmitted diseases and introducing them into areas where they do not normally occur. Recently, a report was published detailing the experience of an Italian traveler who made a trip to India where he had sexual intercourse with a local woman. The traveler subsequently developed painful bilateral inguinal lymphadenopathy. The lymph nodes on the right were significantly larger and more painful than the nodes on the left (9). This case signifies the importance of considering travel experience when evaluating the patient with a genital infection. Physicians should recall that the United States has a relatively liberal policy with regard to foreign travelers when examining patients with genital infection. Many travelers and immigrants tend to visit and dwell in common areas because of familiar customs and language. This increases the possibility of establishing a pool of patients harboring the disease and permitting transmission not only within the restricted population but outside as well.

There are three known serotypes of *C. trachomatis* that are responsible for causing LGV L-1, L-2, and L-3. These serotypes are not responsible for the common cervicitis and salpingitis that occurs in the United States and around the world. Like other serotypes of *C. trachomatis,* these are true bacterial parasites requiring an exogenous source of amino acids and high-energy phosphates to complete their life cycle. The necessary amino acids and adenosine triphosphate are obtained from the host cell. The life cycle is initiated when the infectious particle (elementary body) gains access to a host cell. When inside the cell, the elementary body undergoes a metamorphosis and becomes a metabolically active unit called the reticulate body. (A complete discussion of the life cycle is given in the chapter on *Chlamydia.*) Once the reticulate bodies have depleted the host cell of vital nutrients, they change to infectious particles, and the host cell undergoes lysis releasing the infectious particles.

LGV is primarily transmitted by sexual contact when a mucosal surface comes into contact with an infectious lesion. However, if the patient is shedding infectious material and close nonsexual contact is made, transmission of the bacterium can occur. The disease is usually found among the sexually promiscuous or contracted by individuals traveling to endemic areas who have a sexual encounter with an infected individual. The disease appears to be more prevalent among the lower socioeconomic class. One unique characteristic of this disease is that it may cause a persistent cervical infection, which then may serve as a reservoir for the disease (10). In males, the disease is more often symptomatic than in females; however, females tend to suffer from more severe complications of LGV.

PATHOGENESIS

LGV infection is initiated by attachment of the chlamydial infectious particle to an epithelial cell, which typically occurs when an infectious lesion comes in contact with a mucosal surface. Trauma during sexual intercourse can cause microscopic breaks in the mucosal surface exposing the underlying epithelial cells. A recent study demonstrated a sulfated glycosaminoglycan-dependent mechanism is required for infection. *C. trachomatis,* including LGV biovars, competes for the same receptors on host cells, and this interaction could be inhibited by heparan sulphate. These investigators demonstrated that treating the organism with heparan sulphate lyase (heparintinase) could inhibit host cell attachment (11–14). Once the organism invades the mucosal barrier, it gains entrance to the lymphatic system, and the clinical manifestation of infection is related to the degree of lymphatic involvement and dissemination.

There are three clinically defined stages of LGV. The primary stage is characterized by the development of small papules or vesicles at the site of inoculation. The development of vesicles may make this infection appear to be herpetic. The incubation period is 1 to 3 weeks from the time of exposure. The papule or vesicle may rupture, producing an ulceration that is typically painless (Figs. 12-1 and 12-2). This lesion typically goes unnoticed in the female patient, and in the male, the short duration of the existence of this lesion tends to create a false sense of

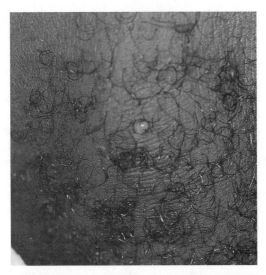

FIG. 12-1. Spontaneous rupture of a papule with drainage of thick pus. (See Color Plate 21 following page 148.)

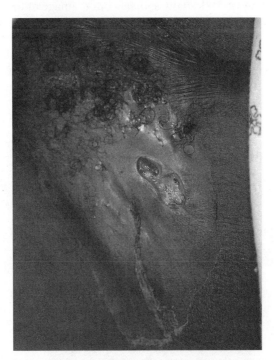

FIG. 12-2. Ulceration of bubo. (See Color Plate 22 following page 148.)

well being in the patient. The most common sites of infection in the female are the labia minora, posterior fourchette, posterior vaginal wall, and cervix. However, other areas of the lower genital tract may be involved. The patient may develop disseminated disease characterized by malaise, myalgias, and hematogenous spread of the organism (15). The patient can also develop pneumonitis, arthritis, hepatitis, and skin lesions (16). *C. trachomatis* has been cultured from the gallbladder, capsule of the liver, and adhesions in the pelvis and abdomen (17). Rare cases of pericarditis and mediastinal lymphadenitis have been reported (18). The organism can be autoinoculated to other mucosal surfaces of the body (e.g., the eye) (11). Inoculation may also occur in the pharynx or mouth via orogenital sex, and proctitis may occur via rectal intercourse (19). The hallmark lesion of the second stage of this disease is the development of enlarged tender lymph nodes leading to the creation of buboes. The patient may have involvement of the deep pelvic nodes and present with fever. When presenting with fever, she may or may not have lymphadenopathy but should, if the history places her at risk, be considered to possibly have syphilis, LGV, or other diseases that may present in a similar fashion. The lymph nodes usually become painful and fluctuant. They may suppurate or spontaneously rupture through the skin (Figs. 12-2 and 12-3). Usually spontaneous drainage of the nodes is accompanied by resolution of pain and fever. The draining pus may contains the microorganism; therefore, *C. trachomatis* can be detected by polymerase chain reaction (PCR), by stains (the organism stains gram negative with Brown-Hopp's tissue Gram stain, faintly blue with hematoxylin and eosin stain, and black with Warthin-Starry silver impregnation stain), and by tissue culture (20). Immunofluorescence stainings can also be used to detect *C. trachomatis* from the aspi-

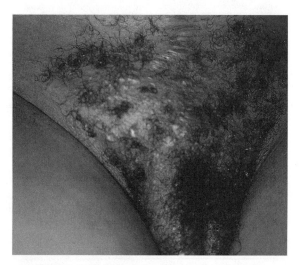

FIG. 12-3. Grove sign. Enlargement of inguinal and femoral lymphonodes separated by inguinal ligament. (See Color Plate 23 following page 148.)

rates of buboes (21). A common complication of aspiration and drainage of the enlarged lymph nodes is the development of chronic draining sinuses (22,23). It is not uncommon for the chain of nodes to become matted together. The direction of spread is dependent on the site of inoculation; for example, if the cervix and upper vagina are involved, then it is likely that the iliac and deep pelvic nodes will become involved. This could create a clinical picture in which the patient presents with pain; fever may or may not be present. On pelvic examination, a markedly tender mass is palpated (24). Frequently, the inguinal and femoral nodes are enlarged because of inflammation and swelling. The involvement of these two chains of lymph nodes, which are located on either side of the inguinal ligament giving rise to the so-called groove sign (Fig. 12-3), which is found in approximately 20% of infected women with stage two disease (10,12).

The third stage of LGV is referred to as the anogenitorectal syndrome and is characterized by proctocolitis and involvement of the perirectal lymph nodes. Initially the patient may present with complaints of anal pruritus, rectal pain, abdominal cramping, tenesmus, and rectal bleeding. Examination reveals an edematous rectal mucosa that is hyperemic and friable. The mucosa may have superficial erosions and small abscesses (25,26). Perirectal abscesses and fissures are common with the development of rectovaginal fistulae (27,28). The patient may develop anorectal stricture or stenosis and resemble a rectal neoplasia (29). Rectal involvement is more common in women but is not usually associated with bubo formation. Therefore, the patient is not likely to seek medical assistance until the disease progresses to a rectal stenosis, a late stage. Rectal stricture and stenosis predisposes to rectal cancer (30).

Rectal involvement may be indicated by a mucoid discharge, which may be purulent if a secondary infection is present. The patient may also develop an obstruction of the perirectal lymphatic system and present with prolapse of the involved lymphatics that resembles hemorrhoids, these are referred to as "lymphorrhoids." The bowel may develop significant lesions, which may undergo spontaneous perforation leading to the development of peritonitis (31). The patient may complain of abdominal pain, described as intermittent or colic in character. The patient may believe she has a degree of constipation and note that when stool is passed it is long and thin, described as "pencil stools." This is caused by the development of granulation tissue, which produces a stricture and is often mistaken for carcinoma. This stricture typically develops 3 to 5 cm above the anocutaneous margin because it is at this level that the perirectal lymphatics are concentrated.

The differential diagnosis of the anogenital syndrome includes rectal carcinoma, extrinsic mass to the rectum, endometriosis, and diverticulitis. An incarcerated inguinal hernia may be mistaken for a bubo. Involvement of the deep pelvic nodes could be mistaken for cervical carcinoma and may mimic the spread of cervical cancer. Lymphorrhoids develop secondary rectal fibrosis that results in obstructions of the lymphatic and venous drainage of the lower rectum. Lymphorrhoids can be confused with hemorrhoids.

DIAGNOSIS

The diagnosis of LGV can be made by culturing the bacterium, serologic testing antibody-antigen immunofluorescence, and PCR (32–34). Overall, genital ulcer disease is clinically easier to diagnose in women than in men. In one study (Table 12-1) of 100 women and 100 men, various genital ulcers were diagnosed (35). The difficulty in establishing a diagnosis on clinical appearance and findings is because of the great similarities in the various causes of genital ulcer disease.

It is possible to culture the serovars responsible for LGV obtained from clinical specimens. However, under the best conditions *C. trachomatis* is recovered in only 30% of infected individuals (36). The original diagnostic test, the Frei test, is no longer used. Currently, the diagnosis is based on clinical presentation and characteristics of the lesion, the complement fixation test, and microimmunofluorescent antigen-antibody interaction. Diagnosis based solely on the clinical characteristics is fraught with potential problems because the lesion, the ulcer or bubo, may resemble one found with chancroid or syphilis. Therefore, treatment, if based solely on clinical diagnosis, should include antimicrobial agents with activity against LGV, chancroid, and syphilis. The complement fixation test cross reacts with other chlamydial antibodies; therefore, it is nonspecific and the diagnosis should not solely be based on this test. A complement fixation titer of greater than 1:674 and a microimmunofluorescent titer greater than or equal to 1:512 are indicative of acute infection. Although the patient with acute LGV usually develops antibodies early in the course of the disease; a negative antibody test does not rule out the disease (37–40). The difficulty in establishing an accurate diagnosis of LGV has been an area of active investigation. One study demonstrated that serologic detection of specific chlamydial antibodies, IgM and IgG, paralleled that of culture in the diagnosis of LGV. The chlamydial specific antibodies were detected using monoclonal antibodies with immunofluorescence. LGV antibodies were detected with enzyme-linked immunosorbent assay (ELISA) using *Salmonella minnesota* mR 595 lipopolysaccharide (LPS) as the antigen and *C. trachomatis* L2 antigen (33).

TABLE 12-1. *Comparative accuracy in the clinical diagnosis of genital ulcer disease in South African men and women*

Diagnosis	Women	Men
Primary syphilis	58%	32%
Secondary syphilis	94%	52%
Donovanosis	83%	38%
Herpes	60%	39%
Chancroid	57%	42%
LGV	40%	66%
Mixed infections	14%	8%

LGV, lymphogranuloma venereum.

TREATMENT

Like all serotypes of *C. trachomatis,* the serotypes that cause LGV are readily susceptible to appropriate antibiotics. Sulfonamides, the agents of choice in the 1930s, should not be used. It has been shown that a large number of patients who received sulfonamides did not achieve microbiologic cure (41). The current recommendations from the CDC are as follows:

Doxycycline 100 mg orally twice a day for 21 days
Tetracycline 500 mg orally four times a day for 21 days
Erythromycin 500 mg orally four times a day for 21 days

Chloramphenicol and rifampin have been demonstrated to be efficacious as well. The recommendations listed apply to all stages of LGV (42). When treating genital ulcer disease, if an accurate diagnosis cannot be established or is not possible, the patient should be treated with antibiotics that are effective against LGV, chancroid, granuloma inguinale, and syphilis. This management should be instituted if a patient visited an area where these diseases are known to be endemic. The patient with genital ulcer disease should also be evaluated for the presence of herpes and human immunodeficiency virus (HIV), because genital ulcer disease is known to place the individual at risk for contracting HIV (43,44).

Although surgery may be indicated to relieve strictures, antibiotic therapy should be tried first because, in some cases, medical therapy alone may relieve stricturing of the rectum. Stricturing resistant to antibiotic therapy develops when the area becomes fibrosed. Aspiration of buboes has been the approach for obtaining a specimen for identification and for draining the infected lymph node. Recently, incision and drainage has been compared with aspiration of fluctuant buboes caused by chancroid. 27 patients were studied (22 men and 5 women) and randomized to incision, drainage, and packing or aspiration. The former method (incision, drainage, and packing) was found to be as effective and may be preferable to aspiration, because the latter (aspiration) often requires multiple aspirations (45).

REFERENCES

1. Kampmeier RH. Early development of knowledge of sexually transmitted diseases. In: Holmes KK, Mardh PA, Sparling PR, et al., eds. *Sexually transmitted diseases.* New York: McGraw-Hill, 1984: 19–29.
2. Mardh PA, Paavonen J, Puolakkainen M. *Chlamydia.* New York: Plenum, 1989:3–5.
3. Frei W. On the skin test in lymphogranuloma inguinale. *J Invest Dermatol* 1938;1:367.
4. Centers for Disease Control. Summary of notifiable diseases, United States 1991. *MMWR* 1991;40:3.
5. Abrams AJ. Lymphogranuloma venereum. *JAMA* 1968;205:199–202.
6. Perine PL, et al. Diagnosis and treatment of lymphogranuloma venereum in Ethiopia. In: *Current chemotherapy and infectious diseases.* Washington DC: American Society for Microbiology, 1980: 1280–1282.
7. Sowmini CN, Gopalan KN, Rao GC. Minocycline in the treatment of lymphogranuloma venereum. *J Am Vener Dis Assoc* 1976;2:19–22.
8. Willcox RR. Importance of the so-called "other" sexually-transmitted diseases. *Br J Vener Dis* 1975; 51:221–226.

9. Monno R, Pastore G, Lamargese V, et al. Lymphogranuloma venereum: a case report in an Italian traveler. *New Microbiol* 1997;20:83–86.
10. Johannisson G, Lowhagen GB, Lycke E. Genital *Chlamydia trachomatis* infection in women. *Obstet Gynecol* 1980;56:671–675.
11. Chen JC, Stephens RS. Trachoma and LGV biovars of *Chlamydia trachomatis* share the same glycosaminoglycan-dependent mechanism for infection of eukaryotic cells. *Mol Microbiol* 1994;11: 501–507.
12. Koteen H. Lymphogranuloma venereum. *Medicine* 1945;24:1.
13. Schacter J. Lymphogranuloma venereum and other oculogenital *Chlamydia trachomatis* infections. In: Hobson D, Holmes KK, eds. *Nongonococcal urethritis and related infections*. Washington DC: American Society for Microbiology, 1977:91–97.
14. Dan M, Rotmench HH, Eylan E, et al. A case of lymphogranuloma venereum of 20 years' duration. Isolation of *Chlamydia trachomatis* from perianal tissue. *Br J Vener Dis* 1980;56:344–346.
15. Sabin AB, Aring CD. Meningoencephalitis in a man caused by the virus lymphogranuloma venereum. *JAMA* 1942;120:1376.
16. Favre M, Hellerstrom S. The epidemiology, etiology and prophylaxis of lymphogranuloma inguinale. *Acta Derm Vererol Suppl (Stockh)* 1954;34:1.
17. Coutts WE. Lymphogranuloma venereum: a general review. *Bull WHO* 1950;2:545.
18. Sheldon WH, Wall M, Slade JR, et al. Lymphogranuloma venereum of supraclavicular lymph nodes with mediastinal lymphadenopathy and pericarditis. *Am J Med* 1948;5:320.
19. Thorsteinsson SB, Musher DM, Min KW, et al. Lymphogranuloma venereum: a cause of cervical lymphadenopathy. *JAMA* 1976;235:1882.
20. Hadfield TL, Lamy Y, Wear DJ. Demonstration of *Chlamydia trachomatis* in inguinal lymphadenitis of lymphogranuloma venereum: a light microscopy, electron microscopy and polymerase chain reaction study. *Mod Pathol* 1995;8:924–929.
21. Viravan C, Dance DA, Ariyarit C, et al. A prospective clinical and bacteriologic study of inguinal buboes in Thai men. *Clin Infect Dis* 1996;22:233–239.
22. Von Haam E, D'Aunoy R. Is lymphogranuloma inguinale a systemic disease? *Am J Trop Med Hyg* 1936;16:527.
23. Prehn DT. Lymphogranuloma venereum and associated disease. *Arch Dermatol Syph* 1937;35:231.
24. Zweizig S, Schlaerth JB, Boswell WD Jr. Computed tomography of lymphogranuloma venereum mimicking cervical cancer. *Comput Med Imaging Graph* 1937;2:97.
25. D'Aunoy R, vonHaam E. Venereal lymphogranuloma. *Arch Pathol* 1991;27:97.
26. Torpin R, et al. Lymphogranuloma venereum in the female. A clinical study of ninety-six consecutive cases. *Am J Surg* 1939;43:688.
27. Mathewson C Jr. Inflammatory strictures of the rectum associated with venereal lymphogranuloma. *JAMA* 1938;110:709.
28. Saad EA, Gouveia OF, Filho PD, et al. Ano-rectal-colonic lymphogranuloma venereum. *Gastroenterology* 1962;97:89.
29. Jeanpretre M, Harms M, Saurat JH. Stenosing anal mass and venereal lymphogranuloma. *Schweiz Med Wochenschr* 1994;124:1587–1591.
30. Chopda NM, Desai DC, Sawant PD, et al. Rectal lymphogranuloma venereum in association with rectal adenocarcinoma. *Indian J Gastroenterol* 1994;13:103–104.
31. Banov L. Rectal stricture of lymphogranuloma venereum: some observations from a five year study of treatment with broad spectrum antibiotics. *Am J Surg* 1954;88:761.
32. Joseph AK, Rosen T. Laboratory techniques used in the diagnosis of chancroid, granuloma inguinale, and lymphogranuloma venereum. *Dermatol Clin* 1994;12:1–8.
33. Deak J, Nedelkovics Z, Foldes J. Comparative studies in the diagnosis of *Chlamydia trachomatis* infections. *Orv Hetil* 1994;135:465–468.
34. Pala S, Risi R, Zicari L, et al. Clinico-diagnostic considerations on various cases of lymphogranuloma venereum. Minerva. *Urol Nefrol* 1996;48:103.
35. O'Farrell N, Hoosen AA, Coetzee KD, et al. Genital ulcer disease: accuracy of clinical diagnosis and strategies to improve control in Durban, South Africa. *Geniturin Med* 1994;70:7–11.
36. Philip RN, Hill DA, Greaves AB, et al. Study of Chlamydia in patients with lymphogranuloma venereum and urethritis attending a venereal disease clinic. *Br J Vener Dis* 1971;47:114–121.
37. Paavonen J. Chlamydial infections. Microbiological, clinical and diagnostic aspects. *Med Biol* 1979; 57:135–151.
38. Schachter J, Smith DE, Dawson CR, et al. Lymphogranuloma venereum. I. Comparison of the Frei test, complement fixation and isolation of the agent. *J Infect Dis* 1969;120:372–375.

39. Kellock DJ, Barlow R, Suvarna SK, et al. Lymphogranuloma venereum: biopsy, serology, and molecular biology. *Genitourn Med* 1997;73:399–401.
40. Wang SP. A simplified method for immunological typing of trachoma-inclusions conjunctivitis-lymphogranuloma venereum organism. *Infect Immunity* 1973;7:356.
41. Jones H, Rake G, Stearns B. Studies on lymphogranuloma venereum. III. The action of sulfonamides on the agent of lymphogranuloma venereum. *J Infect Dis* 1945;76:55.
42. Centers for Disease Control and Prevention. 1993 sexually transmitted diseases treatment guidelines. *MMWR* 1993;42:26.
43. Martin DH, Mroczkowski TF. Dermatologic manifestations of sexually transmitted diseases other than HIV. *Infect Dis Clin North Am* 1994;8:533–582.
44. Goens JL, Schwartz RA, DeWolf K. Mucocutaneous manifestations of chancroid, lymphogranuloma venereum and granuloma inguinale. *Am Fam Physician* 1994;49:415–418.
45. Ernst AA, Marvez-Valls E, Martin DH. Incision and drainage versus aspiration of fluctuant buboes in the emergency department during an epidemic of chancroid. *Sex Transm Dis* 1995;22:217–220.

13

Syphilis

INTRODUCTION

Syphilis is an ancient disease that, like gonorrhea, is referenced in ancient writings including the Bible. This disease was, at one time, considered under control with the number of cases declining and leveling off. However, an increase in the number of cases in the population was recently noted. Among women, the incidence of primary and secondary syphilis remained fairly constant from 1980 to 1986 (Fig.13-1). The initial decrease in the number of cases occurred after the introduction of penicillin in the late 1940s, and this antibiotic continues to be effective in the treatment of syphilis. The increase reported in the mid-1980s paralleled the increase that occurred in the male population (Fig. 13-1). The recent prevalence of human immunodeficiency virus (HIV) brought syphilis back into the forefront. Paralleling the increase in syphilis in the acquired immunodeficiency syndrome (AIDS) patients has been an increase in syphilis in the non-AIDS population. In addition, the number of syphilis cases is also increasing among pregnant women, which is also reflected in an increase in the number of cases of anogenital syphilis.

MICROBIOLOGY

Syphilis is caused by the spirochete, *Treponema pallidum. Treponema* is one of the three genera of the family Spirochaetales that are pathogenic for humans. The other genera are *Borrelia* and *Leptospira.* The genus *Treponema* includes the following species: *T. pallidum; Treponema pertenue,* the causative agent of yaws; and *Treponema carateum,* which is the etiologic agent of pinta.

Treponemes are distinctive among bacteria in that they lack the characteristic cell wall found among the gram-positive and gram-negative bacteria. Therefore, they do not stain when exposed to Gram reagents. The spirochetes are very slender, flexible, and motile organisms, which possess flagellum-like axial filaments located in the periplasmic space between the inner and outer membranes of the cell (1). The filaments originate at the ends of the cell, overlap at the center, and are not connected.

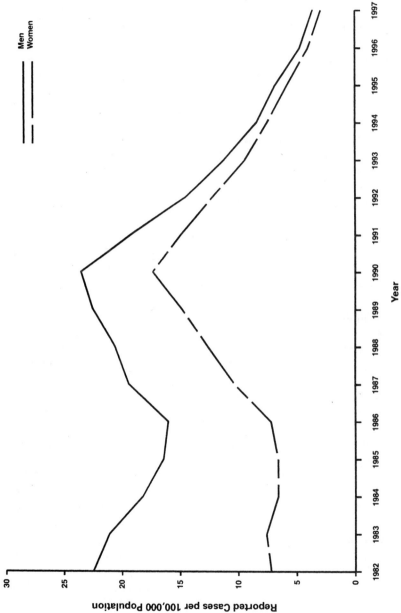

FIG. 13-1. Syphilis (primary and secondary) by sex in the United States from 1982 through 1997. In 1997, the reported rate of primary and secondary syphilis in the United States continued to decline, with rates among both males and females below the Healthy People 2000 objective of 4.0 per 100,000 population. Among men, the rate decreased from 4.7 per 100,000 population in 1996 to 3.6 in 1997. Among women, the rate decreased from 4.0 per 100,000 population in 1996 to 2.9 in 1997.

The slender shape of the spirochetes does not provide enough mass for sufficient refraction of light that prevents them from being seen with ordinary light microscopy. However, they are easily seen by dark-field microscopy or when stained with silver salts. When preparations are examined with the aid of dark-field microscopy, it is noted that the treponemes have a distinctive corkscrew motion as they rotate about their long axis. There is evidence that the organism possesses an outer slime coating that may assist in its virulence and be responsible for the serologic nonreactivity in freshly isolated specimens.

EPIDEMIOLOGY

In the 1940s before the widespread use of penicillin, syphilis was the major cause of morbidity and mortality throughout the world. Syphilis was also responsible for the largest number of admissions to mental institutions with most patients being diagnosed with neurosyphilis. The introduction of penicillin and the institution of public health measures (e.g., contact tracing and treatment of exposed partners) are the major reasons for the decline in the number of patients admitted to mental hospitals for syphilis. Coincident with the steady decline in mortality (in the 1940s there were 15,000 to 20,000 deaths annually, whereas in the early 1980s, there were 300 deaths related to syphilis) was a decline in the number of cases of primary and secondary syphilis (2,3).

The disease peaked during World War II, declined dramatically in the mid-1950s, and plateaued in the heterosexual community. In the 1970s and 1980s, the number of cases began to rise in the homosexual community. This change in the epidemiology of the disease was related to the behavioral practices of a given community or population, which is difficult to alter. Therefore, when the disease develops a strong foothold within a given community, there tends to be an increase in the number of reportable cases. An increase makes an impact on various aspects of the community and, thus, is not restricted to a subset of the population. Eventually, the disease spills into adjacent communities or, via travel, to distant communities because the sexual practices of individuals (i.e., bisexual activity) may allow them to function in both homosexual and heterosexual communities. This results in an increase in the sexually transmitted disease (STD) pool within a community, with individuals sampling this pool periodically and bringing the organisms to individuals who are neither part of nor participate in this pool. Beginning in 1985, there was a significant increase in the number of cases of syphilis in both the homosexual and heterosexual populations (4,5).

The prevalence of syphilis seems to be highest in the southern United States (Fig.13-2). This may be related to the density of the population, use of illicit drugs, and economic conditions. An increase in the number of cases of syphilis was noted in the western United States beginning in 1985, but by 1989 to 1990, the pre-1985 rates for primary and secondary syphilis returned. This was most likely because of a behavioral change in the population initiated by the recognition that HIV and AIDS were acquired through sexual contact. Interestingly, the

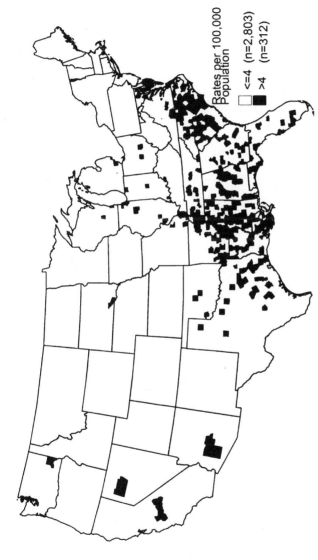

FIG. 13-2. Syphilis (primary and secondary) reported cases per 100,000 population in the United States in 1997. In 1997, the United States rate of primary and secondary syphilis of 3.2 per 100,000 population was below the revised national Healthy People 2000 objective. Forty-one states reported rates below the national objective, and 12 states reported fewer than five cases. The revised Healthy People 2000 objective is ≤4.0 per 100,000 population.

Rates per 100,000
Population

□ <=4 (n=2,803)
■ >4 (n=312)

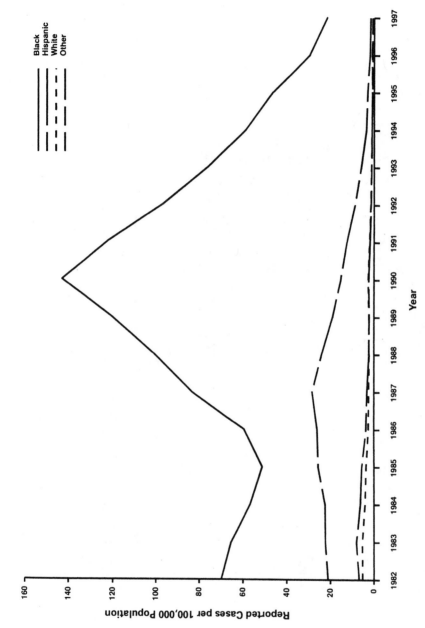

FIG. 13-3. Syphilis (primary and secondary) by race and ethnicity in the United States from 1982 through 1997. In 1997, primary and secondary syphilis rates for all racial and ethnic groups declined. In 1997, however, the rate for non-Hispanic blacks (i.e., 22.0 cases per 100,000 population) was 44-fold greater than that for non-Hispanic whites.

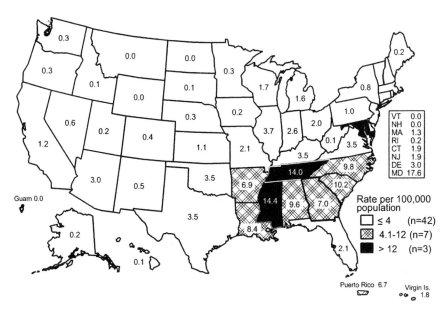

FIG. 13-4. Primary and secondary syphilis rates by state in the United States and outlying areas in 1997. The total rate of primary and secondary syphilis for the United States and outlying areas (including Guam, Puerto Rico, and Virgin Islands) was 3.3 per 100,000 population. The Healthy People year 2000 objective is 4.0 per 100,000 population.

number of syphilis cases in the Midwest remained relatively low until 1987, when a gradual increase began and appears to continue.

When examining the number of primary and secondary cases of syphilis by race and ethnicity, an increased prevalence is found in African Americans (Fig.13-3). This increase reflects the increase seen in Figs. 13-1 and 13-2. The African-American population is denser in the South than in the West. Examining the prevalence of syphilis by individual states (Fig. 13-4), reveals that the highest number of cases is occurring in the South and in Maryland (Figs. 13-2 and 13-4). However, syphilis has been reported to occur in every state in the union.

PATHOPHYSIOLOGY

Syphilis has been studied since the preantibiotic era. Two well-known studies were conducted before the availability of antibiotics, the Tuskeege and Oslo studies (6,7).

These two studies were long-term clinical observations conducted over many years and were designed to monitor the natural course of untreated syphilis. Although much was learned from these studies, they were conducted at a time when there were no safeguards, such as institutional research review boards, to protect human participants.

T. pallidum is primarily transmitted through contact of a syphilis lesion to a mucous membrane. The most common transmission occurs via sexual intercourse, but the disease can also be transmitted via infected blood (by transfusion or transplacentally). However, acquisition of syphilis through transfusion in North America has been eliminated since routine serologic screening of donated blood began. Contributing to the decrease in the risk of syphilis via blood transfusion is the decreased use of whole blood and the increased use of stored blood components. Storage of blood components at 40^0C kills *T. pallidum.*

One third of individuals exposed to an infected individual will become infected (8). There is a high infection rate among individuals who have AIDS and there is concern that the organism may be transmitted by the use of shared needles among intravenous drug abusers who have syphilis. However, the transmission via intravenous needles has not been substantiated.

The organism usually is transmitted from an individual with a chancre when it comes in contact with either the skin or mucous membrane of the sexual partner. If there are breaks in the surface of the exposed tissue or lacerations occur during sexual intercourse in the vagina, rectum, or oral-pharyngeal mucosa, this facilitates entrance of the treponema into the uninfected host. The incubation time is dependent on the inoculum size and ranges between 1 week and 3 months (9). The lesions usually heal spontaneously, within 3 to 6 weeks. The chancre is characteristically painless and typically goes unnoticed in the female patient when present on the genitalia. It is during this stage that dissemination of the spirochetes occurs, resulting in the development of secondary syphilis in 60% to 90% of infected patients. Infected individuals usually develop signs of secondary syphilis within 4 to 10 weeks after developing primary syphilis. Approximately 34% of patients with secondary syphilis will have a primary chancre when the diagnosis is made (10). Recurrent manifestations of secondary syphilis, in the absence of treatment, will reoccur in approximately 25% of patients during the first year. However, symptomatic recurrences in the non-treated patient may occur up to 4 years following primary infection. If the disease is left untreated, it will progress to latent stage, which is not associated with any clinical manifestations. Therefore, secondary syphilis has been divided into two stages: (a) an infectious disease of less than 1 year duration referred to as early latent syphilis and (b) a disease of more than 1 year duration referred to as latent syphilis and not infectious.

In the absence of therapy or with inadequate or inappropriate therapy, the patient's disease may progress to tertiary disease in approximately one third of the cases (7). The manifestations of tertiary syphilis vary with approximately 15% of the patients developing gummas, 10% cardiovascular disease, and 10% neurosyphilis. Gummas may develop within 1 year of acquiring syphilis; therefore, their presence should not automatically lead to the conclusion that the patient has tertiary syphilis. Typically, gummas require 10 to 30 years to develop. Today, tertiary syphilis rarely occurs because many patients who acquire the disease are treated with antibiotics such as penicillin or a cephalosporin for another infection, which is usually effective for the treatment of incubating syphilis. Incubating syphilis would be undetected because there would be neither clinical manifestations nor serologic evidence of infection. However, treatment would be successful because during incubation the numbers would be low and reproduction of the treponemes would be occurring at a low rate. Thus, the antibiotic would be effective. The short-acting penicillins and cephalosporins would maintain a serum level that would be sufficient to kill the treponemes at this stage.

CLINICAL MANIFESTATIONS

Primary Syphilis

Primary syphilis is classically characterized by the presence of a solitary ulceration, termed a chancre, which usually occurs at the site of contact (inoculation). The chancre is painless and, therefore, will not be detected in the female patient when the lesion occurs on the perineum, labia, vaginal introitus, or perianal area. The chancre or ulcer typically has a raised border and an indurated and clean base. The patient usually develops a nontender unilateral or bilateral inguinal lymphadenopathy. It must be emphasized that, although the ulcer tends to be solitary, multiple and atypical lesions do occur. The typical chancre begins as a papule and may resemble a herpetic lesion (11).

In evaluating the patient with a genital ulcer, the physician should consider, in addition to syphilis, any infection that may causes ulcerations (Table 13-1).

It is important to determine if the patient has traveled anywhere because some of these diseases are more prevalent in certain parts of the country and the world. It is not uncommon to find that more than one STD is found to infect an individual; therefore, when an individual is found to have one infectious disease, a second one should be sought. It is estimated that 5% of patients with primary syphilis also have genital herpes (12). Although the chancre of primary syphilis tends to be characteristic, its morphology can be altered by the application of topical medications. The chancre may become secondarily infected and develop a purulent exudate, thereby masking its syphilitic characteristics. Morphologically, it can be altered by the coexistence of an infection such as HIV. The diagnosis is best established by darkfield microscopy of the serum exudate of the

TABLE 13-1. *Ulcerative infectious diseases of the genitalia*

Disease	Cause
Herpes genitalia	Herpes simplex (primarily type II)
Chancroid	*Haemophilus ducreyi*
Lymphogranuloma venereum	*Chlamydia trachomatis* (serotypes L1, L2, & L3)
Granuloma inguinale	*Calymmatobacterium granulomatis*
Ulcerations of bacterial origin	*Streptococcus pyogenes*
	Staphylococcus aureus
Ulcerations of fungal origin	*Candida albicans*
	Blastomyces dermatitidis

chancre. Serologic identification is possible after the infection has been present for at least 3 weeks. If the disease is left untreated or is treated inappropriately, it may progress to the secondary stage.

Although the use of darkfield microscopy is ideal for establishing a diagnosis of primary syphilis, it can also be used for specimens obtained from individuals with secondary and congenital syphilis. The darkfield examination is infrequently performed because the female patient rarely detects the presence of a lesion on the genitalia. In addition, the chancre may develop on the vaginal wall, cervix, or perirectal area and will go unnoticed by the patient. However, darkfield microscopy is seldom employed because many physicians do not have the equipment or training to perform the procedure. Therefore, if a darkfield microscopic examination is desired, the patient must travel to a suitable medical facility to have the procedure performed. This would cause a significant amount of waiting and processing time, not to mention the fact that she would have to be reexamined. Most patients would find this to be unacceptable. An alternative to darkfield microscopy, which requires living organisms, is fluorescent antibody microscopy that does not require the presence of living treponemes. The latter test is conducted using direct fluorescence with Fluorescein isothiocyanate (FITC)-conjugated antibodies to *T. pallidum* or indirect fluorescence using *T. pallidum* specific antibodies (13,14). The most common method used to establish a diagnosis of syphilis is serologic testing. The serologic tests are divided into nonspecific nontreponemal and specific treponemal tests. The treponemal specific test is used to rule out false-positive reactions and not for screening. However, it must be pointed out that false-positive reactions do occur with the treponemal specific test (Table 13-2).

The nonspecific nontreponemal tests commonly used in the United States are the Venereal Disease Reference Laboratory (VDRL) test and the rapid plasma reagin (RPR) test. The first serologic test, developed by Wassermann in 1906, was demonstrated to be a "cholesterol-lecithin-cardiolipin antigen" that reacted with antibodies in the sera of patients with syphilis. Cardiolipin is a normal constituent of the inner membrane of mammalian mitochondria, and antibodies to cardiolipin can be detected in normal sera. Anticardiolipin antibodies can be produced in the absence of treponemal infection, thus giving a false-positive test. In

TABLE 13-2. *Serologic false-positive tests for syphilis*

Recent viral infection
Immunizations
Drug addiction
Malaria
Rheumatoid arthritis
Systemic lupus erythematosus
Other autoimmune disease
Chronic infections
Aging

the absence of diseases, such as collagen vascular disease, the test can be adjusted so that the small amount of antigen present in normal sera is not detected. The VDRL is performed by mixing cholesterol-lecithin-cardiolipin antigen with heated serum obtained from the patient. Clumping on the slide is read as positive; that is, the patient possesses antibody, whereas failure to observe clumping indicates that the patient's serum does not contain antibody. Typically, the test is performed by diluting the patient's serum and the test result is reported as the greatest dilution that produces a positive result (e.g., 1:64, 1:128, 1:256, etc.). Improvements in the sensitivity and specificity of the components of the reaginic antibodies have led to the development of the VDRL and RPR tests. The reagin of these tests should not be confused with the reaginic antibody associated with hypersensitivity reactions, known as allergy-associated IgE antibody. The reagin, nontreponemal test detects the presence of anticardiolipin IgM and IgG antibodies (15).

The VDRL test is not used in most laboratories to screen large numbers of patients and has been replaced by the RPR; however, the VDRL continues to be used when testing cerebrospinal fluid (CSF). When performing the VDRL on CSF, the fluid should not be heated like when the test is performed on serum. The RPR is the most common screening test used today and is performed by placing serum on coated cards and microscopically examining the cards for flocculation. This is a more rapid test because the serum does not have to be heated, microscopic examination is unnecessary, and the test can be performed in an office setting.

The RPR is usually reported as nonreactive or reactive. The VDRL is usually reported as a titer (e.g., 1:16 or 16 dilutions). False-positive titers are usually reported to be less than 1:8, but low titers are commonly found in latent and late syphilis. False-positive titers occur in 1% to 2% of the general population and rise to 10% among intravenous drug users (16–18). False-positive tests are divided into those that become negative within 6 months and those that remain positive after 6 months. The false-positive tests, which revert to negative within 6 months, are usually secondary to other conditions, infectious and noninfectious (Table 13-3).

TABLE 13-3. *Conditions that can yield false-positive nonspecific tests for syphilis*

Infectious	Noninfectious
Mycoplasma pneumonia	Immunizations
Glandular fever	Pregnancy
Viral pneumonia	Autoimmune disease
Hepatitis	Aging
Varicella	Narcotic addiction
Mononucleosis	Malignancy
Measles	
Malaria	
Leprosy	

Persistent false positives are usually because of diseases such as leprosy, autoimmune diseases, aging, narcotic addiction, and malignancy. The presence of persistent false-positive nonspecific nontreponemal tests may precede the onset of underlying disease by several years. Although this result is more common in women than in men, only 15% of women with a false-positive test will develop an autoimmune disease.

Serum that contains large amounts of reaginic antibodies may react weakly or atypically or be nonreactive when used undiluted in the VDRL test. This inhibitory effect has been termed the "prozone reaction" and can be overcome by diluting the serum containing the antibody. The reaction is seen in approximately 1% of the patients with secondary syphilis.

The nonspecific nontreponemal tests should be positive in approximately 76% of patients with primary syphilis. These tests should be positive in 100% of patients with secondary syphilis and approximately 70% in patients with latent and tertiary syphilis.

The specific treponemal tests, *Treponema pallidum* hemagglutination (TPHA) test, the automated qualitative microhemagglutination assay-*Treponema pallidum* (AMHA-TP), the manual qualitative or quantitative micro-hemagglutination assay-*Treponema pallidum* (MHA-TP), and the fluorescent treponemal antibody-absorption test (FTA-ABS), are all directed against the specific detection of treponemal antibodies in the patient's serum. The FTA-ABS or MHA-TP tests are used only to confirm that the patient has syphilis. Once the patient has contracted syphilis and is FTA-ABS or MHA-TP positive, seroconversion to negative rarely occurs. Thus, these tests are of no value in monitoring the effectiveness of therapy. The false-positive rate for the FTA-ABS or MHA-TP tests is less than 1%. Patients with systemic lupus erythematous or drug-induced erythematosus, intravenous drug abusers, recipients of the smallpox vaccine, or pregnant patients can yield a false-positive result. Disease states that are associated with an increase or the production of abnormal immunoglobulins can also produce a false-positive result.

The FTA-ABS is performed by mixing the patient's serum with whole *T. pallidum* that has been fixed to a microscopic slide, then adding fluorescein-tagged anti-human IgG. If antibodies are present in the patient's serum the *T. pallidum* will emit a bright fluorescence. Another common treponemal specific test, MHA-TP, is performed by exposing the patient's serum to erythrocytes coated with the *T. pallidum* antigen. The presence of antibody is detected by agglutination of the antigen-coated erythrocytes. The treponemal specific tests tend to remain positive after successful treatment has been completed, unlike the VDRL and RPR that may revert to negative. The FTA-ABS has a greater sensitivity than the MHA-TP in the early primary stage of syphilis. False-positive results can be obtained because these tests cross react with nonpathogenic treponemal antigens. False-positive results can be reduced by diluting the patient's serum in a material that will absorb antibody produced by nonpathogenic treponemes. This is usually done by using an absorbent prepared from *Treponema phagedenas* (14).

Secondary Syphilis

Secondary syphilis usually begins 4 to 10 weeks after the chancre has appeared. This is the systemic phase of syphilis and is usually preceded by the onset of flulike symptoms. The patient typically develops myalgias, arthralgias, malaise, and fever. The patient often develops a generalized nontender lymphadenopathy. The most characteristic lesion of secondary syphilis is the development of a nonpruritic, maculopapular rash, which typically occurs on the trunk, limbs, soles of the feet, and palms of the hands (Figs. 13-5 and 13-6). The rash may become pustular, nodular, eczematous, or plaque-like, and the patient may develop a chancre as seen in Figs. 13-7 and 13-8. The familiar genital, perineum, or perianal lesions referred to as condylomata lata occurs in 10% to 20% of infected patients. Condylomata lata must be distinguished from condylomata acuminata because the former is highly infectious. Condylomata lata are typically flat, have the appearance of a mound with a broad base, and are fleshy and smooth. Condylomata acuminata are typically heaped up and pyriforme and may be moist or dry. Other associated lesions of secondary syphilis, although infrequently observed, are alopecia, syphilitic hepatitis, and immune complex nephritis. Central nervous system (CNS) involvement can occur during secondary syphilis, for example, aseptic meningitis, cranial neuropathies, and eye involvement. It is not uncommon for the patient to present with fever, inguinal lymphadenopathy, and no other signs or symptoms (Fig. 13-9). This must be distinguished from HIV, mononucleosis, and other viral syndromes.

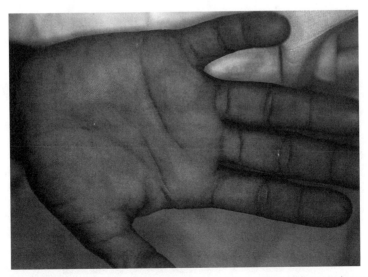

FIG. 13-5. Maculopapular rash on the palms of the hand in a patient with secondary syphilis. (See Color Plate 24 following page 148.)

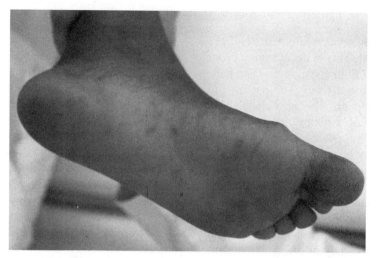

FIG. 13-6. Maculopapular rash on the sole of the foot of a patient with secondary syphilis. (See Color Plate 25 following page 148.)

The duration of this stage of secondary syphilis, commonly referred to as early latent syphilis, is 1 to 2 years. If this stage of disease is undetected or not treated appropriately, most patients will progress to late latent syphilis. This concept is important because it has direct bearing on treatment. In primary and early latent syphilis, the treponemes are dividing rapidly and, therefore, susceptible to a single dose of long-acting penicillin. It is also important to understand that if

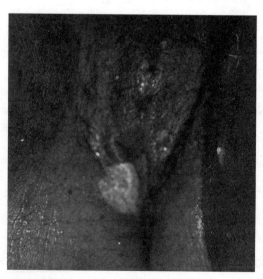

FIG. 13-7. Chancre on the inferior aspect of labia in a patient with secondary syphilis. (See Color Plate 26 following page 148.)

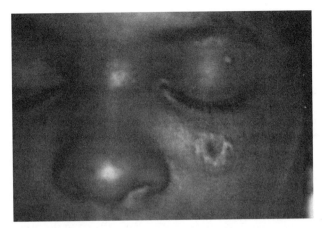

FIG. 13-8. Chancre of secondary syphilis occurring on the face of the patient. Lesion is secondarily infected. (See Color Plate 27 following page 148.)

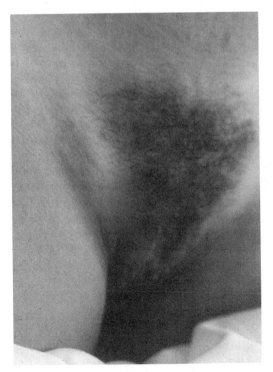

FIG. 13-9. Bilateral inguinal adenopathy of patient with secondary syphilis. Patient had temperature of 102°F and a VDRL of 1:128. (See Color Plate 28 following page 148.)

a patient is treated with ceftriaxone for gonorrhea this agent will also be effective against incubating syphilis when administered in a single dose. However, a single dose of ceftriaxone 250 mg may not be effective in the treatment of primary and early latent secondary syphilis. The pregnant patient with primary and early latent secondary syphilis should be treated with long-acting penicillin, benzathine penicillin. Pregnant patients allergic to penicillin should undergo desensitization and subsequently treated with sequential doses of penicillin to maintain an effective serum level to be effective against the slowly growing treponemes. Individuals with syphilis of 1- to 2-years duration are likely to have recurrent manifestations of the disease and are likely to transmit the infection. Individuals who have had their disease for greater than 2 years are considered to have late latent syphilis, are less likely to develop characteristic lesions, and are likely to transmit the disease to their sexual partners.

All patients with syphilis of unknown duration, including pregnant ones, should always be considered to have at least late latent secondary syphilis. There is no way to determine the exact duration of infection, especially if the patient does not recall ever having a lesion. Therefore, it is appropriate to treat the patient with sequential doses of penicillin; 1.2 million units of benzathine penicillin, administered in each buttock, once a week for 3 weeks. The total dose administered is 7.2 million units of benzathine penicillin.

Tertiary Syphilis

Tertiary syphilis is the most confusing stage because many of its manifestations (e.g., CNS involvement) may occur at all stages of syphilis. Laboratory evidence of CNS involvement may be frequently found in the earlier stages of syphilis. Examination of CSF in the syphilitic patient may be no different from that of the nonsyphilitic patient. In addition, the CNS fluid in the untreated asymptomatic syphilitic patient may not be different from that found in the patient with neurosyphilis. Depending on the duration of untreated syphilis, approximately 30% to 70% of individuals with CNS involvement will have abnormal CSF findings (15). The CSF findings in the syphilitic patient are typically a leukocytosis, elevated protein concentration, and a reactive VDRL. A reactive CSF-VDRL is the best test available in establishing a diagnosis of neurosyphilis (16). This test has a sensitivity of 30% to 70% (17,18). The CSF-VDRL will be positive in 25% of patients with secondary syphilis, whereas the test will be positive in a lower percentage of patients with latent syphilis, suggesting that the CSF abnormalities will resolve in untreated patients (18). A false-positive CSF-VDRL results from blood contamination of CSF; therefore, in the absence of blood in the CSF, a positive CSF-VDRL indicates either past or present involvement of the CSF. Patients with reactive CSF-VDRL will always have a positive direct treponemal test when performed on the CSF. A nonreactive CSF FTA-ABS, TPHA, or MHA-TP rules out neurosyphilis (19).

Clinical tertiary syphilis can present with gummata, which occurs in the skin, subcutaneous tissue, and bone. Gummata can develop anywhere in the body; however, when they occur in bone they cause significant pain. If they develop in the liver, the patient often presents with jaundice and can progress to hepatic failure.

Patients who develop cardiovascular syphilis typically develop an aortic aneurysm associated with aortic regurgitation and coronary ostial stenosis. It is believed that typical cardiovascular involvement is the result of undetected or untreated syphilis. Neurosyphilis was characteristically manifested by the presence of paresis and tabs dorsalis. However, since the use of antibiotic treatment, the most common manifestations of neurosyphilis are neuro-ophthalmic findings or seizures (20,21).

Syphilitic meningitis may become noticeable within 2 years of acquiring the infection and can be diagnosed because the patient typically develops headaches, neck stiffness, photophobia, nausea, vomiting, and confusion (22).

CNS involvement may occur early if syphilis is untreated (23). When treated appropriately, individuals with CNS involvement will have resolution of the infection, and some individuals may resolve spontaneously without treatment (24–26). Infected individuals who are untreated and have persistent CSF abnormalities are likely to develop clinical manifestations of neurosyphilis (27).

Analysis of CSF is used to determine if the patient has neurosyphilis. A normal CSF is characterized by an opening pressure of less than 180 mm of H_2O. Polymorphonuclear leukocytes are typically not found, but when white blood cells (WBCs) are found they are usually mononuclear cells. Glucose concentration in CSF is 60% that of the blood level. Normal CSF values have been reported in patients with clinically active symptomatic neurosyphilis (28–31). Among patients left untreated and followed for 10 years, approximately 16% developed clinical neurosyphilis (32–34).

Although the CSF may remain normal in a number of infected individuals who progress to neurosyphilis, it is unlikely that treated patients whose CSF remains normal for up to 2 years following treatment would develop neurosyphilis (35–37). This finding was confirmed in another study in which patients were followed for up to 5 years after treatment; less than 1% of the patients with normal CSF findings developed neurosyphilis (36). Dattner reported that CSF following treatment of neurosyphilis may show the following:

1. Permanent arrest, the cell count returns to normal (less than 9 WBCs/mm^3) within 6 months of treatment, total protein trends toward normal, and the serologic abnormalities may take years to revert to negative
2. Temporary arrest, the cell count declines or returns to normal and other findings show improvement, but this is followed by recurrence of a pleocytosis and an elevation of protein within 2 years
3. Failure to arrest progression, the CSF pleocytosis persists for more than 6 months without improvement in other quantitative CSF tests (36)

Neurosyphilis is described as consisting of four major syndromes: meningeal neurosyphilis, meningovascular neurosyphilis, parenchymatous neurosyphilis, and gummatous neurosyphilis. All four syndromes result from meningeal inflammation; therefore, meningeal involvement is found in all four syndromes (38,39). Vascular involvement, endarteritis, may cause meningovascular disease, which results in progressive vascular narrowing leading to obstruction and thrombosis. Meningovascular syphilis typically occurs within 4 to 10 years of the initial infection, whereas parenchymatous syphilis occurs 10 to 25 years after the onset of the primary infection and is associated with progressive irreversible deterioration in connection with neuronal loss, demyelination, and gliosis.

Neurosyphilis has been categorized as symptomatic and comprises up to one third of the cases of diagnosed neurosyphilis. The frequency of asymptomatic neurosyphilis decreases after 2 years in patients with untreated infection. This indicates either a progression to symptomatic disease or spontaneous resolution. The progression from asymptomatic to symptomatic neurosyphilis is more likely to develop in patients whose CSF findings are moderately to severely abnormal (40).

Symptomatic neurosyphilis consists of meningeal syphilis, meningovascular syphilis, parenchymal syphilis, general paresis, tabes dorsalis, and gummatous syphilis. Meningeal involvement is commonly found in patients with early syphilis and in 25% to 40% of patients with untreated secondary syphilis. Although a significant number of infected individuals may develop meningeal syphilis only a small percentage, in one study 6% of infected patients, develop severe disease (41). Patients with meningeal neurosyphilis present with headache, confusion, nausea, vomiting, and a stiff neck. Typically, these patients do not have an elevated body temperature. CSF analysis reveals an abnormal cell count (more than 10 WBCs/mm^3), protein greater than 45 mg/dL, and a mild hypoglycorrhachia (glucose less than 30 mg/dL).

Meningovascular syphilis occurs following a localized arteritis with a subsequent thrombosis and infarction leading to the development of focal neurologic signs. The peak incidence of meningovascular syphilis occurs approximately 4 to 7 years after primary infection. There has not been a significant change in the occurrence of this disease from the preantibiotic to the antibiotic era (42,43). Onset of the disease may be abrupt, insidious, or episodic. The patient may develop headache, vertigo, insomnia, memory loss, and mood disturbances. Deficits are most frequent in the distribution of the middle cerebral artery (62%) and basilar artery (12%) (44). Involvement of the spinal arterial vessels results in hemiparesis or hemiplegia and aphasia, as well as seizures (44,45).

The characteristic changes that occur in meningovascular syphilis take place in the meningeal compartment, as reflected by CSF findings, and in the vascular compartment. The CSF findings are typically abnormal with a lymphocytosis (more than 10 WBCs/mm^3) and protein greater than 45 mg/dL. The histologic changes reflect a lymphocytosis and plasma cell infiltration of the vasa vasorum and adventitia of large and medium vessels referred to as Heubner's arteritis (45).

Since the introduction of penicillin, parenchymal neurosyphilis has become a relatively rare complication of syphilis. Tabes dorsalis and general paresis, although rarely seen, tend to occur especially in countries where antimicrobial therapy is not readily available. General paresis, or paretic neurosyphilis, was described in 1946 as a chronic condition brought about by a spirochetal meningoencephalitis affecting the function of the cerebral cortex (44). This results in impairment of both the mental and physical functions of the patient. Neurosyphilitic paresis, left untreated, becomes manifested in 10 to 20 years after primary syphilis, and has been referred to as general paralysis of the insane, general paresis, and dementia paralytica (42,45,46). The key to this stage of syphilis is that it may mimic every type of mental disorder. It is insidious in its onset with an early decrease in cognitive function with an inability to concentrate, the loss of higher integrative function, and an increase in irritability. The patient may also exhibit signs of mania, depression, and other psychosis. Progression of this stage of disease is characterized by increasing signs of dementia and development of seizures (47). Nontreponemal tests are positive in 95% to 100% of cases, and specific treponemal tests are positive in 100% of cases. CSF evaluation is always abnormal; lymphocytosis with 10 to 200 WBCs/mm^3 and protein 45 to 100 mg/dL. Nontreponemal tests are rarely nonreactive (48,49).

Tabes dorsalis, or locomotor ataxia, is rarely encountered in most countries today but accounted for 30% of syphilis patients in the pre-penicillin era (46). This stage of disease usually occurs 15 to 25 years after primary infection. The disease begins with the acute onset of sharp pains in the lower extremities, paresthesias, decreased deep tendon reflexes, progressive ataxia (characterized by a wide slapping walking associated with sensory loss that leads to Charcot joints), trophic ulcers referred to as mal perforans, and bowel and bladder incontinence. The patient develops abnormalities of the pupils as well as optic nerve atrophy. These pupil abnormalities are very common, occurring in 94% of patients with tabes dorsalis. Approximately 48% of patients develop a small irregular pupil that does not react to light but constricts normally to accommodation-convergence. Development of proprioceptive nerve fiber loss results in areflexia and hypotonia (44).

Patients with tabes dorsalis, unlike patients with an advanced stage of syphilis, do not typically have abnormal CSF findings. In a study reported in 1970, 60% of patients with tabes dorsalis had normal CSF findings (50).

Another characteristic of neurosyphilis is the development of a localized mass of granulation tissue referred to as gummas (51–54). A gumma is an area of necrosis surrounded by the intermingling of connective tissue and epithelioid cells as well as giant cells. The periphery of the gumma is characterized by a marked inflammatory response of lymphocytes, plasma cells, and giant cells; vascular infiltrate; and a noticeable absence of spirochetes. Gummas typically develop in the pia mater and may invade the brain or spinal cord.

The introduction of penicillin has caused a significant change in the clinical presentation of neurosyphilis. Interestingly, this change is thought to be the result not solely of the introduction of penicillin and treatment of syphilis but also because of the use of antimicrobial agents for the treatment of unrelated infections (43,55). Holtson (54), who studied the occurrence of neurosyphilis in the preantibiotic and postantibiotic era, studied the natural history and clinical manifestations of neurosyphilis. He found that in the postantibiotic era the clinical manifestations of neurosyphilis have become modified, more monosymptomatic, and often subtle. Several authors have also concluded that the use of oral antibiotics for treatment of various infections has modified neurosyphilis by partially treating an unknown neurosyphilis (42,55).

TREATMENT

Primary and early secondary syphilis are best treated with benzathine penicillin, 2.4 million units administered in two equally divided doses (1.2 million units) in each buttock. Nonpregnant infected women who are allergic to penicillin may be treated with doxycycline 100 mg orally twice daily for 15 days or tetracycline 500 mg orally four times a day for 15 days. Erythromycin should not be used because of the high failure rate (56). The concern over using an oral regimen is the patient's failure to be compliant in taking the full course of prescribed therapy. Patients who fail to complete their prescribed course of medication raise several concerns (Table 13-4).

These individuals serve as undetected sources of transmission because they often believe that they are cured of the infection even though they have not finished their medication. This is one of the reasons that it is extremely important that patients being treated for syphilis be monitored with regard to their treatment to determine its success or failure. Syphilis is a curable disease and, therefore, should not progress to advanced disease or result in congenital infection.

Patients diagnosed with late latent syphilis or infection of unknown duration should receive benzathine penicillin 2.4 million units administered intramuscularly in two equally divided doses weekly for 3 weeks to provide a total dose of 7.2 million units of penicillin. Patients who are allergic to penicillin and are not pregnant may be treated with oral doxycycline 100 mg twice daily for 30 days or tetracycline 500 mg four times a day for 30 days. An extended course of therapy is required in the latent stage of syphilis because the treponemes are much slower to replicate in the later stages of the disease. Therefore, it is necessary to maintain an adequate serum level of antibiotic over a prolonged period. This regimen may also be used for the patient with tertiary disease if there are no indications of neurosyphilis. Women known to have or suspected of having neurosyphilis can be treated with one of the regimens listed in Table 13-5.

Patients who are known to be contacts of individuals with syphilis should be treated with 1.2 million units of benzathine penicillin administered intramuscu-

---

TABLE 13-4. *Potential complications in failure of patient's compliance in taking medication for treatment of syphilis*

Remains infectious
Serves as a vector of transmission to sexual partners
If pregnant, can serve as a vector of transmission to fetus
Disease can advance

TABLE 13-5. *Antibiotic regimens for treatment of neurosyphilis*

Aqueous crystalline penicillin G 12 to 24 million units daily administered IV, in divided doses or by constant infusion for 14 days

Procaine penicillin G 2 to 4 million units administered intramuscularly daily in conjunction with probenecid 500 mg four times a day for 14 days

Amoxicillin 2 g orally three times a days plus probenecid 500 mg orally three times a day for 14 days

larly in each buttock for a total of 2.4 million units, administered one time. If the patient has already been treated for gonorrhea with ceftriaxone this should be adequate for the treatment of incubating syphilis.

All patients treated for syphilis should be monitored for response to the treatment by performing a VDRL or RPR test at 3, 6, and 12 months after therapy has been completed. Individuals who have been successfully treated can be detected by noting a fourfold or greater decrease in their titer. Patients who fail to demonstrate a significant change in VDRL or RPR titer may be considered either treatment failures or reinfected. These individuals should be treated with 7.2 million units of penicillin as described for late latent syphilis. Approximately 2% of the course of therapy with penicillin or other beta-lactam antibiotics will result in an allergic reaction. There have been several hundred deaths associated with allergic reactions in the treatment of syphilis because individuals develop anaphylaxis (57–59).

PREGNANCY AND SYPHILIS

Congenital syphilis has increased dramatically since 1986 when there were approximately 50 cases of congenital syphilis per 100,000 cases of primary and secondary syphilis in women. In 1988, there were 350 reported cases of congenital syphilis per 100,000 cases of primary and secondary syphilis in women in New York City. In the United States, the number of cases of congenital syphilis rose from 1985 to 1991, and then there was a steady decline (Fig. 13-10).

Mothers giving birth to infants with congenital syphilis were more likely to use drugs, particularly cocaine/crack, and their infants tended to be of low birthweight, preterm, and not infected. Syphilitic mothers were less likely to obtain prenatal care (Table 13-3) (56).

Prevention of congenital syphilis requires a program designed to prevent infection of the mother, assist with early recognition of the disease, institute of penicillin therapy, desensitize penicillin-allergic pregnant women, and provide a follow-up program. A program of prevention is dependent on meticulous surveillance and not assumptions that a particular patient or population is less likely to acquire the disease. Primary prevention begins by obtaining a detailed history and educating the patient of the necessity to obtain accurate information with regard to her sexual behavioral practices; the behavior of her sexual partner, documentation of past treatment for STDs; the latest episode of a STD; the use of

Rate (per 100,000 live births)

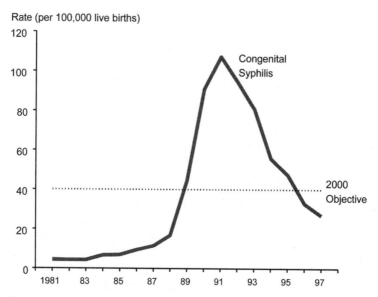

FIG. 13-10. Congenital syphilis rates for infants less than 1 year of age in the United States from 1981 through 1997 and the Healthy People year 2000 objective. The surveillance case definition for congenital syphilis changed in 1988.

drugs regardless of which ones used; and a recent screen for gonorrhea, chlamydia, syphilis (VDRL), hepatitis B, and HIV. Individuals who have a documented STD during pregnancy should be screened for syphilis in each trimester. A VDRL should be performed on all pregnant women admitted to labor and delivery, and the infant should be tested shortly after birth. If at all possible, the screening performed during the prenatal period should be accomplished at the time of the first prenatal visit. If the patient has behavior that places her at risk, a repeat VDRL should be done in each trimester. Ideally, the results should be known before the patient leaving the office, and, if positive, treatment should be administered. However, because this does not occur, the patient should be asked to return as soon as the results are known, so that appropriate treatment may be instituted. The treatment should not be delayed until the patient's next visit because this delay may result in infection of the fetus.

Because alternative treatments to penicillin have not been documented to be efficacious in preventing congenital syphilis, penicillin remains the antibiotic of choice. Pregnant patients allergic to penicillin should not be treated with an alternative antibiotic but should undergo desensitization to penicillin. Penicillin sensitivity has proven to be an effective method in determining which individuals are truly allergic to penicillin. Skin testing with penicilloyl determinant coupled to polylysine, as well as other penicillin derived determinants, is a quick and inexpensive method for determining if the patient is allergic to penicillin. Patients who relate a suspected history of penicillin allergy and have a negative skin test have not manifested an anaphylactic reaction, whereas 67% of patients with a positive skin test developed allergic reactions when administered penicillin. Approximately 1% of individuals with a history of penicillin allergy and a negative skin test developed cutaneous reactions (60–64). Penicillin testing is important because serious allergic reactions such as laryngeal edema, significant hypotension, bronchospasm, and cardiac irregularities occur in 2% to 13% of penicillin-allergic patients. Approximately 9% of anaphylactic reactions result in death (65,66). Thus, desensitization can be useful in treating significant infections in patients who are allergic to penicillin. This technique has been useful in the treatment of syphilis, listeriosis, and *Streptococcus viridans* endocarditis in pregnant and nonpregnant patients (67,68).

PENICILLIN ALLERGY SKIN TESTING AND DESENSITIZATION

The antigens to be tested are penicilloyl polylysine, benzylpenicillin G, and benzylpenicillin acid (69–72). A prick test is performed with the antigens, histamine, and saline on the volar aspect of the forearm. The antigens are prepared in the following concentrations, 10 mol/L and 10^{-2}mol/L. The patient is first tested with the diluted concentration of antigen and if negative is then tested with the more concentrated antigen. Amounts are then used to produce a wheal, 5 mm × 5 mm, which is considered to be the loading dose. The production of a wheal, by the prick test, that measures 7 mm × 7 mm is considered positive. If an intradermal test is used and a wheal measuring 2 mm × 2 mm is produced within 15 minutes, this should be considered positive. A positive test should preclude further testing (72–74).

Desensitization can be accomplished by administering penicillin elixir (Table 13-6). The first dose is 100 units and is doubled every 15 minutes until

TABLE 13-6. *Oral desensitization protocol for patients allergic to penicillin[a]*

Penicillin V suspension dose	Units/mL	mL	Cumulative Units	dose (units)	Dosing interval (min)
1	1,000	0.1	100	100	15
2	1,000	0.2	200	300	15
3	1,000	0.4	400	700	15
4	1,000	0.8	800	1,500	15
5	1,000	1.6	1,600	3,100	15
6	1,000	3.2	3,200	6,300	15
7	1,000	6.4	6,400	12,700	15
8	10,000	1.2	12,000	24,700	15
9	10,000	2.4	24,000	48,700	15
10	10,000	4.8	48,000	96,700	15
11	80,000	1.0	80,000	176,000	15
12	80,000	2.0	160,000	336,000	15
13	80,000	4.0	320,000	656,000	15
14	80,000	8.0	640,000	1,296,700	15

[a]Adapted from Wendel GD Jr, Stark BJ, Jamison RB, et al. Penicillin allergy and desensitization in serious infections during pregnancy. *N Engl J Med* 1985;312:1229–1232, with permission.

1,396,700 units of penicillin have been administered. An intravenous line should be established before commencing the desensitization and maintained for 24 hours after the last dose of penicillin is administered. The patient's vital signs and clinical response should be closely monitored. A physician, as well as resuscitation equipment and personnel, must be readily available. If mild cutaneous reactions occur, they should be left to resolve on their own, or diphenhydramine 25 mg can be administered intravenously. If a serious reaction occurs, the procedure should be discontinued, or the last dose that did not cause a reaction should be readministered (75).

Intravenous desensitization can be accomplished by making a penicillin G solution at a concentration of 0.01 units/mL. The first dose is administered in a concentration of 5 units of penicillin over a 30-minute infusion. If no reaction occurs, the dose is increased 10 to 50 units until 100,000 units/mL is reached.

The most serious reaction that can occur in penicillin-allergic patients is anaphylaxis, which usually occurs within a few minutes of administering penicillin intramuscularly or intravenously. Anaphylaxis is unlikely to occur following oral intake of penicillin. Fatalities are estimated to occur in one to two cases following 100,000 injections. The more immediate the onset of anaphylaxis, the more severe the episode. Initially the patient becomes unconscious and develops severe hypotension, pulses cannot be detected, and the patient develops apnea. Patients who develop a reaction over a long period develop anxiety and a feeling of impending death. These individuals develop edema of the face, bronchospasm, urticaria, and arthralgias and may become febrile. The most common allergic response is a delayed reaction. This usually occurs several days after the penicillin has been administered, either by injection or orally, and is heralded by urticaria. It may be accompanied by arthralgias, joint effusions, facial edema, and fever.

Patients receiving procaine penicillin may experience an allergic reaction to the procaine. There are two types of reactions: anxiety and hyperventilation. The patient who develops an anxiety reaction usually feels as though she is going to die. Along with these feelings are hallucinations, disorientation, and depersonalization. These patients often become aggressive and there is concern for their own safety; therefore, they may require restraints. The patients who develop hyperventilation often experience hypertension, tachycardia, and vomiting. This reaction is more commonly seen when procaine penicillin has been mistakenly administered intravenously, which is associated with microembolization of the lungs and brain. Patients who experience a procaine reaction should be treated with supportive care and close monitoring of vital signs.

PREVENTION AND MANAGEMENT OF ADVERSE REACTIONS TO PENICILLIN

Patients who give a history or suspect a positive history of being allergic to penicillin should not be given this antibiotic until they have been tested for sensitivity to penicillin. Patients treated with intramuscular penicillin should remain for a period of observation of not less than 15 minutes. An emergency resuscitation cart should be readily available. The following should also be available:

1. Adrenaline solution 1:1000
2. Injectable antihistamine 10 to 20 mg
3. Injectable hydrocortisone 100-mg ampoules
4. Aminophylline 25 mg/mL
5. An airway
6. Ambu bag
7. Oxygen

Patients who develop anaphylaxis should be treated without delay. The patient should be placed in Trendelenburg position. An airway should be established immediately, and adrenaline 1:1000 solution should be administered in 0.5 to 1 mL (500 to 1,000 μg) doses intramuscularly. The adrenaline can be repeated in 10 minutes if the initial response has been unsatisfactory. An antihistamine (10 to 20 mg) should be administered intravenously. Hydrocortisone 100 mg can be administered intramuscularly or intravenously. If there is evidence of bronchospasm, aminophylline should be administered in a dosage of 250 mg in 10 mL of saline and infused intravenously over 20 minutes. Patients not responding successfully should be observed in the hospital for at least 24 hours because they may experience a recurrence.

Jarisch-Herxheimer Reaction

Pregnant women treated with penicillin should be monitored for the development of the Jarisch-Herxheimer reaction. This is an acute reaction characterized by fever, malaise, chills, vasodilation noted by flushing, tachycardia, hyperventilation, and hypertension. If present, skin and mucosal lesions are intensified. The reaction typically occurs within 12 hours of the administration of penicillin. Pregnant patients who have experienced this reaction have also been found to have an intrauterine demise. Therefore, it is imperative that the patients be monitored for a minimum of 12 hours following the administration of penicillin. The patient's vital signs and fetal heart rate should be monitored using continuous electronic fetal monitoring.

The mechanism of the Jarisch-Herxheimer reaction is not completely understood. It is thought that there is an intense antibody response following the massive killing of treponemes, which results in a release of treponemal antigens. It is also thought that this leads to an allergic reaction. The reaction occurs in 50% of the treated cases of primary syphilis, 90% of secondary cases, 25% of early latent cases, and rarely in late syphilis (68,76,77). When the reaction occurs in early syphilis, it is usually mild and often misinterpreted as a reaction to penicillin because typical presentation is a rash. Patients with neurosyphilis may experience serious reactions such as general paresis, violent psychosis, and seizures. Patients with cardiovascular syphilis may experience sudden death.

MANAGEMENT OF THE TREATED PATIENT

Every patient treated for syphilis, regardless of the antibiotic chosen, must be monitored to determine the effectiveness of treatment. It is also necessary to monitor the patient who acquires syphilis, or any STD, because it is an indication of the behavior of the patient that places her at risk for reinfection. This is also important because the patient may not be placing herself directly at risk; she may be at risk because of her partner's sexual behavior.

The patient should undergo repeat serologic testing, VDRL or RPR, at 1, 3, 6, and 12 months following treatment. Typically, a patient who becomes infected will be serologically positive, VDRL or RPR and FTA-ABS, within 4 to 6 weeks after being infected. Patients successfully treated for primary and early secondary syphilis will usually become seronegative (VDRL or RPR) within 1 year. Patients with late secondary syphilis will demonstrate a decrease in titer, usually at least a four-fold decrease in dilution (e.g., from 1:128 to 1:16) but may or may not eventually become negative. Once a decrease in serologic titer has been demonstrated, these patients, unless reinfected, must be followed by annual testing until the titer becomes fixed (e.g., 1:4) or negative. Individuals who demonstrate a four-fold increase in titer, even though they may be completely asymptomatic, should be considered either reinfected or treatment failures and should receive a full course of treatment (a total of 7.2 million units of penicillin intramuscularly). In addition, their partners must be contacted and treated. The specific treponemal, FTA-ABS or MHA-TP, will remain positive and, therefore, should not be used to determine whether or not the treatment was successful.

Patients treated for neurosyphilis must be monitored for life. The patient should have an initial evaluation of the CSF; CSF evaluation should be repeated 4 weeks after the completion of therapy. Patients who demonstrate a positive response to therapy should have the test repeated in 3 and 6 months. The patient who continues to improve should have a repeat examination of the CSF in 1 year.

Patients suspected of having neurosyphilis should have a spinal tap and examination of CSF. The CSF of a patient with neurosyphilis should demonstrate a cell count greater than 5×10^6 cells/L, total protein greater than 40 mg/dL, and, in some cases, a positive FTA-ABS (78). Associated conditions, such as nonsyphilitic meningitis caused by the meningococcus, tuberculosis, HIV, or benign lymphocytic meningitis, or successfully treated syphilis can also interfere with the analysis of CSF, including the FTA-ABS test. Patients with syphilis who suffer a subarachnoid hemorrhage or have cerebral cancer can also have a false-positive FTA-ABS of the CSF. This is because of the transudation of specific antibodies developed to *T. pallidum,* secondary to breaks in the blood-brain barrier.

CONGENITAL SYPHILIS

For many years, it was believed that *T. pallidum* could not penetrate the placenta before 18 weeks' gestation. Dippel (79), in 1944, reported that treponemes could not be detected in fetuses of less than 18 weeks. Silverstein (80) hypothesized that fetal immunoincompetence may explain the lack of apparent clinical involvement and the high success of treatment noted before 18 weeks. Clinically, it is important for the physician to detect syphilis as early as possible to prevent progression of the disease in the maternal compartment, congenital infection, and transmission to sexual contacts. Remember, congenital infection should not occur in any patient who is receiving prenatal care throughout the pregnancy (81).

The number of cases of primary and secondary syphilis have risen significantly since 1986 (7 to 8 per 100,000 population). In 1987 there were approximately 10 per 100,000 cases rising to a peak in 1990 of approximately 16 per 100,000 with a declining incidence in 1996 of less than 5 per 100,000 (Fig. 13-11). Coincident with this increase in disease in the general population has been a noticeable rise in the number of cases of congenital syphilis (82) (Fig. 13-10). The increase in the number of cases of congenital syphilis occurs predominantly in association with crack cocaine use and HIV disease (Table 13-7).

The degree of severity of fetal infection is dependent on the inoculum received and the gestational age when maternal infection occurs. The significant fact is that when there is a large inoculum the maternal treponema is likely to occur and, as a result, the fetus is at significant risk of becoming infected. In conjunction with the maternal treponema, it is unlikely that there will be sufficient time for the mother to manifest an antibody response. Therefore, there will not be enough time for maternal IgG to cross the placenta and offer the fetus any protection. The fetus may be overwhelmed and die in utero, as commonly occurs

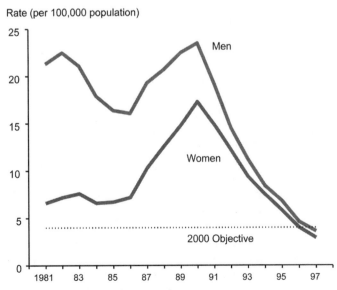

FIG. 13-11. Primary and secondary syphilis rates by gender in the United States from 1981 through 1997 and the Healthy People year 2000 objective.

TABLE 13-7. *Maternal risk factors for acquiring syphilis*

Multiple sex partners
Prostitution
Unmarried and sexual active
Lower socioeconomic class
Use of illicit drugs
Individual <25 years of age, unmarried, and sexually active
No or incomplete prenatal care
Poorly educated

when the fetus is less than 20 weeks gestation. Thus, pregnancy outcome is related to the gestational age at which infection occurs, and infection can result in abortion, preterm labor, preterm birth, low birthweight, nonimmune hydrops, stillbirth, congenital infection, or neonatal death. Therefore, most infants born with congenital infection acquired the disease from their mother who either had primary or secondary syphilis, which correlates to a stage in the disease at which there is a high number of spirochetes present and there is likely to be a treponema (83).

The patient's history is very important in determining the possible time of infection or exposure, especially in those individuals who experience spontaneous abortion. It is highly likely that an infected woman would go unnoticed. Individuals who have undetected syphilis and become pregnant are likely to experience an intrauterine fetal demise close to term. If these individuals are not screened and achieve a subsequent pregnancy, the infant will bear the stigma of congenital syphilis. The explanation for this is the patient will have a decrease in the number of treponemes but maintain a significant number of organisms to cause congenital infection. If the patient gives birth to a female infant, this individual, should she become pregnant when reproductively mature, will not in all likelihood give birth to an affected child. After a 4-year period following the initial disease, it is unlikely that the patient will continue to have circulating treponemes.

The evaluation of the pregnant patient should begin with an RPR or VDRL at the initial visit. If the patient has any risk factors, repeat screening should occur in each trimester. If the screening test is positive, then FTA-ABS should be performed. If the confirmatory test is positive, the patient should be notified and asked to come to the office within 24 hours for treatment. If the patient is in the first trimester, embryonic or fetal viability should be documented. Regardless of the status of the pregnancy, treatment should be instituted. If the patient is in the second or third trimester, an ultrasound should be performed to establish the well-being of the fetus and to rule out hydrops (Table 13-8).

Typical ultrasonographic findings of a fetus with hydrops are skin thickening of greater than 5 mm, placenta greater than 4 mm in thickness, ascites, pericardial effusions, and polyhydramnios (84,85). Oligohydramnios may also occur in association with fetal hydrops and carries a grave prognosis. The mortality rate associated with fetal nonhydrops ranges from 50% to 98% (85–87). Grave prog-

TABLE 13-8. *Infectious causes of fetal hydrops*

Syphilis
Chaga's disease
Leptospirosis
Cytomegalovirus
Herpes simplex
Parvovirus B19
Rubella
Congenital hepatitis

nostic findings associated with nonimmune hydrops are a generalized lymphangiectasis and fetal structural abnormalities.

SUMMARY

Although syphilis is a curable disease and it may be preventable, it is unlikely that it will be totally prevented. This is mainly because individuals will continue to practice behavior that exposes them to infected sexual partners. Syphilis is an extremely interesting disease because of its multiple presentations. Therefore, it is not often thought of when a patient is evaluated for a medical illness. Because of the silent nature of primary infection in women, the disease usually progresses to secondary infection before the clinical manifestations may be noticed by the patient. However, because the clinical manifestation can resolve spontaneously, the patient is likely to believe that the disease has vanished. Thus, the physician should determine the degree of risk for each individual patient. This does not require a great deal of time because the patients will automatically fall into groups—the group at significant risk are those who are unmarried and sexually active. This is not to say that the married patient may not be at risk, but if the marriage is stable, the risk should be essentially nonexistent.

Congenital syphilis should not occur in patients receiving prenatal care. Pregnant women found to have a STD should be screened for STDs, including syphilis, in each trimester. Women who do not seek prenatal care or who fail to complete all of their prenatal visits should also be considered at risk.

Individuals who are treated should not be considered as cured unless they have been followed in a systematic fashion. This is necessary to determine if the treatment was successful and had eradicated the disease, if treatment failed, or if reinfection occurred. The most efficient mechanism to follow treated patients is to monitor the RPR or VDRL titer and to look for a significant decrease in titer (1 : 4 dilution or higher). Pregnant patients diagnosed with syphilis who are allergic to penicillin must undergo desensitization and then treatment with penicillin.

REFERENCES

1. Berg HC. How spirochetes may swim. *J Theor Biol* 1976;56:269–273.
2. Brandt AM. Dr. Erlich's magic bullet. In: *No magic bullet: a social history of venereal disease in the United States since 1880.* New York: Oxford University Press, 1987:171.

3. Brandt AM. Shadow of the land. In: *No magic bullet: a social history of venereal disease in the United States since 1880.* New York: Oxford University Press, 1987:129.
4. Anonymous. Continuing increase in infectious syphilis—United States. *MMWR* 1988;37:35–38.
5. Anonymous. Relationship of syphilis to drug use and prostitution—Connecticut and Philadelphia, Pennsylvania. *MMWR* 1988;37:755–758.
6. Rockwell DH, Yobs AR, Moore MB. The Tuskegee study of untreated syphilis. *Arch Intern Med* 1964; 114:792.
7. Clark EG, Danbolt N. The Oslo study of the natural course of untreated syphilis: an epidemiologic investigation based on re-study of the Boeck-Bruusgaard material. *Med Clin North Am* 1964;48:613.
8. Schroeter AL, Turner RH, Lucas JB, et al. Therapy for incubating syphilis. Effectiveness of gonorrhea treatment. *JAMA* 1971;218:711–713.
9. Mangnuson HJ, Thomas EW, Olansky S. Inoculation of syphilis in human volunteers. *Medicine* 1956; 35:33.
10. Mindel A, Tovey SJ, Timmins DJ, et al. Primary and secondary syphilis, 20 years experience. 2. Clinical features. *Genitourin Med* 1989;65:1–3.
11. Chapel TA, Brown WJ, Jefferies C, et al. How reliable is the morphological diagnosis of penile ulcerations. *Sex Transm Dis* 1977;4:150–152.
12. Chapel TA, Brown WJ, Jefferies C, et al. The microflora of penile ulcerations. *Infect Dis* 1978;137: 50.
13. Kellogg DS Jr, Mothershed SM. Immunofluorescent detection of *Treponema pallidum. JAMA* 1969;207:938–941.
14. Hook EW III, Roddy RE, Lukehart SA, et al. Detection of *Treponema pallidum* in lesion exudate with a pathogen-specific monoclonal antibody. *J Clin Microbiol* 1985;22:241–244.
15. Kukehart SA. Syphilis. In: Wentworth BB, ed. *Diagnostic procedures for bacterial infections.* Washington, DC: American Public Health Association, 1987:519.
16. Cohen P, Stout G, Ende N. Serologic reactivity in consecutive patients admitted to a general hospital. A comparison of the FTA-ABS, URDL, and automated reagin tests. *Arch Intern Med* 1969;124: 364–367.
17. Jaffe HW, Larsen SA, Jones OG, et al. Hemagglutination tests for syphilis antibody. *Am J Clin Pathol* 1978;70:230–233.
18. Wentworth BB, Thompson MA, Peter CR, et al. Comparison of a hemagglutination treponemal test for syphilis (HATTS) with other serologic methods for the diagnosis of syphilis. *Sex Transm Dis* 1978;5:103–114.
19. Hooshmand H, Escobar MR, Kopf SW. Neurosyphilis. A study of 241 patients. *JAMA* 1972;219: 726–729.
20. McLeish WM, Pulido JS, Holland S, et al. The ocular manifestations of syphilis in the human immunodeficiency virus type 1-infected host. *Ophthalmology* 1990;97:196–203.
21. Simon RP. Neurosyphilis. *Arch Neurol* 1985;42:606–613.
22. Chesney AM, Kemp JE. Incidence of spirochaeta pallida in cerebrospinal fluid during early stage of syphilis. *JAMA* 1924;83:1725.
23. Lukehart SA, Hook EW III, Baker-Zander SA, et al. Invasion of the central nervous system by *Treponema pallidum*: implications for the diagnosis and therapy. *Ann Inter Med* 1988;109:855–862.
24. Merit HH, Adams RD, Solomon HC. *Neurosyphilis.* New York: Oxford, 1946.
25. Wile UJ, Stokes JH. Prognosis of general paresis after treatment. *Lancet* 1968;2:1370.
26. Moore JE, Hopkins HH. Asymptomatic neurosyphilis VI. The prognosis of early and late asymptomatic neurosyphilis. *JAMA* 1930;95:1637.
27. Byrne TN, Bose A, Sze G, et al. Syphilitic meningitis causing paraparesis in an HIV-negative woman. *J Neurol Sci* 1991;103:48–50.
28. Hooshmand H, Escobar MR, Kopf SW. Neurosyphilis: a study of 241 patients. *JAMA* 1972;219:726.
29. Kolar OJ, Burkhart JE. Neurosyphilis. *Br J Vener Dis* 1977;53:221–225.
30. Smikle MF, James OB, Prabhakar P. Diagnosis of neurosyphilis: a critical assessment of current methods. *South Med J* 1988;81:452–454.
31. Hahn RD. Some remarks on the management of neurosyphilis. *J Chron Dis* 1961;13:1.
32. Hahn RD, Clark EG, Felsovany A, et al. Asymptomatic neurosyphilis: prognosis. *Am J Syph Gonorrhea Vener Dis* 1946;30:513.
33. Hahn RD, Culter JC, Curtis AC, et al. Penicillin treatment of asymptomatic central nervous system syphilis I. Probability of progression to symptomatic neurosyphilis. *Arch Dermatol* 1956;74:355.
34. Moore JE, Kemp JE. The treatment of early syphilis II. Clinical results in 402 patients. *Bull Johns Hopkins Hosp* 1926;39:16.

35. Adams RD, Victor M. *Principles of neurology.* New York: McGraw-Hill, 1981.
36. Dattner B, Thomas EW, Demello L. Criteria for management of neurosyphilis. *Am J Med* 1951;10: 463.
37. Izzat NN, Bartruff JK, Clicksman JM, et al. Validity of the VDRL test on cerebrospinal fluid contaminated by blood. *Br J Vener Dis* 1971;47:162–164.
38. Meritt HH, Moore M. Acute syphilitic meningitis. *Medicine (Baltimore)* 1935;14:119.
39. Simon RP. Neurosyphilis. *Arch Neurol* 1985;42:606.
40. Musher DM. Evaluation and management of an asymptomatic patient with a positive VDRL reaction. In: Remington JS, Schwartz MN, eds. *Current clinical topics in infectious disease.* New York: McGraw-Hill, 1988.
41. Jordan KG. Modern neurosyphilis—a critical analysis. *West J Med* 1988;149:47–57.
42. Hahn RD, Clark EG. Asymptomatic neurosyphilis: a review of the literature. *Am J Syph Gonorrhea Vener Dis* 1946;30:305.
43. Dans PE, Cafferty L, Otter SE, et al. Inappropriate use of the cerebrospinal fluid Venereal Disease Research Laboratory (VDRL) test to exclude neurosyphilis. *Ann Intern Med* 1986;104:86–89.
44. Hahn RD, Webster B, Weikhardt G, et al. Penicillin treatment of general paresis (dementia paralytica). *Arch Neurol Psych* 1959;81:557.
45. Johns DR, Tiernay M, Parker SW. Pure motor hemiplegia due to meningovascular neurosyphilis. *Arch Neurol* 1987;44:1062–1065.
46. Swartz M. Neurosyphilis. In: Holmes KK, Mardh PA, Sparling PF, et al., eds. *Sexually transmitted diseases,* 2nd ed. New York: McGraw-Hill, 1990:231.
47. Burke AW. Syphilis in a Jamaican psychiatric hospital. A review of 52 cases including 17 of neurosyphilis. *Br J Vener Dis* 1972;48:249–253.
48. Ch'ien L, Hathaway BM, Isreal CW. Seronegative dementia paralytica: report of a case. *J Neurol Neurosurg Psych* 1970;33:376–380.
49. Towpik J, Nowakowska E. Changing patterns of late syphilis. *Br J Vener Dis* 1970;46:132–134.
50. Aho K, Sievers K, Salo OP. Late complications of syphilis. A comparative epidemiological and serological study of cardiovascular syphilis and various forms of neurosyphilis. *Acta Derm Venerol (Stockh)* 1969;49:336–342.
51. Kaplan JG, Sterman AB, Horoupian D, et al. Luetic meningitis with gumma: clinical, radiographic and neuropathologic features. *Neurology* 981;31:464–467.
52. Fleet WS, Watson RT, Ballinger WE. Resolution of gumma with steroid therapy. *Neurology* 1986;36:1104–1107.
53. Kulla L, Russell JA, Smith TW, et al. Neurosyphilis presenting as a focal mass lesion: a case report. *Neurosurgery* 1984;14:234–237.
54. Holtson JR. Modern neurosyphilis: a partially treated chronic meningitis. *West J Med* 1981;135:191.
55. Willcox RR. Treatment of neurosyphilis. *Bull WHO* 1981;59:655.
56. Anonymous. Congenital syphilis—United States, 1983–1985. *MMWR* 1986;35:625–628.
57. Schroeter AL, Lucas JB, Price EV, et al. Treatment of early syphilis and reactivity of serologic tests. *JAMA* 1972;221:471–476.
58. Sogn DD. Penicillin allergy. *J Allergy Clin Immunol* 1989;74:589.
59. Parker CW. Drug allergy. In: Parker CW, ed. *Clinical immunology.* Philadelphia: WB Saunders, 1980:1219.
60. Shapiro J. Hypersensitivity to penicillin acid derivatives in humans with penicillin allergy. In: *Proceedings of the world forum on syphilis and other treponematoses.* DHEW Publication No. 997, 328. Washington, DC: Department of Health, Education, and Welfare, 1964.
61. Green GR, Rosenblum AH, Sweet LC. Evaluation of penicillin hypersensitivity: value of clinical history and skin testing with penicilloyl-polylysine and penicillin G. *J Allergy Clin Immunol* 1977;60: 339–345.
62. Sullivan TJ, Wedner HJ, Shatz GS, et al. Skin testing to detect penicillin allergy. *J Allergy Clin Immunol* 1981;68:171–180.
63. Levine BB, Zolov DM. Prediction of penicillin allergy by immunological tests. *J Allergy* 1969;43: 231–244.
64. Idsoe O, Guthe T, Wilcox RR, et al. Nature and extent of penicillin side-reactions with particular reference to fatalities from anaphylactic shock. *Bull WHO* 1968;38:159–188.
65. Stark BJ, Earl HS, Gross GN, et al. Acute and chronic desensitization of penicillin-allergic patients using oral penicillin. *J Allergy Clin Immunol* 1987;79:523–532.
66. Wendel GD Jr, Stark BJ, Jamison RB, et al. Penicillin allergy and desensitization in serious infections during pregnancy. *N Engl J Med* 1985;312:1229–1232.

67. Ziaya PR, Hankins GD, Gilstrap LC III, et al. Intravenous penicillin desensitization and treatment during pregnancy. *JAMA* 1986;256:2561–2562.
68. Young EJ, Weingerten NM, Baughn RE, et al. Studies on the pathogenesis of the Jarisch-Herxheimer reaction: development of an animal model + evidence against a role for classical endotoxin. *J Infect Dis* 1982;146:606.
69. Parker JW, Shapiro J, Kern M, et al. Hypersensitivity to penicillin acid derivatives in human beings with penicillin allergy. *J Exp Med* 1962;115:821.
70. Rytel MW, Klion FM, Arlender TR, et al. Detection of penicillin hypersensitivity with penicilloyl-polylysine. *JAMA* 1963;186:894.
71. Mendelson LM, Ressler C, Rosen JP, et al. Routine elective penicillin allergy skin testing in children and adolescents: study of sensitization. *J Allergy Clin Immunol* 1984;73:76–81.
72. Brown BC, Price EV, Moore MB. Penicilloyl-polylysine as an intradermal test of penicillin sensitivity. *JAMA* 1964;189:599.
73. Lentz JW, Nicholas L. Penicilloyl-polylysine intradermal testing for penicillin hypersensitivity. *Br J Venereal Dis* 1970;46:457–460.
74. Budd MA, Parker CW, Worden CW. Evaluation of intradermal skin tests in penicillin hypersensitivity. *JAMA* 1964;190:115.
75. Gadde J, Spence M, Wheeler B, et al. Clinical experience with penicillin skin testing in a large inner-city STD clinic. *JAMA* 1993;270:2456–2463.
76. Shenep JL, Feldman S, Thornton D. Evaluation of endotoxemia in patients receiving penicillin therapy for secondary syphilis. *JAMA* 1986;256:388–390.
77. Sexually Transmitted Disease Surveillance, 1991. U.S. Department of Health and Human Services, Centers for Disease Control, Atlanta, GA.
78. Jaffe HW, Kabins SA. Examination of cerebrospinal fluid in patients with syphilis. *Rev Inf Dis* 1982;4 (Suppl):S842.
79. Dippel AL. The relationship of congenital syphilis to abortion and miscarriage and the mechanism of intrauterine protection. *Am J Obstet Gynecol* 1944;47:369.
80. Silverstein AM. Congenital syphilis and the timing of immunogenesis in the human fetus. *Nature* 1962;294:196.
81. Harter H, Benirschke K. Fetal syphilis in the first trimester. *Am J Obstet Gynecol* 1976;124:705–711.
82. Anonymous. Primary and secondary syphilis—United States, 1981–1990. *MMWR* 1991;40:314–315, 321–323.
83. Centers for Disease Control. Congenital syphilis—New York, 1986–1988. *MMWR* 1989;38:825.
84. Fiumara NJ. Treating syphilis with tetracycline. *Am Fam Physician* 1982;26:131–133.
85. Chinn DH. Ultrasound evaluation of hydrops fetalis. In: Callen PW, ed. *Ultrasonography in obstetrics and gynecology.* Philadelphia: WB Saunders, 1988:277.
86. Mahony BS, Filly RA, Callen PW, et al. Severe nonimmune hydrops fetalis: sonographic evaluation. *Radiology* 1984;151:757–761.
87. Fleischer AC, Killam AP, Boehm FH, et al. Hydrops fetalis: sonographic evaluation and clinical implications. *Radiology* 1981;141:163–168.

14

Hepatitis

Viral hepatitis continues to be a significant problem around the world, and in addition to the human immunodeficiency virus type-1 (HIV-1), viral hepatitis is a major public health concern. There are five hepatotropic viruses, A, B, C, D, and E. Hepatitis B (HBV) and hepatitis C (HCV) are the viral infections, in this class, of most concern. The acute illness caused by these viral agents is similar but differs from one another in virology, epidemiology, and chronic sequelae. Several other viruses have been demonstrated to cause hepatitis, but these viral agents are not hepatotropic (Table 14-1).

The five hepatotropic viruses do not belong to the same family and are not of similar size (Table 14-2). However, they are relatively small viruses, ranging in size from 27 nm to 45 nm.

Although hepatitis A (HAV) has not been shown to be sexually transmitted, as HBV and HCC have, a discussion of HAV is included for completeness.

HEPATITIS A

HAV is a common infection in the United States and the seroprevalence rate is estimated to be 40%. In developing and undeveloped counties, the seroprevalence rate approaches 100% (1). The mode of transmission is the fecal to oral route—contamination of food and water. HAV is diagnosed by a blood test that is positive for IgM HAV. IgM antibodies to HAV can be detected up to 12 months following infection. Declining IgM levels are usually coincident with rising IgG antibodies to HAV. Once an individual develops IgG antibodies to HAV, he or she can remain positive for life. In developing countries, however, individuals acquiring infection in early childhood may not have detectable antibodies when they achieve adulthood. This suggests that to maintain immunity an individual may have to experience repeated exposure to the virus (2). False-positive IgM antibodies to HAV have been found in individuals with a positive rheumatoid factor.

HAV most commonly occurs in children and young adults. The incubation period, following acquisition of the virus, is 15 to 45 days, with an average of 25 days. The virus is taken in orally and gains entrance to the liver. The virus repro-

TABLE 14-1. *Nonhepatotropic viral agents known to cause hepatitis*

Rubella
Cytomegalovirus
Herpes simplex
Epstein-Barr
Coxsackie A and B
Yellow fever virus
Measles virus
Adenovirus
Echovirus

duces in hepatocytes, gains entrance to the bloodstream inducing a viremia, and simultaneously enters the biliary system (3,4). By entering the biliary system, the virus is able to reach the feces for dissemination. The infected patient sheds virus and experiences a viremia before developing an elevation in liver enzymes. Infectivity ceases coincident with the development of humoral antibodies (5,6).

Following infection with a significant viral inoculum and an incubation period of 15 to 45 days, the patient experiences clinical symptoms consistent with hepatitis. The typical signs and symptoms of viral hepatitis are general malaise, nausea, fever, loss of appetite, development of jaundice, and markedly elevated liver enzymes. Children and infants do not usually develop symptomatic infection, whereas adults frequently manifest symptoms and signs of acute hepatitis. There is a rise in IgM, IgA, and, subsequently, IgG levels coincident with the onset of clinical disease. The rise in IgM and IgA levels precedes the IgG rise, and IgM and IgA levels remain elevated for approximately 1 month before declining. They can, however, be detected for up to 12 months. IgG antibodies begins to reach detectable levels shortly after the appearance of IgM and IgA antibodies.

Treatment of HAV has, until recently, been the administration of human immune serum globulin obtained from individuals infected with the virus. Human immune serum contains significant amounts of antibodies to HAV (7). HAV has been the most common type of hepatitis in the United States with approximately 25,000 reported cases per year (23 per 100,000 population) (8). The incidence of HAV worldwide is estimated to be 1,400,000 cases annually (9). The cost to treat HAV in the United States is estimated at $200 million (10).

TABLE 14-2. *Hepatitis viral families*

Virus	Family	Genome	Envelope
A	Picornaviridae	ssRNA	Not Present
B	Hepadnaviridae	dsDNA	Present
C	Flaviviridae	ssRNA	Present
D	Viroid (satellite virus)	ssRNA	Not Present
E	Caliciviridae	ssRNA	Not Present

ss, single stranded; ds, double stranded.

Therefore, the best approach is to prevent infection, which is accomplished by the vaccination of susceptible individuals. An inactivated HAV vaccine has been developed and is licensed in the United States. The vaccine contains HAV strain HM175, grown MRC-5 cells (human diploid cells), and was purified via sterile filtration, ultrafiltration, and column chromatography (11). Inactivation of the virus is accomplished by incubating in 250 µg/mL formaldehyde at 37°C for 15 days (12). The vaccine was tested in 104 clinical studies completed by 1993. These studies were conducted in 27 countries, involved 50,677 individuals, and administered more than 120,000 doses of vaccine (13). The vaccine was found to be safe, well tolerated, and highly immunogenic in all age groups tested (from 2 years old and older). Seroconversion was 100% after 1 month following initial vaccination, and antibody titers persisted for 1 year in adults and after two doses in children (13). This vaccine can be administered with other vaccines and does not interfere with conferring immunity. This is important for travelers who must receive multiple vaccines (e.g., polio, tetanus and diphtheria, HBV, yellow fever, typhoid, and cholera).

HEPATITIS B

Introduction

Hepatitis is an ancient disease first described by Hippocrates in the fifth century B.C. Hippocrates described an epidemic of jaundice cases, many of which were caused by hepatitis, most likely HAV and HBV. Epidemics of jaundice continued to be described throughout history, especially during the wars of the nineteenth and twentieth centuries. In 1833, Lurmann (14) observed that hepatitis was transmitted by blood or blood products during the administration of the smallpox vaccine. Several other episodes of hepatitis have been documented to occur in groups of individuals receiving various blood products or vaccines (15,16) (Table 14-3). This is because these immunizations contain human serum that contains HBV.

Several studies conducted in the 1930s and 1940s revealed that this disease was caused by two viruses. MacCallum and Bauer (17,18), in 1947, proposed that infectious hepatitis be referred to as HAV and homologous serum hepatitis

TABLE 14-3. *Hepatitis B associated with other conditions placing the patient at risk*

Risk groups
Diabetics
Individuals with an STD
Individuals with tuberculosis
Individuals receiving a blood transfusion
Immunizations
Individuals inoculated with mumps or measles convalescent-phase serum
Yellow fever vaccine

be referred to as HBV. Further investigations established significant differences between HAV and HAV. Krugman et al. referred to types of viral hepatitis, MS-1 and MS-2 (19–21). Studies with human volunteers revealed that MS-1, or HAV, was acquired via the fecal-oral route and had an incubation period of 15 to 45 days. MS-2, or HBV, was transmitted percutaneously and had a longer incubation period than HAV. The incubation period was found to be 40 to 108 days.

Blumberg et al. (22) demonstrated that an immunoprecipitin was present in the serum of a leukemic Australian aborigine and termed this antigen the Australian antigen. This antigen was detected among other individuals of varying populations and was frequently found in those individuals who had received blood products (23–25). The Australian antigen was demonstrated to be associated with acute HBV. This discovery led to the development of specific tests for identifying individuals with HBV infection (26,27). Subsequently, other antigens were discovered that enabled physicians to follow the course of the disease (Table 14-4).

The cause of HBV was established in 1970 by electron microscopy (27). It was subsequently established that these particles, referred to as Dane particles, were HBV. Soon afterwards, specific tests were developed to distinguish between HAV and HBV. A third virus (later identified as HCV) detected was referred to as non-A and non-B hepatitis. A new antigen was detected in the serum of patients with chronic liver disease and is referred to as the delta antigen (28). This antigen was a core protein of a defective virus, hepatitis D (HDV), which requires HBV to replicate. This was a significant and important discovery because prevention of HBV can also prevent HDV and the morbidity and mortality associated with this disease (29).

TABLE 14-4. *Hepatitis nomenclature[a]*

Abbreviation	Term	Definition
HBV	Hepatitis B virus	Etiologic agent of "serum" hepatitis; referred to as Dane particle
HBsAg	Hepatitis B surface antigen	Surface antigen(s) of HBV detectable in large quantities of serum; several subtypes identified
HBcAg	Hepatitis B core antigen	Core antigen of HBV; no commercial test available
HBeAg	Hepatitis B e antigen	Soluble antigen; correlates with HBV replication, high titer HBV in serum, and infectivity of serum
Anti-HBs	Antibody to HBsAg	Indicates past infection and immunity to HBV, passive antibody from HBIG, or response to HBV vaccine
Anti-HBc	Antibody to HBcAg	Indicates prior infection at some undefined time in past
Anti-HBe	Antibody to HBeAg	Presence in serum of persons with chronic HBV infection indicates low titer of HBV
HBIG	Hepatitis B immune globulin	Contains high titers of antibody to HBsAg

[a]Mahoney FJ. Update on diagnosis, management, and prevention of hepatitis B virus infection. *Clin Microbiol Rev* 199;12:351–366, with permission.

TABLE 14-5. *Risk factors for HBV infection*

Sexual intercourse with bisexual men
Sexual intercourse with multiple sex partners
Sexual intercourse with intravenous drug users
Intravenous drug use
Household contacts with individuals with chronic HBV infection
Individuals receiving blood or blood products
Occupation that exposes an individual to blood and other body fluids
Institutionalized persons

HBV, hepatitis B virus.

Epidemiology

HBV infection occurs worldwide with varying prevalence, ranging from less than 2% [low hepatitis B surface antigen (HBsAg)] to greater than 8% (high HBsAg) of the population being exposed to the virus. It is estimated that 45% of the world's population live in areas where HBV infection is high (8% or higher) (30). In areas where infection is high (8% or higher), the lifetime risk of acquiring HBV infection exceeds 60%. In these endemic areas, infection usually occurs at the time of birth or during early childhood (31–33).

Infection tends to cluster in households where chronically infected individuals, like a mother or sibling, reside (34). Success of perinatal transmission is dependent on the mother's hepatitis B e antigen (HBeAg) positive status. A pregnant woman who is HBsAg positive, HBeAg positive, and anti-HBeAg negative has a 70% to 90% chance of transmitting the infection to her neonate if the infant is not given immunoprophylaxis (35,36). If a mother is HBsAg positive and HBeAg negative, the risk of perinatal transmission of HBV to her neonate is 5% to 20%. Infants who escape infection at birth remain at risk because of subsequent exposure to infected individuals in the family (37).

The prevalence of HBV in the United States is low (less than 2%), except for in Alaska and the Hawaiian Islands where it is high (8% or higher). The prevalence in these areas is similar to that observed in the Amazon basin of South America, Africa, Asia (excluding Japan and India), and the Middle East (38–40). Risk factors for the acquisition of HBV are listed in Table 14-5.

HEPATITIS C

Introduction

HCV, formerly known as non-A, non-B hepatitis, is the primary cause of chronic liver disease and liver failure in the world (41,42). The main vector of transmission was thought to be via transfusion of blood and blood products. This conclusion was reached because studies to determine the prevalence of HCV were performed mostly on blood donors. Studies were not performed on random persons within the population or on specific populations (43,44). Current estimates indicate that 2.7 million people in the United States have chronic HCV (45).

Epidemiology

HCV is a worldwide problem because individuals find travel between countries to be easy and contact with individuals through sharing of equipment or intimacy is common (Fig. 14-1). Therefore, infection among travelers becomes an issue when developing programs for prevention. It is estimated that there are 100 million cases of HCV in the world (46). In the United States alone there are 100,000 new cases of HCV per year (47–49). Approximately 20% to 30% of individuals infected with HCV will develop cirrhosis, placing them at risk to acquire liver cancer and become candidates for liver transplants (50–52). There are at least 30,000 deaths annually in the United States because of HCV, making this disease the ninth leading cause of death in the country (48).

Liver failure resulting from cirrhosis occurs in a significant number of patients with HCV infection alone and in those who abuse alcohol or become infected with HIV (53). In the United States and in countries where liver transplants are performed, HCV-induced end-stage liver disease is the most common cause for orthotopic liver transplantation. Among renal transplant patients, chronic liver disease caused by HCV is the second most common cause of death (54,55). Chronic liver disease resulting in death is more commonly associated with HCV infection than with HBV.

HCV infection in a population of blood donors is less than 1.5%, and the risk of transfusion-associated infection is approximately 1 in 103,000 units of blood

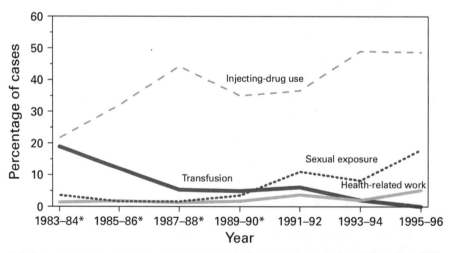

FIG. 14-1. Reported cases of acute hepatitis C by selected risk factors in the United States from 1983 to 1996. *Data presented for non-A, non-B hepatitis. (U.S. Department of Health and Human Services, Centers for Disease Control, Atlanta, GA.)

(56). Transmission of HCV can also occur through heterosexual intercourse, but this was believed to be relatively uncommon (57,58). The presence of HIV seems to increase the risk of HCV transmission from males-to-females by a factor of five (59). The prevalence of HCV in conjunction with HIV ranges from 9% to 40% (60). A significant contributing factor to acquisition of HCV and HIV is intravenous (IV) drug use. The prevalence of HCV among individuals with HIV (who use illicit drugs intravenously) is between 52% and 90% (60). There is also a high prevalence of HCV among hemophiliacs, in whom rates of 60% to 85% have been reported (61). Interestingly, the prevalence of HCV in IV drug abusers and hemophiliacs is similar whether or not the patient is coinfected with HIV. This finding strengthens the argument that IV drug abuse or blood contamination in individuals sharing needles is a common vector for transmission of HCV. Thus, the debate over the transmission of HCV has continued since the virus was first described 20 years ago. Alter et al. (45) performed antibody tests for HCV on serum samples obtained from 21,241 individuals 6 years of age and older. The overall prevalence was 1.8% corresponding to approximately 3.9 million cases of HCV infection in the United States (45). Approximately 74% were found to be positive for HCV RNA indicating that 2.7 million individuals in the United States have chronic HCV infection (45).

African Americans have a higher prevalence of HCV infection than whites and Hispanics (Fig. 14-2). In the general population, the highest prevalence rates of HCV occur in individuals 30 to 49 years of age, and the highest inci-

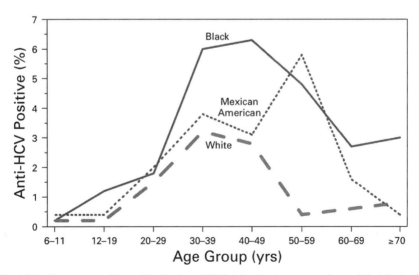

FIG. 14-2. Prevalence of hepatitis C virus (HCV) infection by age and race/ethnicity in the United States from 1988 to 1994. (From *Third National Health and Nutrition Examination Survey*, U.S. Department of Health and Human Services, Centers for Disease Control, Atlanta, GA, with permission.)

dence of acute HCV occurs in 20 to 39 year olds. Interestingly, 15% to 20% of patients with acute HCV have a history of sexual exposure and no other risk factors. Approximately 66 % of these individuals have a sex partner who is anti-HCV-positive, and 33% have more than two sexual partners 6 months before the onset of their illness (62). Women who have sex with a male partner who is anti-HCV positive are more likely to contract HCV then a negative male who has sex with an anti-HCV positive female (46). The transmission of HCV appears to be similar to other sexually transmitted disease (STD) in that transmission from males to females is more likely than from females to males. Increased transmission from males to females is likely to be caused by two conditions: (a) eversion of the endothelial columnar epithelium, which results in a significant increase in the surface area of this receptive tissue, and (b) microscopic lesions of the vaginal epithelium, which are a result of sexual intercourse.

Analysis revealed that the most common risk factors independently associated with acquisition of HCV are illegal drug use and high-risk sexual behavior (45) (Table 14-6). Two other factors that affect acquisition of HCV are economic level below the poverty level, and age older than 16 years (divorced or separated). However, the most important factors were illegal drug use and high-risk sexual behavior. Interestingly, cocaine and marijuana use are not directly involved in acquisition, but both practices can lead to use of IV drugs and high-risk sexual behavior. Cocaine users often share nasal tubes. This apparatus can traumatize the nares, thus leading to contamination with blood (63). Among individuals found to be HCV positive who also use cocaine, it is not uncommon for them to also use IV drugs. Most IV drug users who are HCV positive also admit to using cocaine and marijuana (46).

Sexual behavior affects the individual's risk for acquiring STDs in general. Concerning HCV infection, sex at an early age was likely to place the individual at greater risk because he or she is more likely to have a greater number of sexual partners in a lifetime. Likewise, the individual who is a serious user of illegal drugs is more likely to have multiple sexual partners during his or her lifetime. The prevalence of HCV was higher in the group of individuals who had sex at an early age, had at least 50 sexual partners, and had genital herpes simplex infection (45). This study also found that individuals who were positive for HBV

TABLE 14-6. *Risk factors associated with HCV infection*

Marijuana (≥100 times) and cocaine use
IV drug use
Multiple sex partners (≥50 in a lifetime)
Income below the poverty level
Education ≤12th grade
Divorced or separated

HCV, hepatitis C virus.

TABLE 14-7. *Estimated average prevalence of hepatitis C virus (HCV) infection in the United States by various characteristics and estimated prevalence of persons with these characteristics in the population*

Characteristic	HCV-infection prevalence %	(range, %)	Prevalence of persons with characteristic, %
Persons with hemophilia treated with products made before 1987	87	(74–90)	<0.01
Injecting-drug users			
Current	79	(72–86)	0.5
History of prior use	No Data		5
Persons with abnormal alanine aminotransferase levels	15	(10–18)	5
Chronic hemodialysis patients	10	(0–64)	0.1
Persons with multiple sex partners (lifetime)			
≥50	9	(6–16)	4
10–49	3	(3–4)	22
2–9	2	(1–2)	52
Persons reporting a history of sexually transmitted diseases	6	(1–10)	17
Persons receiving blood transfusions before 1990	6	(5–9)	6
Infants born to infected mothers	5	(0–25)	0.1
Men who have sex with men	4	(2–18)	5
General population	1.8	(1.5–2.3)	NA[a]
Health care workers	1	(1–2)	9
Pregnant women	1	—	1.5
Military personnel	0.3	(0.2–0.4)	0.5
Volunteer blood donors	0.16	—	5

[a]Not applicable.

were six times more likely to be positive for HCV compared with individuals without HBV infection (10.2% vs. 1.6%).

HCV infection in health care workers secondary to needle stick injuries can result in infection. However, this is a relatively rare occurrence and does not constitute a major mechanism of acquisition of HCV infection (64,65). Table 14-7 lists characteristics common to individuals found to be HCV positive.

Perinatal transmission of HCV occurs in 5% to 30% of cases (66). There is a three-fold increase in transmission of HCV if the mother is coinfected with HIV (67). Most neonates born to HCV-positive mothers do not have detectable levels of HCV RNA until after an intermediate period of time (68).

Management

The best defense against contracting HCV is to take measures to prevent transmission of the virus. Because the main routes of acquisition are illegal drug use and high-risk sexual behavior, eradication of this disease will await the development of a vaccine. Modifying individual behavioral practices is an extremely difficult task. Women should insist that the male wears a condom, or they can use the female condom themselves. Although this is not foolproof, it does offer a significant degree of protection.

Individuals infected with HCV can be treated with the combination of interferon alfa-2b and ribavirin. Treatment with interferon alfa-2b alone has demonstrated that 40% of patients will manifest improvement (i.e., normalization of serum aminotransferase), and HCV RNA cannot be detected in the serum (69–72). However, short-course therapy usually results in relapse shortly after cessation of therapy. Increasing therapy to 12 to 24 weeks increases the duration of response, but there was a significant relapse rate (73–76).

Ribavirin is a nucleoside analog that is used for the treatment of respiratory syncytial virus (RSV) in high-risk infants. It has also been used to treat RSV in pregnant women (77). Ribavirin has been shown, *in vitro,* to inhibit RSV, influenza virus, and herpes simplex virus (78). Treatment with ribavirin alone does not alter the serum HCV RNA levels in patients with chronic HCV. However, ribavirin does reduce the serum alanine transferase concentrations (79–81). Improvement in treatment of HCV infection has been achieved by administering a combination of interferon alfa-2b and ribavirin. In one study comparing the combination against interferon alfa-2b alone, the combination proved to be more effective. Among patients receiving interferon and ribavirin for 24 weeks, 31% responded favorably. In those that received treatment for 48 weeks, 38% responded favorably compared with 13% who received interferon alfa-2b alone ($p < 0.001$), (82) (Table 14-8). The relapse rate in the combination group was 42% in the group that received treatment for 24 weeks and 24% for those treated for 48 weeks. This was compared with 80% for those treated for 24 weeks with interferon alone and 46% for those treated for 48 weeks (82). Histologic improvement occurred in all groups. However, the group that received combination therapy was more likely to demonstrate improvement when pretherapy and posttherapy liver biopsies were compared (82).

Patients initially treated with interferon alfa-2b alone have a significant relapse rate. A second course of interferon can be administered to these patients, but only 20% to 50% will maintain a sustained response (83–85). Davis et al. (86) demonstrated that patients treated with interferon alone who had relapsed could safely be treated with the combination interferon alfa-2b and ribavirin. They also reported that serum HCV RNA was undetectable in 82% (141/173) of the patients treated with combination therapy compared with 47% (80/172) of patients treated with interferon alone, $p < 0.001$ (CC18). The serum HCV RNA levels were undetectable throughout the follow-up period (24 weeks) in 49 (84%) of the patients compared with 5 (8%) of the patients treated with interferon alone (86). The serum alanine transferase levels were normal in 89% (154/173) of the patients in the group receiving combination therapy compared with 57% (98/172) of the group receiving only interferon, $p < 0.001$ (86). Thus, the studies by McHutchison, Davis, and their respective colleagues demonstrate that the combination of interferon alfa-2b and ribavirin is well tolerated and effective as either an initial treatment or for patients previously treated with interferon.

TABLE 14-8. *Virologic and biochemical responses at the end of treatment and follow-up[a]*

Response	Interferon		Interferon and ribavirin	
	24 wk	48 wk	24 wk	48 wk
Virologic				
End of treatment				
No. with response/				
Total no. treated	66/231	54/225	121/228	115/228
Percent (95% CI)	29(23–34)	54(18–30)	53(47–60)[b]	50(44–57)[b]
End of follow-up				
No. with response/				
Total no. treated	13/231	29/225	70/228	87/228
Percent (95% CI)	6(3–9)	13(9–17)	31(25–37)[b]	38(32–45)[b,c]
Biochemical				
End of treatment				
No. with response/				
Total no. treated	56/231	62/225	133/228	83/228
Percent (95% CI)	24(19–30)	28(22–33)	58(52–65)	65(54–67)
End of follow-up				
No. with response/				
Total no. treated	25/231	35/225	72/228	83/228
Percent (95% CI)	11(7–15)	16(11–20)	32(25–38)[b]	36(30–43)[b]

[a]A virologic response was defined as the absence of serum HCV RNA (limit of detection, 100 copies per milliliter), and a biochemical response was defined as a normalization of the serum alanine aminotransferase concentration. Responses were assessed in the last week of treatment and 24 weeks later. CI denotes confidence interval.

[b]$p < 0.001$ for the comparison with either interferon group.

[c]$p = 0.05$ for the comparison with 24 weeks of interferon and ribavirin.

Table taken from McHutchison JG, Gordon SC, Schiff ER, et al. Interferon alfa-2b alone or in combination with ribavirin as initial treatment for chronic hepatitis C. *N Engl J Med* 1998;339:1487, with permission.

Both agents are associated with significant adverse effects and patients should be monitored appropriately. Ribavirin can accumulate in red blood cells and cause hemolysis (81). Most common side effects of the treatment regimen were nausea, shortness of breath, and a rash (Table 14-9). There were no serious side effects reported by the patients or detected by the physicians.

SUMMARY

HCV is an RNA virus and is primarily acquired via illegal IV drug use and high-risk sexual behavior. HCV RNA can be detected in the blood of an infected individual 1 to 3 weeks after exposure. All infected individuals are likely to develop liver injury, and this can be detected by demonstrating a rise in the serum alanine aminotransferase concentration in the serum. Infected adults tend to be asymptomatic and anicteric. Approximately 20% to 25% of infected individuals develop malaise, anorexia, fatigue, and jaundice. Antibody to HCV can be detected within 3 months in 90% of infected individuals. It is estimated that 85% of infected individuals will go on to develop chronic hepatitis, with 20% of these individuals developing cirrhosis. One percent to 5% of individuals with

TABLE 14-9. *Rates of symptoms during treatment[a]*

Symptom	Interferon (N = 172) (%)	Interferon + ribavirin (N = 173) (%)
Influenza-like		
Headache	54	55
Fatigue or asthenia	39	46
Myalgia	39	44
Arthralgia	23	21
Fever	33	32
Rigors	21	26
Gastrointestinal		
Anorexia	13	20
Nausea	20	35[b]
Diarrhea	18	12
Psychiatric		
Depression	11	16
Insomnia	23	20
Respiratory		
Cough	9	10
Dyspnea	6	14[c]
Pharyngitis	9	11
Dermatologic		
Alopecia	18	21
Rash	5	13
Pruritus	6	13

[a]Table taken from Davis GL, Esteban-Mur R, Rustgi V, et al. Interferon alfa-2b alone or in combination with ribavirin for the treatment of relapse of chronic hepatitis C. *N Engl J Med* 1998;339:1497, with permission.
[b]$p = 0.002$ for the comparison with interferon alone.
[c]$p = 0.02$ for the comparison with interferon alone.

chronic hepatitis will develop hepatocellular carcinoma 20 years after the initial diagnosis. Individuals who develop cirrhosis have an increased rate of developing hepatocellular carcinoma.

REFERENCES

1. Alter MJ, Mast EE. The epidemiology of viral hepatitis in the United States. *Gastroenterol Clin North Am* 1994;23:437–453.
2. Melnick JL. History and epidemiology of hepatitis A virus. *J Infect Dis* 1995;171(Suppl 1):S2–8.
3. Cohen JI, Feinstone S, Purcell RH. Hepatitis A infection in a chimpanzee: duration of viremia and detection of virus in saliva and throat swabs. *J Infect Dis* 1989;160:887–890.
4. Stapleton JT, Lemon SM. Hepatitis A and hepatitis E. In: Hoeprich PD, Jordan MC, Ronald AR, eds. *Infectious diseases, a treatise on infectious process,* 5th ed. Philadelphia: JB Lippincott, 1994: 790–800.
5. Gust ID, Feinstone SM. *Hepatitis A.* Boca Raton, FL: CRC Press, 1988.
6. Gerety RJ. *Hepatitis A.* Orlando, FL: Academic Press, 1984.
7. Stokes J Jr, Neefe JR. The prevention and attenuation of infectious hepatitis by gamma globulin: preliminary note. *JAMA* 1945;127:144–145.
8. Centers for Disease Control. Centers for Disease Control hepatitis surveillance. *MMWR CDC Surveillance Summ* 1990;53:1–35.
9. Hadler SC. Global impact of hepatitis A infection changing patterns. In: Hollinger FB, Lemon SM, Margolis H, eds. *Viral hepatitis and liver disease. Proceedings of the 1990 international symposium on viral hepatitis and liver disease: contemporary issues and future prospects.* Baltimore: Williams & Wilkins, 1991:14–20.

10. Institute of Medicine. The prospects for immunizing against hepatitis A virus. In: *New vaccine development: establishing priorities. Vol II. Diseases of importance in developing countries.* Washington DC: National Academy Press, 1986:197–206.
11. Andre FE. Hepburn A, D'Hondt E. Inactivated candidate vaccines for hepatitis A. *Prog Med Virol* 1990;37:72–95.
12. Peetermans J. Production, quality control and characterization of an inactivated hepatitis A vaccine. *Vaccine* 1992;10(Suppl 1):99–101.
13. Clemens R, Safary A, Hepburn A, et al. Clinical experience with an inactivated hepatitis A vaccine. *J Infect Dis* 1995;171(Suppl 1):S44–49.
14. Lurmann A. Eine icterus Epidemic. *Berlin Klin Wochenschr* 1855;22:20–23.
15. Flaum A, Malmros H, Person E. Eine nosocomiale icterus-epidemic. *Acta Med Scand* 1926;16: 544–548.
16. Neefe JR, Gellis SS, Stokes. Homologous serum hepatitis and infectious (epidemic) hepatitis: studies in volunteers bearing on immunological and other characteristics of etiologic agents. *Am J Med* 1946;1:3–22.
17. MacCallum FO, Bauer DJ. Homologous serum hepatitis. *Lancet* 1947;2:691–692.
18. MacCallum FO, Bauer DJ. Homologous serum jaundice transmission experiments with human volunteers. *Lancet* 1944:1:622–627.
19. Giles JP, McCollum RW, Berndtson LW Jr, et al. Relation of Australia-SH antigen to the willowbrook MS-2 strain. *N Engl J Med* 1969;281:119–122.
20. Krugman S, Giles JP. Viral hepatitis, type B (MS-2-strain). Further observations on natural history and prevention. *N Engl J Med* 1973;288:755–760.
21. Krugman S, Giles JP, Hammond J. Infectious hepatitis. Evidence for two distinctive clinical, epidemiological, and immunological types of infection. *JAMA* 1967;200:365–373.
22. Blumberg BS, Alter HJ, Visnich S. Landmark article February 15, 1965: a "new" antigen in leukemia serum. *JAMA* 1984;252:252–257.
23. Blumberg BS, Gerstley BJ, Hungerford DA, et al. A serum antigen (Australian antigen) in Down's syndrome, leukemia, and hepatitis. *Ann Intern Med* 1967;66:924–931.
24. Blumberg BS, Mazzur K, Hertzog K, et al. Australian antigen in Solomon Islands. *Hum Biol* 1974; 46:239–262.
25. Prince AM. An antigen detected in the blood of patients during incubation of serum hepatitis. *Proc Natl Acad Sci U S A* 1968;60:814–821.
26. Blumberg BS. Australia antigen and the biology of hepatitis B. *Science* 1977;197:17–25.
27. Prince AM, Ikram H, Hopp TP. Hepatitis B virus vaccine: identification of HBsAg/a and HBsAg/d but not HbsAg/y subtype antigenic determinants on a synthetic immunogenic peptide. *Pro Natl Acad Sci U S A* 1982;79:579–582.
28. Dane DS, Cameron CH, Briggs M. Virus-like particles in serum of patients with Australia-antigen-associated hepatitis. *Lancet* 1970;1:695–698.
29. Rizzetto M, Canese MG, Arico S, et al. Immunofluorescence detection of new antigen-antibody system (delta/anti-delta) associated to hepatitis B virus in liver and serum of HBsAg carriers. *Gut* 1977: 18:997–1003.
30. Mahoney FJ. Update on diagnosis, management, and prevention of hepatitis B virus infection. *Clin Microbiol Rev* 1999;12:351–366.
31. Hu MD, Schenzle D, Deinhardt F, et al. Epidemiology of hepatitis A and B in Shanghai area: prevalence of serum markers. *Am J Epidemiol* 1984;120:404–413.
32. Hyams KC, al-Arabi MA, al-Tagani AA, et al. Epidemiology of hepatitis B in the Gezira region of Sudan. *Am J Trop Med Hyg* 1989;40:200–206.
33. Mahoney FJ, Woodruff BA, Erben JJ, et al. Effect of a hepatitis B vaccination program on the prevalence of hepatitis B virus infection. *J Infect Dis* 1993;167:203–207.
34. Lok AS, Lai CL, Wu PC, et al. Hepatitis B virus infection in Chinese families in Hong Kong. *Am J Epidemiol* 1987;126:492–499.
35. Stevens CE, Neurath RA, Beasley RP, et al. HBeAg and anti-HBe detection with radioimmunoassay: correlation with vertical transmission of hepatitis B virus in Taiwan. *J Med Virol* 1979;3:237–241.
36. Xu ZY, Liu CB, Francis DP, et al. Prevention of perinatal acquisition of hepatitis B virus carriage using vaccine: preliminary report of a randomized double-blind placebo-controlled and comparative trial. *Pediatrics* 1985;76:713–718.
37. Beasley RP, Hwang LY. Postnatal infectivity of hepatitis B surface antigen-carrier mothers. *J Infect Dis* 1983;147:185–190.
38. McMahon BJ, Alberts SR, Wainwright RB, et al. Hepatitis B related sequelae: prospective study in 1400 hepatitis B surface antigen-positive Alaska native carriers. *Arch Intern Med* 1990;150: 1051–1054.

39. Wong DC, Purcell RH, Rosen L. Prevalence of antibody to hepatitis A and hepatitis B viruses in selected populations of the South Pacific. *Am J Epidemiol* 1979;110:227–236.
40. Toukan AU, Sharaiha ZK, Abu-el-Rub OA, et al. The epidemiology of hepatitis B virus among family members in the Middle East. *Am J Epidemiol* 1990;132:220–232.
41. Choo QL, Kuo G, Weiner AJ, et al. Isolation of a cDNA clone derived from a blood-borne non-A, non-B viral hepatitis genome. *Science* 1989;244:359–362.
42. Kuo G, Choo QL, Alter MJ, et al. An assay for circulating antibodies to a major etiologic virus of human non-A, non-B hepatitis. *Science* 1989;244:362–364.
43. Alter MJ. Epidemiology of hepatitis C in the West. *Semin Liver Dis* 1995;15:5–14.
44. Mansell CJ, Locarnini SA. Epidemiology of hepatitis C in the East. *Semin Liver Dis* 1995;15:15–32.
45. Alter MJ, Kruszon-Moran MS, Nainan OV, et al. The prevalence of hepatitis C virus infection in the United States, 1988 through 1994. *N Engl J Med* 1999;341:556–562.
46. Alter MJ. Epidemiology of hepatitis C. *Hepatology* 1997;26(3 Suppl 1):62S–65S.
47. Alter MJ, Sampliner RE. Hepatitis C: and miles to go before we sleep. *N Engl J Med* 1989;321: 1538–1540.
48. Anonymous. Management of hepatitis C. National Institutes of Health Consensus Development Conference Panel Statement. *Hepatology* 1997;26(3 Suppl 1):2S–10S.
49. Heintges T, Wands JR. Hepatitis C virus: epidemiology and transmission. *Hepatology* 1997;26: 521–526.
50. Takahashi M, Yamada G, Miyamoto R, et al. Natural course of chronic hepatitis C. *Am J Gastroenterol* 1993;88:240–243.
51. Tremolada F, Casarin C, Alberti A, et al. Long-term follow-up of non-A, non-B (type C) post-transfusion hepatitis. *J Hepatol* 1992;16:273–281.
52. Yano M, Kumada H, Kage M, et al. The long-term pathological evolution of chronic hepatitis C. *Hepatology* 1996;23:1334–1340.
53. Ostapowicz G, Watson KJ, Locarnini SA, et al. Role of alcohol in progression of liver disease caused by hepatitis C virus infection. *Hepatology* 1998;27:1730–1735.
54. Rao KV, Andersen RC. Long-term results and complications in renal transplant recipients. Observations in the second decade. *Transplantation* 1988;45:45–52.
55. Grotz WH, Peters TH, Schlayer HJ, et al. Immunosuppressive therapy and hepatitis C virus infection: the clinical course of liver disease. *J Mol Med* 1996;74:407–412.
56. Schreiber GB, Busch MP, Kleinman SH, et al. The risk of transfusion-transmitted viral infections. *N Engl J Med* 1996;334:1685–1690.
57. Wyld R, Robertson JR, Brettle RP, et al. Absence of hepatitis C virus transmission but frequent transmission of HIV-1 from sexual contact with doubly-infected individuals. *J Infect* 1997;35:163–166.
58. Hallam NF, Fletcher ML, Read SJ, et al. Low risk of sexual transmission of hepatitis C virus. *J Med Virol* 1993;40:251–253.
59. Eyster ME, Alter HJ, Aledort LM, et al. Heterosexual co-transmission of hepatitis C virus (HCV) and human immunodeficiency virus (HIV). *Ann Intern Med* 1991;115:764–768.
60. Zylberberg H, Pol S. Reciprocal interactions between human immunodeficiency virus and hepatitis C virus infections. *Clin Infect Dis* 1996;23:1117–1125.
61. Brettler DB, Mannucci PM, Gringeri A, et al. The low risk of hepatitis C virus transmission among sexual partners of hepatitis C-infected hemophilic males: an international, multicenter study. *Blood* 1992;80:540–543.
62. Thomas DL, Zenilman JM, Alter HJ, et al. Sexual transmission of hepatitis C virus among patients attending sexually transmitted disease clinics in Baltimore—an analysis of 309 sex partnerships. *J Infect Dis* 1995;171:768–775.
63. Conry-Cantilena C, VanRaden M, Gibble J, et al. Routes of infection, viremia, and liver disease in blood donors found to have hepatitis C virus infection. *N Engl J Med* 1996;334:1691–1696.
64. Thomas DL, Factor SH, Kelen GD, et al. Viral hepatitis in health care personnel at The Johns Hopkins Hospital: the seroprevalence of and risk factors for hepatitis B virus and hepatitis C virus infection. *Arch Intern Med* 1993;153:1705–1712.
65. Panlilio AL, Shapiro CN, Schable CA, et al. Serosurvey of human immunodeficiency virus, hepatitis B virus, and hepatitis C virus infection among hospital-based surgeons. *J Am Col Surg* 1995;180: 16–24.
66. Thomas DL, Villano SA, Riester KA, et al. Perinatal transmission of hepatitis C virus from human immunodeficiency virus type1-infected mothers. Women and Infants Transmission Study. *J Infect Dis* 1998;177:1480–1488.
67. Novati R, Thiers V, Monforte AD, et al. Mother-to-child transmission of hepatitis C virus detected by nested polymerase chain reaction. *J Infect Dis* 1992;165:720–723.

68. Roudot-Thoraval F, Pawlotsky JM, Thiers V, et al. Lack of mother-to-infant transmission of hepatitis C virus in human immunodeficiency virus-seronegative women: a prospective study with hepatitis C virus RNA testing. *Hepatology* 1993;17:772–777.

69. Davis GL, Balart LA, Schiff ER, et al. Treatment of chronic hepatitis C with recombinant interferon alfa. A multicenter randomized controlled trial. *N Engl J Med* 1989;321:1501–1506.

70. Di Bisceglie AM, Martin P, Kassianides C, et al. Recombinant interferon alfa therapy for chronic hepatitis C. A randomized, double-blind, placebo-controlled trial. *N Engl J Med* 1989;321:1506–1510.

71. Tine F, Magrin S, Craxi A, et al. Interferon for non-A, non-B chronic hepatitis. A meta-analysis of randomised clinical trials. *J Hepatol* 1991;13:192–199.

72. Poynard T, Leroy V, Cohard M, et al. Meta-analysis of interferon randomized trials in the treatment of viral hepatitis C: effects of dose and duration. *Hepatology* 1996;24:778–789.

73. Poynard T, Bedossa P, Chevallier M, et al. A comparison of three interferon alfa-2b regimens for long term treatment of chronic non-A, non-B hepatitis. *N Engl J Med* 1996;334:1143–1152.

74. Lin R, Roach E, Zimmerman M, et al. Interferon alfa-2b for chronic hepatitis C: effects of dose increment and duration of treatment on response rates. Results of the first multicentre Australian trial. *J Hepatol* 1995;23:487–496.

75. Shiffman ML, Hoffmann CM, Luketic VA, et al. Improved sustained response following treatment of chronic hepatitis C by gradual reduction in the interferon dose. *Hepatology* 1996;24:21–26.

76. Carithers RL Jr, Emerson SS. Therapy of hepatitis C: meta-analysis of interferon alfa-2b trials. *Hepatology* 1997;26(3 Suppl 1):83S–88S.

77. Kirshon B, Faro S, Zurawin RK, et al. Favorable outcome following treatment with amantadine and ribavirin in pregnancy complicated by influenza pneumonia. *J Reprod Med* 1988;33:399–401.

78. Patterson JL, Fernandez-Larsson R. Molecular mechanisms of action of ribavirin. *Rev Infect Dis* 1990;12:1139–1146.

79. Dusheiko G, Main J, Thomas H, et al. Ribavirin treatment for patients with chronic hepatitis C: results of a placebo-controlled study. *J Hepatol* 1996;25:591–598.

80. Di Bisceglie AM, Shindo M, Fong TL, et al. A pilot study of ribavirin therapy for chronic hepatitis C. *Hepatology* 1992;16:649–654.

81. Bodenheimer HC Jr, Lindsay KL, Davis GL, et al. Tolerance and efficacy of oral ribavirin treatment of chronic hepatitis C: a multicenter trial. *Hepatology* 1997;26:473–477.

82. McHutchison JG, Gordon SC, Schiff ER, et al. Interferon alfa-2b alone or in combination with ribavirin as initial treatment for chronic hepatitis C. *N Engl J Med* 1998;339:1485–1492.

83. Alberti A, Chemello L, Noventa F, et al. Therapy of hepatitis C: re-treatment with alpha interferon. *Hepatology* 1997;26(3 Suppl 1):137S–142S.

84. Picciotti A, Brizzolara R, Campo N, et al. Two year interferon retreatment may induce a sustained response in relapsing patients with chronic hepatitis C. *Hepatology* 1996;24(Suppl):273A(abst).

85. Toyoda H, Nakano S, Takeda I, et al. Retreatment of chronic hepatitis C with interferon. *Am J Gastroenterol* 1994;89:1453–1457.

86. Davis GL, Esteban-Mur R, Rustgi V, et al. Interferon alfa-2b alone or in combination with ribavirin for the treatment of relapse of chronic hepatitis C. *N Engl J Med* 1998;339:1493–1499.

Subject Index

Page numbers followed by *f* refer to figures; page numbers followed by *t* refer to tables

A

Ablative therapy, condylomata acuminata and, 179

Abscess. *See also* Intraabdominal abscess; Liver abscess; Perirectal abscess; Splenic abscess
bacteria combinations and, 101
E. coli and, 72
E. faecalis and, 72
granuloma inguinale and, 94
Trichomonas vaginalis and, 127

Actinomyces, Trichomonas vaginalis and, 128

Acute infection, HIV acquisition associated with, 193

Acyclovir
herpes simplex virus and, 157, 158*t*
HIV and, 200

Adenosine triphosphate (ATP), chlamydia and, 28

Adenovirus, *Trichomonas vaginalis* and, 128

Adnexa, pelvic inflammatory disease (PID) and, 63

Adrenaline, anaphylaxis and, 237

Age, gonorrhea and, 4

AIDS (acquired immunodeficiency syndrome)
case definition of, 189*t*
CD4 lymphocyte count and, 189, 192*t*
chancroid and, 95
genital herpes and, 146
natural history of, 188–190
revised classification for, 190*t*
treatment of, 195

Alcohol, hepatitis C (HCV) and, 250

Allergy, metronidazole (Flagyl), 125

Altered vaginal microflora (AVM)
algorithm for evaluation and management of, 105*f*
environment pH vs bacterial growth in, 98*t*
healthy vaginal ecosystem (HVE) and, 97
infections of genital tract and, 97, 98
overview of, 102–107

risk factors of, 106
sexual activity and, 110

Amniocentesis, transplacental migration of virus and, 169

Amniotomy,
HIV and, 198

Amoxicillin/clavulanic acid (Augmentin), pelvic inflammatory disease (PID) treatment and, 73

Ampicillin
gonorrhea and, 8
granuloma inguinale and, 94
pelvic inflammatory disease (PID) treatment and, 74

Anaphylaxis
allergic reactions in treatment of syphilis and, 233
penicillin and, 236, 237

Anogenital condylomata acuminata, treatment regimens for, 180*t*

Anogenital syndrome, differential diagnosis of, 209

Anogenitorectal syndrome
characteristics of, 209
lymphogranuloma venereum (LGV) and, 208*f*, 209

Antibiotics
cervicitis and, 20
diagnosis of pelvic inflammatory disease (PDI) and, 68
gonorrhea and, 6, 7
lymphogranuloma venereum (LGV) and, 211
pelvic inflammatory disease (PID) and, 53
vulvovaginal candidiasis (VVC) and, 133, 139, 142

Antifungal agents
HIV and, 199
vulvovaginal candidiasis (VVC) and, 140*t*

Antigen test, screening with, 36

Antigens, HIV, lymphoid tissue and, 195–196